EVALUATION, TREATMENT AND PREVENTION OF MUSCULOSKELETAL DISORDERS

3rd Edition

Volume One • Spine

H. Duane Saunders, MS PT
Robin Saunders, MS PT

with guest authors

Steven L. Kraus, PT OCS
Allyn Woerman, MMS PT

and contributions from

Daniel T. Wolfe, GDMT PT
John P. Tomberlin, PT OCS

•

The Saunders Group
4250 Norex Drive
Chaska, Minnesota 55318

Library of Congress Number 84-091301

ISBN Number 1-879190-06-0

Cover Design: Audrey Saunders
Copy Editor and Layout Design: Clarke Stone

Printed in the United States of America.

Authors and Contributors

Steven L. Kraus, PT OCS
Clinic Director
Plantation Shops
2770 Lenox Rd
Suite 102
Atlanta, GA 30324

H. Duane Saunders, MS PT
President
The Saunders Group
4250 Norex Drive
Chaska, MN 55318

Robin Saunders, MS PT
Director
Saunders Therapy Centers
2334 University Av W
Suite 170
St. Paul, MN 55114

John Tomberlin, PT OCS
Clinic Director
Physical Therapy Associates
600 7th St SE
Cedar Rapids IA 52401

Allyn Woerman, PT MMS
Director of Clinics
Olympic Sports and Spine Rehabilitation
8011 112th St Court E
Puyallup, WA 98373

Daniel T. Wolfe, MT PT
Director
Saunders Therapy Centers
6550 York Av S
Suite 520
Edina, MN 55435

ACKNOWLEDGMENTS

One just doesn't sit down and write a textbook like this. It is like a back injury, in a way, because it results from the cumulative effects and influences of many things over many months and years. It is a result of encounters with patients/clients, health care professionals and business/industry professionals who have an interest in spinal disorders. I am truly indebted to all of you who have challenged, criticized, encouraged and supported me. This especially means my daughter, Robin, who has contributed the bulk of the new material in this edition, and to Allyn Woerman and Steve Kraus for their contributions.

I wish to thank my wife, Bonnie, and our children for allowing me to take many extra hours for all of my "physical therapy projects." Their understanding and help has been invaluable to me. I also want to thank Beth Solheim and others here at The Saunders Group for helping me develop a business organization that is the vehicle that permits me to accomplish my professional goals. This textbook is one of the results.

H. Duane Saunders

CONTENTS

CHAPTER 5 TREATMENT OF THE SPINE BY DIAGNOSIS   99

CHAPTER 6 TREATMENT OF THE SPINE BY PROBLEM   145

CHAPTER 7 EVALUATION AND TREATMENT OF PELVIC GIRDLE DYSFUNCTIONS
by Allyn L. Woerman, MMSc PT   161

CHAPTER 8 EVALUATION AND MANAGEMENT OF TEMPOROMANDIBULAR DISORDERS
by Steven L. Kraus, PT OCS   193

SECTION 1
Laying the Foundation

CHAPTER 1

INTRODUCTION

FOREWORD BY H. DUANE SAUNDERS, MS PT

This book is the result of the twenty-nine years of experience I have gained from clinical practice, my association with physicians, fellow physical therapists, other health care practitioners, professionals from business and industry, intensive self-study and attendance of many educational seminars and courses. My clinical practice experience ranges from the hospital and nursing home when I was younger to many years in industrial and sports outpatient clinics and, more recently, to industrial consultation.

I have seen many changes occur in my lifetime and my career has evolved in response to these changes. I expect it to continue to change in the future. Almost all the change I have witnessed has been good change. While we still have many problems with the way we care for our patients, we have accomplished a great deal.

We now know how to prevent and treat most musculoskeletal disorders. Perhaps the most frustrating obstacle now is the difficult task of communicating this information to everyone who needs to know it, such as business/industrial and health care professionals, the insurance industry and mostly to patients and workers.

Today, most patients treated by a physical therapist soon realize that physical therapy is not just the application of modalities and exercises, but the application of a comprehensive, systematic approach to the patient's problem. The physical therapist's new role involves the areas of patient evaluation, problem assessment, treatment planning, application of treatment techniques, reassessment, modification of the treatment program, rehabilitation, education, motivation and prevention.

The above definition of the "new role" of physical therapists may be presumptuous. One could argue that physical therapists are not yet fully deserving of this role. In the real world, some therapists continue to use passive modalities as their primary form of treatment. On the other hand, we have accomplished a great deal in the past few years. For the first time in history, we are beginning to find answers to the problems that were once so frustrating to us all. Many of these answers have to do with the simple, common sense ideas that we have often overlooked because we have tried to find a "scientific" answer to what we have incorrectly defined as a complicated, complex problem. This textbook will address some concepts and misconceptions that have brought us to where we are and to what should be expected of the physical therapist today.

Regardless of the area of medical practice (primary care, specialists, chiropractic or physical therapy) there is concrete evidence that many traditional approaches to low back problem management have failed. Many reasons for our failures have been suggested.[1] The greatest reason has been that many of our efforts have been limited to the acute phase only, treating the <u>symptoms</u> such as pain, inflammation and muscle guarding with little or no effort made to evaluate and treat <u>function</u> or to *address the problems which caused the disorder to occur in the first place.* And, to make matters worse, much of the treatment given is passive and does not involve the active participation or interest of the patient. Rest, medication, physical therapy modalities, manipulation and surgery are all passive forms of treatment and do not require the patient's active participation. Recognition of the reasons for our past failures has helped lead to a new, positive approach to evaluation and treatment of low back pain.

Several years ago a simple wrist fracture was casted from the base of the patient's fingers to the middle of the upper arm for several weeks. Heart attack patients were put to bed for several weeks. Ten to fourteen days of bed rest was routine after childbirth and most patients were confined to bed for days or weeks after surgery. Over the years we have found that in most cases bed rest and immobilization was not necessary and in fact, it was often harmful and was actually responsible for many of the complications once attributed to the original medical condition. Have we learned this valuable lesson when it comes to back care? Or, are we treating our back pain patients with methods we abandoned many years ago with other types of patients? This textbook examines this question in depth and proposes a more aggressive philosophy of managing back pain patients.

I do not have a great capacity for academic achievement. I believe my accomplishments have been because of hard work, persistence, a dissatisfaction and frustration with the way we have cared for our patients and a willingness to try new ideas before passing judgment.

Nine years ago I published the first edition of this book and, although it was an amateurish publication in many ways, I was extremely pleased with the reception my colleagues gave it. With very little promotion, that edition sold over 7,000 copies in less than two years and many schools of physical therapy adopted it as a textbook for their programs. Seven years ago the second edition, which has sold over 30,000 copies, was published. I have enjoyed much satisfaction from that publication and many opportunities have arisen because of it. Some allopathic and osteopathic physicians and many chiropractors have shown interest in the book. All this pleases me very much and has encouraged me to undertake this third edition. When I finished the second edition, I felt that it truly said what I wanted to say and how I wanted to say it - at least, at that time. The third edition is now necessary because we have learned more and improved our skills.

I have always been impressed with the desire we physical therapists have shown to improve our skills and with the sincerity we demonstrate in our approach to patient management. I have been disappointed, however, with our lack of professional esteem. I am frustrated that we have not achieved the level of practice and recognition that our skills and knowledge should empower. But we are improving. If this book contributes in some way to the continued improvement of patient care and the raising of standards of practice in physical therapy and health care in general, my goals will have been accomplished.

ABOUT <u>EVALUATION, TREATMENT AND PREVENTION OF MUSCULOSKELETAL DISORDERS</u>

This text is intended for students and clinicians who are interested in a common-sense, integrated approach to spinal disorders. Those readers who are familiar with the second edition of <u>Evaluation, Treatment and Prevention of Musculoskeletal Disorders</u> will notice several changes in the third edition. One exciting change is the reorganization of the text into two volumes. Conditions involving the extremities are now covered in greater detail in Volume Two, <u>Extremity Disorders</u>, which was co-authored by John P. Tomberlin, PT CSCS, and Duane. John is responsible for most of the new material.

Volume One, <u>Spinal Disorders</u>, is completely updated and reorganized into an easier-to-follow format. Robin Saunders, MS PT, joins Duane as co-author. A unique way of integrating different treatment approaches is introduced. All experienced clinicians know that a definitive diagnosis cannot always be made. Furthermore, even a patient with a clear diagnosis will not always respond as expected to the appropriate treatment. The treatment approaches discussed in this text help the clinician with this challenging dilemma. Depending upon the evaluation results, a physical therapist can choose a treatment approach based on either the patient's diagnosis, or the patient's treatable problems that the therapist finds in the evaluation. Therefore, the spinal treatment section of this text is divided accordingly.

The third edition also contains more detailed information on spinal rehabilitation, prevention and work hardening programs, a more complete evaluation and treatment scheme for sacroiliac/pelvic dysfunctions, new mobilization techniques and a new section on exercise. Allyn L. Woerman, MMSc PT, authors <u>Basic Spinal Biomechanics</u> and <u>Evaluation and Treatment of Pelvic Girdle Dysfunctions</u>, Chapters 2 and 7. Steven L. Kraus, PT OCS, authors Chapter 8, <u>Evaluation and Treatment of Temporomandibular</u>

<u>Disorders</u>. The authors sincerely appreciate the contribution these excellent clinicians have made to the third edition. The authors also wish to recognize and thank John P. Tomberlin and Daniel T. Wolfe, GDMT PT, for their expertise and advise on neural tension testing and spinal mobilization techniques.

Volume One is organized into four sections, containing fourteen chapters:

Section One, *Laying the Foundation*, contains the introductory material, including spinal biomechanics and a discussion of evaluation and treatment philosophy.

Section Two, *Evaluation and Treatment*, is divided into five chapters which cover evaluation and treatment of the spine, sacroiliac joint and pelvis, and the temporomandibular joint.

Section Three, *Specific Treatment Techniques*, contains chapters on mobilization, spinal traction, spinal orthoses, exercise and spinal rehabilitation. Chapter 12, "Exercise," is completely new and contains drawings of our favorite spinal exercises, along with indications for their uses. Chapter 13, "Spinal Rehabilitation," discusses general rehabilitation philosophy, as well as Work Hardening and Work Conditioning programs and Functional Capacity Evaluations.

Finally, Section Four, *Prevention*, covers preventive philosophy and techniques for industry.

The reader will find the third edition of <u>Evaluation, Treatment and Prevention of Musculoskeletal Disorders</u> a refreshing change from some textbooks that approach physical therapy evaluation and treatment from a very didactic and philosophically restrictive perspective. It is not our intent to teach a particular school of thought, but to develop the reader's ability to solve problems and make appropriate clinical decisions. If we have helped the student and clinician develop a common-sense, integrated approach to evaluation and treatment, then we have accomplished our purpose.

REFERENCES

1. Quebec Task Force. Scientific Approach to the Assessment and Management of Activity Related Spinal Disorders. Spine 12:7S, 1987.

CHAPTER 2

BASIC SPINAL BIOMECHANICS
By Allyn L. Woerman, MMSc PT

INTRODUCTION

The purpose of this chapter is not to provide the reader with an academic or detailed picture of the biomechanics or applied anatomy of the spine. Some areas are controversial and some speculations and findings vary greatly among researchers. The complexity of the spine and its relative inaccessibility compared to the extremities has made it very difficult to study. Therefore, this chapter will present material essential to understanding concepts presented elsewhere in this text. The reader is referred to the bibliography for more complete works on spinal biomechanics and related topics.

The reader may notice a bias toward osteopathic terminology. I have found the osteopathic literature contains excellent descriptions of normal and abnormal biomechanics and a comprehensive, common sense evaluation and treatment philosophy. Where appropriate, I have borrowed osteopathic terms and describe their usage as necessary to give the reader a clear picture of the pertinent concepts presented here.

Tensegrity

Kapandji makes a good comparison between the vertebral column and the mast of a ship in that the spine must be able to rigidly support the trunk on the pelvis, yet provide flexibility and movement.[12] This dual role of the spine has sometimes been referred to as "tensegrity." The spine meets these contradictory requirements through a system of muscular and ligamentous tighteners at all levels which link the shoulder girdle to the pelvis (much like the main yard and the guy ropes on a sailing ship). When these forces are in balance, the spine is straight and the pelvis and shoulders are level (rigidity). However, when the pelvis is not level, as when the body rests on one limb, the vertebral column is forced to bend (plasticity) (Fig 2-1). Since the spine is made of multiple components superimposed on one another, it will first bend in the lumbar region (convex toward the resting limb), then try to compensate by bending concavely in the thoracic region and again convexly in the cervical area. The muscular/ligamentous tighteners will actively and automatically adapt to these changes to maintain

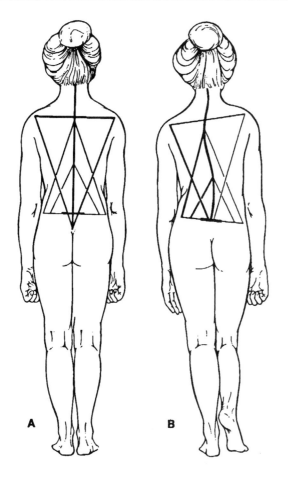

Figure 2-1. Tensegrity: A) Rigidity and B) Plasticity (adapted from Kapandji[12]).

rigidity, shortening on one side and lengthening on the other. This automatic postural accommodation is under the influence of the extrapyramidal system and is geared to maintaining the eyes in the horizontal plane.

Physiological Curves

Viewed from the front or back, the spine is straight. However, viewed from the side, the spine has four curves (Fig 2-2):

1) Sacral - the fused sacrum is convex posteriorly

2) Lumbar - concave posteriorly

3) Thoracic - convex posteriorly

4) Cervical - concave posteriorly

These curves reciprocate and balance one another in such a way that in the normal spine, if a plumb line were dropped from the atlanto/occipital joint at the top of the column, it would intersect the center of motion at the lumbosacral junction at the bottom. If dropped

further, the plumb line would intersect the hip joint. These curves not only provide balance, they provide added strength for the vertebral column to withstand axial compressive loads. Engineers have calculated that the presence of the three curves in the spine (excluding the sacrum) increases the resistance of the spine to compression ten times compared to a column with no curves at all. These curves can also be shown to influence the function of the spine as a whole. Spines with exaggerated curves tend to be more dynamic and spines with reduced or flattened curves tend to be more static[12] (Fig 2-3).

FUNCTIONAL COMPONENTS OF THE VERTEBRAL COLUMN

In this section, the intervertebral disc and certain muscles and ligaments will be discussed with some detail, while other functional components of the vertebral column will not. It is not the intent to underemphasize certain components, but to emphasize those components that have particular clinical significance to the rest of this textbook. The reader is referred to Janet Travell's[19] text for a more detailed explanation of the role of the muscles in biomechanical dysfunction.

Each spinal segment (i.e., two adjacent vertebræ with the intervertebral disc between) may be divided into an active portion and a passive portion. The vertebral bodies are the passive portion while the disc, the intervertebral foramen, articular processes, ligaments and muscles are the active portion.[12] Each segment, through the vertebral arches, forms a first class lever system where the articular processes (facets) are the fulcrum (Fig 2-4). Axial compressive loads are applied through the vertebral column with direct and passive absorption of some force at the disc and indirect and active absorption by the ligaments and muscles.

The Intervertebral Disc

The anatomy and biomechanics of the intervertebral disc will be discussed in great length here because understanding its function is essential to understanding certain evaluation and treatment concepts presented later in this textbook. The intervertebral disc consists of two portions: an inner gelatinous center called the nucleus pulposus, and an outer structure made up of layers of concentric fibers called the annulus fibrosis (Fig 2-5). The nucleus, which tends to be spherical in shape, is basically water with a mucopolysaccharide matrix and is hydrophilic; that is, it has the ability to absorb water. During the day, the compressional forces of the upright position

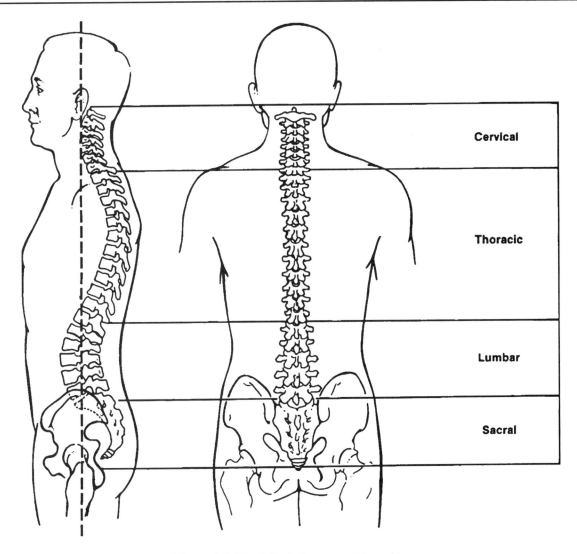

Figure 2-2. Physiological curves of the spine.

cause water to be lost from the nucleus. This is why one tends to be shorter at the end of the day than when first arising in the morning. It is during the recumbent, non-weight bearing position overnight when the nucleus imbibes water, thus increasing its height. The aging process diminishes the ability of the nucleus to imbibe fluid. There is a transitional area between the nucleus and the innermost of the annular rings where the gel of the nucleus is interspaced between these first few rings.[12,8]

The fibers of the annulus are oriented diagonally and alternate their direction between layers in a crisscross (X) fashion. The inner fibers are more obliquely oriented and the outer fibers are more vertical. This arrangement is very much like a bias-ply tire where the crisscross pattern allows for strength and flexibility. The inner fibers of the annulus are quite weak in comparison to the outer. The annular rings are firmly attached superiorly and inferiorly to adjacent

vertebral bodies and the vertebral endplates and serve to maintain the nucleus under constant pressure and in a central position. In the adult, the disc is considered to be both avascular and aneural except for some sensory innervation in the outermost layers of the annulus.[8]

The disc is flexible, allowing motion in all directions, and serves to dissipate forces and stresses transmitted to it, especially vertical or compressive loads. The disc may thus be likened to a shock absorber. Forward bending (flexion) of the spine causes compressive forces to be placed upon the anterior portion of the vertebral body and the disc, thus exerting a posterior force on the nucleus pulposus. This action is analogous to the squeezing of a water-filled balloon on one end, with the fluid moving away from the compressive force. Backward bending of the spine (extension) produces the opposite effect on the disc.[2,16] Sidebending produces a force which is opposite to the

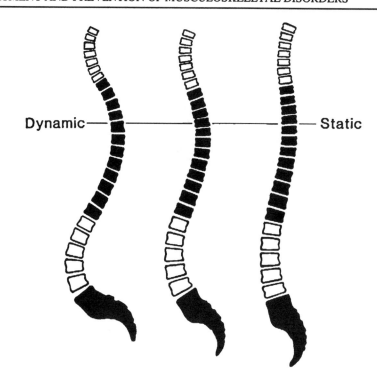

Figure 2-3. Dynamic and static spines. An increase in the normal curves tends to make the spine more flexible or dynamic. A spine with flattened curves tends to be less flexible or static.

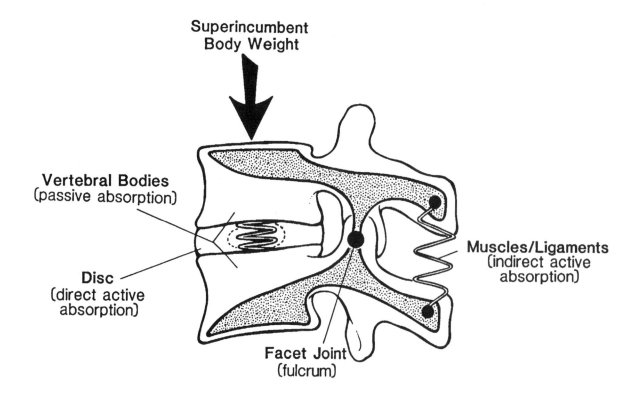

Figure 2-4. The spinal segment as a first class lever system, showing active and passive portions (adapted from Kapandji[12]).

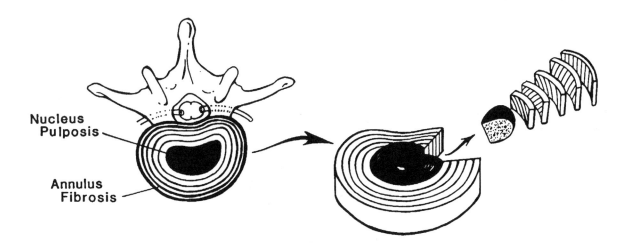

Figure 2-5. Intervertebral disc.

direction of the sidebend (Fig 2-6). In the healthy disc, the annular rings tend to resist displacement of the nuclear gel, thus maintaining the nucleus in its proper shape and location. In the unhealthy disc where the annular fibers have torn, usually in a radial manner, the nuclear gel is permitted to migrate, thus setting the stage for the clinical manifestations of the herniated disc.

Rotation, a compressive force, causes an increase in intradiscal pressure and tends to narrow the joint space. When rotation occurs, the annular fibers that are oriented in the direction of the rotatory movement become taut, while the fibers that are oriented in the opposite direction tend to slacken. This situation puts the disc in a vulnerable position for injury, particularly if it is also under a load (Fig 2-7). Intradiscal pressure is greatly affected by body position and activities. Nachemson has published important data concerning intradiscal pressures in various body positions and under various loads[15] (Fig 2-8). Knowledge of these pressures is important to the physical therapist when designing activity and exercise programs for patients with disc problems. Note that sitting and forward bending (flexion) of the spine tend to cause greater intradiscal pressures than the upright standing posture.

Extrinsic Muscular and Ligamentous Influences

Quadratus Lumborum

The quadratus lumborum lies in the anterior compartment of the lumbar fascia. It arises from the transverse process of L5, the iliolumbar ligament and from a short length of the adjoining iliac crest. It attaches to the transverse processes of L1-L4 and to the inferior border of the 12th rib (Fig 2-9). The quadratus lumborum functions as a stabilizer of the lumbar spine and can act as an elevator of the ilium and lateral bender of the lumbar spine. Acting bilaterally, the quadratus lumborum extends the lumbar spine and assists forced exhalation and coughing. The two quadratii, working simultaneously, can be synergistic or antagonistic in function.

Iliopsoas

The iliacus and psoas muscles share a common insertion and have similar actions. Thus, the combined mass is often called the iliopsoas. The iliacus arises from the iliac fossa, the inner lip of the iliac crest and the anterior sacroiliac ligament. The psoas arises from the lateral and anterior portions of the lumbar vertebræ. Both muscles insert onto the lesser trochanter (Fig 2-10). The primary functions of the iliopsoas are hip flexion and internal hip rotation. The psoas portion can help with lumbar extension and plays a significant role in maintaining upright stance. The psoas and sometimes the iliacus are active during sitting and standing. Both are active during ambulation. The iliacus portion is very active through the last 60° of a full sit-up.

Piriformis

The piriformis arises from the sacrum, passes laterally through the sciatic notch and attaches to the upper border of the greater trochanter (Fig 2-11). The piriformis functions as a lateral rotator of the hip when the hip is extended in non-weight bearing. It can also function as an abductor of the hip when the hip is flexed to 90°. In weight bearing, the piriformis restrains vigorous or excessive internal rotation of the hip.

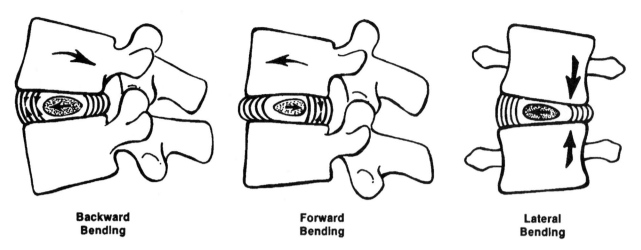

Backward Bending

Forward Bending

Lateral Bending

Figure 2-6. Effects of forward, backward and sidebending on the nucleus pulposus (adapted from Kapandji[12]).

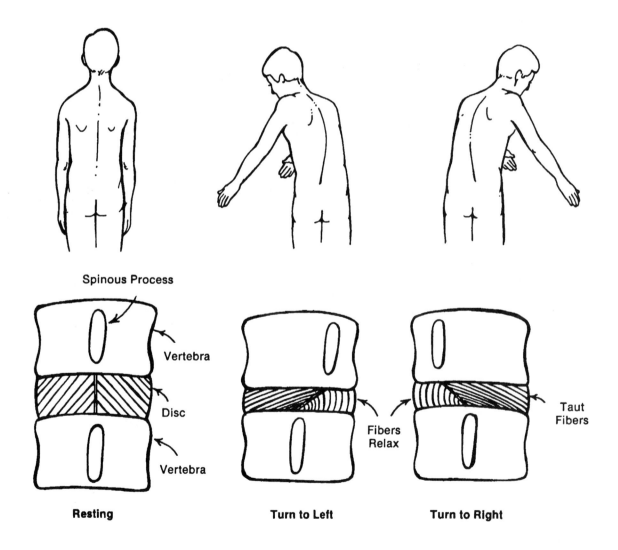

Figure 2-7. Effects of rotation on the intervertebral disc.

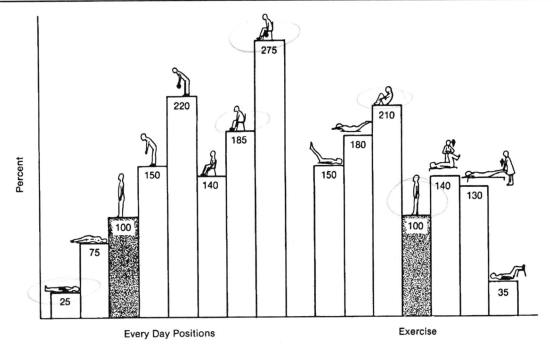

Figure 2-8. Intradiscal pressures as they relate to body positions and activities (adapted from Nachemson[15]).

Iliolumbar Ligaments

The iliolumbar ligaments, under the influence of the quadratus lumborum and iliopsoas deserve special notice as they affect both the lumbar spine and sacrum. In other words, movements of L4 and L5, through the pull of the iliolumbar ligaments and the action of the quadratus lumborum and iliopsoas, will affect the SI joint. Conversely, movements of the sacrum and ilium can influence the movements and position of L4 and L5.

The iliolumbar ligaments have two bands: the superior band runs from the transverse process of L4 to the iliac crest; the inferior band runs from the transverse process of L5 to the iliac crest, the anterior surface of the SI joint and the lateral sacral ala (Fig 2-12). During sidebending of the spine, these ligaments tighten contralaterally and slacken ipsilaterally. During flexion, the superior band tightens and the inferior band slackens. During extension, the reverse takes place.[12]

Because of this direct ligamentous influence between the L4 and L5 segments and the SI joint, these areas must be adequately examined when dysfunction exists. For example, an posteriorly rotated innominate on the left will tighten the iliolumbar ligaments ipsilaterally and tend to sidebend L4 and L5 to the left and also rotate them to the right. Thus, restriction of lumbar movement in sidebending right and rotation may be observed with this dysfunction.[18]

NORMAL BIOMECHANICS OF THE SPINE AND SACROILIAC JOINTS

Fryette's Laws

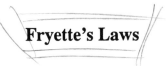

Before looking at spinal movement specifically, certain "laws" of movement must be understood. These laws were first described by Fryette in the early part of this century.[13]

Law I: If the segments are in "neutral" (or Easy Normal) without locking of the facets (erect standing posture), rotation is in the *opposite* direction of sidebending. Simply stated, if the spine is sidebent to the right, rotation of the spine occurs to the left. This mechanical phenomenon is true for the normal physiological motion in lumbar and thoracic regions (Fig 2-13).

Law II: If the segments are in full flexion or extension with the facets engaged (or locked), rotation and sidebending occur to the *same* side. Thus, if one bends forward bends (flexes) and sidebends to the right, rotation of the spine will occur to the right. This occurs in the lumbar and thoracic regions but is considered non-physiological movement. Law II also applies to the cervical area, but is normal physiological motion in this region.

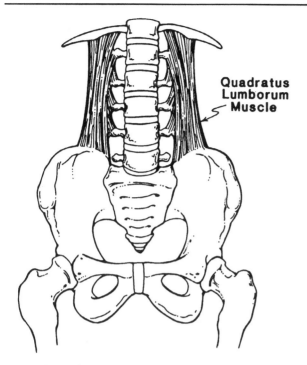

Figure 2-9. The quadratus lumborum muscle.

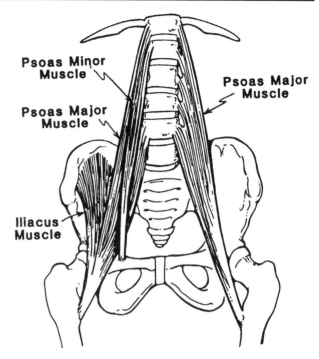

Figure 2-10. The psoas and iliacus muscles with their common insertions make up the iliopsoas.

Law III: If motion is introduced into a segment in any plane, motion in the other planes is *reduced*. This means that since vertebral movements are usually coupled (concomitant), movement into one plane lessens the range of movement available in the other two planes.

Spinal Motion, General Comments

Movement in the spine generally takes place about an axis situated slightly posterior to the center of the intervertebral disc. This axis moves slightly anterior with spinal flexion and slightly posterior with spinal extension.[12] The facet joints, sometimes referred to as zygoapophyseal or apophyseal joints, guide and limit these motions. The facet joints are diarthrodial joints complete with synovial membrane and capsule, and are highly innervated. The plane of the facet joint determines the direction and amount of movement possible between segments. These movements may generally be thought of as gliding movements. The nucleus, due to its spherical shape, functions like a ball-bearing or a swivel.[12] This capacity facilitates the gliding of the facets. Thus, in three-dimensional space, the spinal segment has six degrees of freedom[11] (Fig 2-14). In other words, a vertebral body can move in the following six ways:

1. Along the longitudinal axis of the spine, i.e., under compression or distraction effects;

2. Rotation in the transverse plane around the longitudinal axis of the spine;

3. Forward and backward in the transverse plane, i.e., a degree of gliding or translation movement;

4. Sidebending to either side in the frontal plane around a sagittal axis;

5. Lateral gliding or translation in the transverse plane;

6. Forward and backward bending around the frontal axis, i.e., flexion and extension.

It must be recognized that spinal movement is complex and intricate and that normal physiological movement occurs through coupling of two or more of these possible movements simultaneously.

Depending on whether the trunk movement is primarily one of sidebending or of rotation, the concomitant movements will involve greater or lesser degrees of forward/backward bending versus compression/distraction of facets. For example, in the lumbar spine, if one rotates left, distraction (widening of the joint space) occurs on the left and compression (squeezing together) occurs on the right. If one sidebends left, the left facet will glide inferiorly (close) while the right facet will glide superiorly (open). Thus, if the left facet should become restricted, the

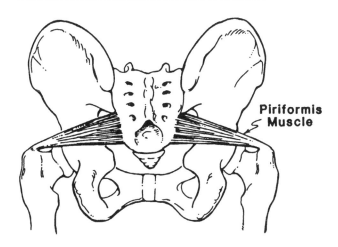

Figure 2-11. The piriformis muscle.

loss of motion would be most noticeable in rotation left and sidebending right. Cyriax calls this the capsular pattern of motion restriction for the spine.[4]

The importance of understanding the normal physiological motions of the spine comes with the realization that one can override these movements voluntarily. One can make the spine move in ways contrary to its natural tendency for motion. This has great implication in the mechanics of injury and for subsequent treatment.

Generally speaking, spinal joints oriented in the sagittal plane and moving about a frontal axis produce

the gross motions of flexion and extension; joints oriented in the horizontal plane moving about a vertical axis produce rotation; and the joints oriented in the frontal plane moving about an anterior-posterior axis produce sidebending. It should be remembered that movement of the spine is described as the superior portion of the segment moving relative to the inferior portion of the segment.

Spinal Motion at Specific Joints

Atlanto/Occipital Joint — The A/O joints, which are condyloid in nature, are oriented in the horizontal plane and move primarily about a frontal axis, producing motion in the sagittal plane. Nodding the head on the cervical spine is the most free movement with approximately 10° occurring in flexion and 25° in extension. Only small amounts of sidebending and rotation take place at the A/O joints due to the concave-convex relationships of the joint surfaces. This small rotational movement is of clinical significance and can be easily palpated at the end of range.

During flexion of the head and neck all cervical vertebræ move simultaneously. The atlas may be thought of as performing a "meniscus-like" function during movements of the head on the neck. In the normal physiological motion of flexion, where the entire cervical spine is free to move, the occipital condyles roll forward on the atlas while the atlas itself glides backward, tilting upward slightly so that the

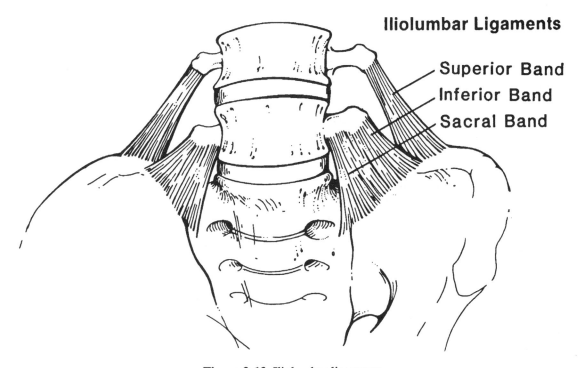

Iliolumbar Ligaments

Superior Band
Inferior Band
Sacral Band

Figure 2-12. Iliolumbar ligaments.

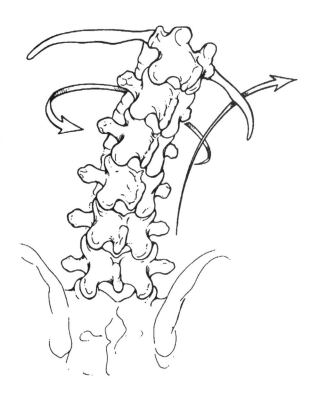

Figure 2-13. Fryette's Law I: Sidebending and rotation occur in opposite directions.

atlas and occiput approximate.[11] If the cervical spine is stabilized, either through pathological processes or by voluntary action, the occipital condyles glide backward on the atlas while the atlas moves slightly forward and cranially, moving the odontoid with it. Thus, the occiput and posterior arch of the atlas tend to move apart in this situation.

Atlanto/Axial Joint — The A/A joint (C1-2) is a plane joint whose surfaces are oriented in the horizontal plane with a vertical axis as its primary axis of movement. The presence of the odontoid process of the axis, which projects through the ring of the atlas, provides a pivot joint which further facilitates rotation at this level. Nearly one-half of the entire range of cervical rotation occurs at the A/A joint, approximately 40° to either side, with 50° or so recruited in the lower segments. There are only small amounts of motion available to the A/A joint in the sagittal (flexion-extension) and frontal (sidebending) planes.

C2-C6 Segments — The facet joint planes of these segments are oriented between the horizontal and dorsal planes. These surfaces tend to separate during forward bending, approximate during backward bending and move asymmetrically in rotation and sidebending. For example, in sidebending to the right, the right facet joints will close and the left facet joints

will open. Remembering that Fryette's Law II is true for the cervical spine, the segmental action of sidebending right will occur with rotation to the right. According to Kapandji, this combined movement of sidebending and rotation totals 50°. Total range of motion in flexion and extension for these segments is 100-110°. When combined with the movement of the upper cervical spine, the total range of motion is 130°.[12]

Uncovertebral Joints — The uncovertebral joints (Joints of Von Lushka) are formed by the articulations of the uncinate processes of the inferior vertebral body (superolateral plateau) and the semi-lunar facets of the superior vertebral body (inferolateral plateau). These joints are cartilaginous and encapsulated. During flexion and extension, these joints slide relative to each other, guiding the vertebral bodies into this A/P movement. During sidebending and rotation, the contralateral joint tends to open while the ipsilateral joint tends close. These joints can be of significant in cervical pathology, especially spinal stenosis and degenerative joint disease.[8,12]

C7-T3 Segments — These segments represent a transitional zone between the cervical lordosis and the thoracic kyphosis. Forward and backward bending are not great and all ranges are diminished (not necessarily in a graduated manner). The facet joints become somewhat more vertically oriented into the frontal plane.

T3-T10 Segments — The thoracic spine is characterized by narrow disc spaces and elongated spinous processes. These spinous processes gradually become nearly vertical in their frontal plane orientation throughout the spine. This elongation of the spinous processes limits the amount of extension possible at each segment. In forward bending, the nearly vertical facets separate superiorly, but this is somewhat restricted. Sidebending and rotation occur in much the same manner as in the cervical spine. Both sidebending and rotation are limited by the bony thorax. It should be noted that all thoracic vertebræ (except T12) have three demi-facets on each side for the articulations of the ribs.

T11-L1 Segments — These segments represent a transitional zone between the thoracic kyphosis and the lumbar lordosis. While the facet joints remain vertically oriented, they begin to change from the frontal to the sagittal plane. Thus, the T12 vertebra has its superior facets in the frontal plane and its inferior facets in the sagittal plane to match those of L1. The discs also begin to increase in height. General mobility in this area is somewhat greater in comparison to the rest of the thoracic spine.

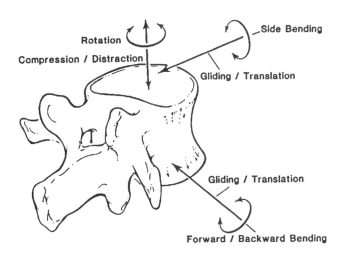

Figure 2-14. Six degrees of freedom of movement of a spinal segment (adapted from Grieve[11]).

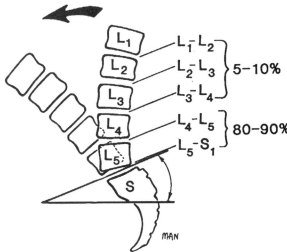

Figure 2-15. Percentage of total flexion of the lumbar spine by segment (adapted from Cailliet[2]).

L1-L4 Segments — The lumbar facet joints are vertically oriented in the sagittal plane. Thus flexion/extension is facilitated while sidebending and rotation are limited by apposition of the facets.

Lumbosacral Junction (L5-S1) — The facet joints abruptly change their orientation from the sagittal plane somewhat obliquely into the frontal plane. This tight apposition of the facet surfaces limits sidebending and rotation to one or two degrees but does not similarly restrict flexion/extension. Cailliet[2] states that 75% of the total amount of lumbar flexion/extension takes place at the lumbosacral junction with 20% at L4-L5. The remaining 5% of motion is at the remaining segments L1-L3 (Fig 2-15). Farfan, however, believes that the greatest flexion/extension range occurs at L4-L5 (10° extension and 12° flexion) with slightly less at the lumbosacral junction.[6]

Regardless of the amount of motion existing at the L5-S1 segment, the tight apposition of the facet surfaces provides the main counterbalance to the tremendous shear forces which are present at the lumbosacral junction (Fig 2-16). The normal lumbosacral angle is 140° with a sacral inclination angle of 30°. The arrangement produces shear forces of 50% of the superincumbent body weight. If the sacral inclination angle increases to 40°, the shear increase to 65%. An increase to 50° produces a 75% shear force. It should also be remembered that the orientation of the auricular surfaces of the sacroiliac joint will influence this angle. Should the posterior arch become fractured at the pars interarticularis, the condition of *spondylolysis* results. Should the spondylolysis be bilateral and the anterior elements begin to separate from the posterior

elements, the condition of *spondylolisthesis* results. Thus, the integrity of this joint is of primary importance.

The total range of motion of the spine is summarized in Figure 2-17. The values given are for the normal adult.[12,11] One should keep in mind that motion will vary by age with the greatest amount available in the 2-13 year age group, and the least available in the 65-77 year age group.[10]

Normal Sacroiliac Movements

The fact that the sacroiliac joints move is not a matter of conjecture. Adequate documentation exists in a variety of literature to demonstrate the certainty of their movement both in vivo and in vitro. How much they actually do move varies according to the sample studied and the methodology of the researchers.[1-7] However, Gray's Anatomy states that the sacroiliac joint moves 5 to 6 mm in flexion/extension movement.[8]

In osteopathic literature, the sacroiliac joint is considered to be two joints: iliosacral (IS) - the innominates moving on the sacrum; and sacroiliac (SI) - the sacrum moving within the ilia. Functionally and from a treatment standpoint, these distinctions are meaningful, even though they are one and the same articulation.[13]

The sacrum itself is wedge shaped and fits vertically between the wings of the two iliac bones. It is suspended between the ilia by strong, dense ligaments. The wedge shape of the sacrum facilitates a self-locking mechanism of the sacrum within the ilia

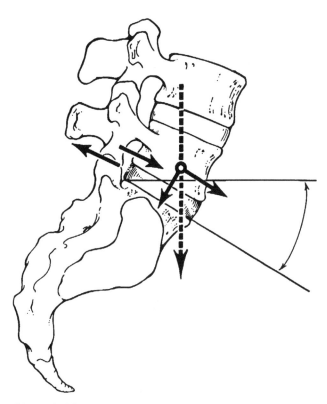

Figure 2-16. Resistance of L5-S1 facet joints to shear forces at the lumbosacral junction (adapted from Kapandji[12]).

with the ligaments tightening as heavier weight is be imposed on it from above.[12]

With the possible exception of the piriformis, movement of the SI joint is not directly produced by muscular action. Motion of the SI joint is indirectly imposed by actions, movements, and stresses of adjacent and other body parts[16] (Fig 2-18).

The SI joint is auricular (ear-like) in shape with corresponding parts between the sacrum and the iliac portions of the joint. The joint surfaces are irregular and characterized by peaks and valleys. Generally, there is a long crest running through the center of the iliac portion of the joint and a corresponding trough on the sacral portion.[12] According to Weisel, the cranial

portion of the sacral articular facet is longer and narrower than it caudal portion. He reports that there is a central depression at the junction of these segments and an elevation at the edge of each segment[20] (Fig 2-19).

Kapandji describes the movements of nutation and counternutation (flexion and extension) of the sacrum within the ilia about a transverse axis posterior to the joint at the sacral tuberosity at the insertion of the sacroiliac ligaments.[12] During nutation (flexion), movement of the sacral promontory is anterior and inferior (the coccyx moves posteriorly), the iliacs approximate and the ischial tuberosities move apart. Conversely, during counternutation (extension), the sacral promontory moves posterior and superior (the coccyx moves anteriorly), the iliacs move apart and the ischial tuberosities approximate. These movements occur naturally during forward bending and backward bending as part of the lumbo-pelvic rhythm.

The following anatomical considerations affect SI joint function and stability:

1) the lateral distance of the pelvic outlet is larger in females

2) the bone density in the female pelvis is less

3) the SI joints are located farther from the hip joints, creating a longer lever arm in females

4) females have smaller SI joint surfaces

5) females have flatter SI joint surfaces

6) the iliac crests are farther apart in the female

7) the vertical dimension of the pelvis is smaller in females.[1, 4, 8, 11, 12]

Another factor contributing to the function of the rest of the spine is the horizontal/vertical orientation of the sacrum within the ilia. A more vertical sacrum usually results in a flattened lumbar spine, which increases compression forces on it. A more horizontally oriented sacrum increases lumbar curving and also

	Rotation	Sidebending	Flexion	Extension
Upper Cervical C1-2	40°	5 – 8°	10°	10 – 20°
Cervical C3-7	50°	35 – 45°	40°	75°
Thoracic T1-12	35°	20°	24 – 48°	12 – 24°
Lumbar L1-5	5°	20°	40 – 43°	30 – 40°

Figure 2-17. Spinal range of motion by region.

increases shear forces at the lumbosacral junction. The vertical sacrum is associated with the static spine and the horizontal sacrum with the dynamic spine previously described (Fig 2-20).

Axes of Movement

Other movements of the sacrum and ilia are possible about any of several axes. Mitchell, Moran, and Pruzzo[13] describe the following axes and movements (Fig 2-21):

1) Superior Transverse Axis - runs through the second sacral segment horizontally. This is known as the Respiratory Axis and is actually a fulcrum formed by the attachments of the posterior sacroiliac ligaments and the thoracodorsal fascia. As one inhales and exhales, the sacrum extends (counternutates) and flexes (nutates);

2) Middle Transverse Axis - located at the second sacral body and is the principle axis of normal sacroiliac movement (nutation/counternutation);

3) Inferior Transverse Axis - runs transversely through the inferior pole of the sacral articulation and extends laterally through the PSIS. It is the principle axis of normal iliosacral motion;

4) Transverse Pelvic Axis - runs transversely through the symphysis pubis about which the innominates rotate allowing movement in an anteroposterior direction during locomotion (see Gait and Sacroiliac Joint Function).

5) Right and Left Oblique Axes - these axes run through the superior end of the articular surface of the sacrum obliquely to the opposite Inferior Lateral Angle (ILA). Each axis is named for its site of origin at the sacral base. Because iliosacral motion is conjoined with the pubis, the sacrum must make adaptive movements about these oblique axes alternately.

Thus, one can see that multiple actions of the sacrum and ilia are possible given the number of axes of motion described above. It is simplistic to think of sacroiliac joint motion only in terms of anteroposterior movements.

Normal iliosacral (IS) movements are usually anteroposterior rotations of one innominate with respect to the other about the Inferior Transverse Axis of the sacrum and the Transverse Pelvic Axis. Other movements of the innominates on the sacrum are possible, but do not normally occur except as seen in dysfunctional states.

Gait and Sacroiliac Joint Function

The following is a synopsis of an article by Mitchell on this topic.[14] The cycle of movement of the pelvis in walking is described in sequence as though the patient were starting to walk by advancing the right foot first:

1. Trunk rotation in the thoracic region occurs to the left, accompanied by left sidebending of the lumbar spine, forming a convexity to the right.

2. The body of the sacrum begins a torsional movement to the left, locking the lumbosacral junction and shifting the body weight to the left sacroiliac. This locking mechanism establishes movement of the sacrum on the left oblique axis. As the sacrum can now turn torsionally to the left, the sacral base must also move down on the right to conform to the lumbar convexity that was formed on the right.

3. As the right leg accelerates forward through action of the quadriceps, tension accumulates at the junction of the left oblique axis and the inferior transverse axis and eventually locks. As the body weight swings forward, slight anterior movement is

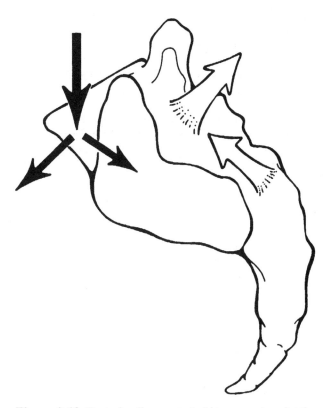

Figure 2-18. Posterior ligaments (white arrows) resist the force of body weight on the sacroiliac joint (adapted from Kapandji[12]).

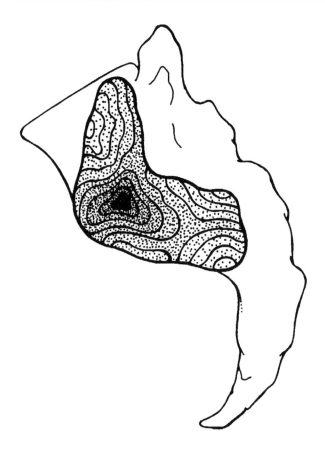

Figure 2-19. Irregular auricular surface of the sacrum, showing central depression. There is a corresponding surface on the left ilium (adapted from Kapandji[12]).

increased by the backward thrust of the resting left leg as the right heel strikes the ground.

4. Tension in the right hamstrings begins with heel-strike. As the body weight moves forward and upward toward the right crest of femoral support, there is a slight posterior movement of the right innominate on the inferior transverse axis. This movement is also increased by the forward thrust of the propelling leg action. This ilial rotational movement is also influenced, directed, and stabilized by the torsional movement of the pubic symphysis on this transverse axis. Also at heel-strike, the right piriformis contracts to fixate the left oblique axis at the inferior lateral angle, thus allowing for a left forward torsion of the sacrum on the left oblique axis (left-on-left forward torsion). From the standpoint of total pelvic movement, one might consider the transverse pubic symphyseal axis as the postural axis of rotation for the entire pelvis.

5. As the right heel strikes the ground, trunk rotation and accommodation begin to reverse themselves. At midstance, as the left foot passes the right and the body weight passes over the crest of the

femoral support, accumulating forces move to the right oblique axis, which then allows the left sacral base to move forward and torsionally to the right. The cycle of movements is then repeated in identical fashion on the left.

Lumbo-Pelvic Rhythm

There is an interconnection of movement between the spine and the pelvis. This is especially true in the total forward bending of the spine: there is a synchronous movement in a rhythmic ratio of the lumbar spine to that of pelvic rotation about the hips.

During forward bending, the lumbar curve reverses itself from concave to flat to slightly convex. At the same time, there is a proportionate degree of pelvic rotation about the hips while the amount of movement at each lumbar level is different (more at L5-S1 and L4-5 and less at the other levels). The rhythm between levels should be so smooth and precise that at every point in the forward bending arc, there will be balance between lumbar reversal and pelvic rotation[2] (Fig 2-22). Obviously, the ability of a person to forward bend will thus be influenced by this balance or lack of it. Many factors such as facet restriction, degenerative joint disease or tight hamstring muscles can influence this balance. Thus, to achieve full, non-pathological

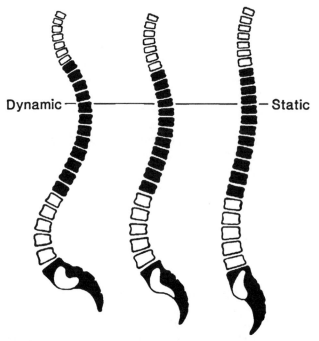

Figure 2-20. Orientation of the sacroiliac joint and its effect on the spine, producing dynamic or static types of function and posture (adapted from Kapandji[12]).

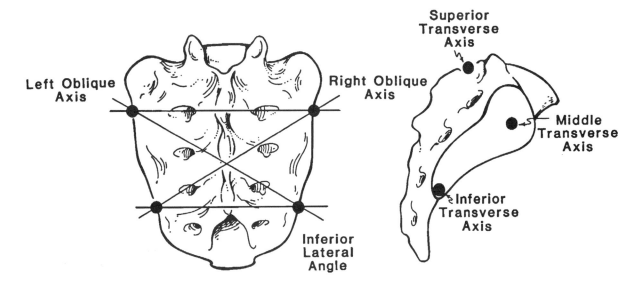

Figure 2-21. Multiple axes of the sacroiliac joint (adapted from Mitchell, Moran and Pruzzo[13]).

forward bending, the lumbar spine must fully reverse itself and the pelvis must rotate to its full extent. The sacrum also moves within the ilia during this action of forward bending. Initially, the sacrum nutates (flexes) but as motion in the lumbar spine is recruited and the pelvis rotates anteriorly over the hips, the sacrum begins to counternutate (extend) within the ilia. Tethering of the pelvis by the hamstrings completes the counternutation movement.

At the same time that these movements occur in the sagittal plane, there is a backward movement of the pelvis on the hips in the horizontal plane. This represents a shift in the pelvic fulcrum so that the center of gravity is maintained over the feet, otherwise the person would fall forward.

As the person returns to the standing position, just the converse occurs: the lumbar spine becomes concave, the pelvis derotates and also shifts forward. The same degree of smoothness and rhythm should be achieved with extension as well as with forward bending.

DYSFUNCTIONAL BIOMECHANICS OF THE SPINE AND SACROILIAC JOINTS

Type I and Type II Restrictions of the Spine

In osteopathic terminology, Fryette's Laws translate into categories of dysfunction. For example, Law I = Type I restrictions and Law II = Type II restrictions. Type I restrictions are usually multisegmental (3 or more segments) and Type II restrictions are unisegmental.

Type I restrictions are also referred to as "accommodating," "adapting," or "neutral" and occur in response to Type II restrictions, anatomic and/or functional asymmetries, sacroiliac dysfunctions, postural problems, etc. Scoliosis is an example of a condition involving Type I dysfunctional mechanics because it involves multiple segments; sidebending and rotation occur in opposite directions; and it may occur in response to some other factor (leg length discrepancy, pelvic obliquity, asymmetrical muscle balance, etc.). The principle restriction to spinal motion with Type I restrictions is sidebending.

Type II restrictions are also referred to as "non-accommodating," "non-adapting," or "non-neutral" lesions and are usually traumatic in nature. For example, in the lumbar spine, normal accommodation is according to Type I mechanics (i.e., a long leg will produce a concavity in the lumbar spine to the same side). But an injury such as a slip and fall or a twist will often produce the single segment Type II restriction: the vertebra will sidebend and rotate in the same direction. A Type II lesion in the lumbar spine will restrict the segment above and below it. Flexion and extension are the active motion components most affected by the Type II restriction.

Dysfunctional Mechanics of the Sacroiliac Joint

The following discussion describes a model for sacroiliac dysfunction as taught by osteopathic

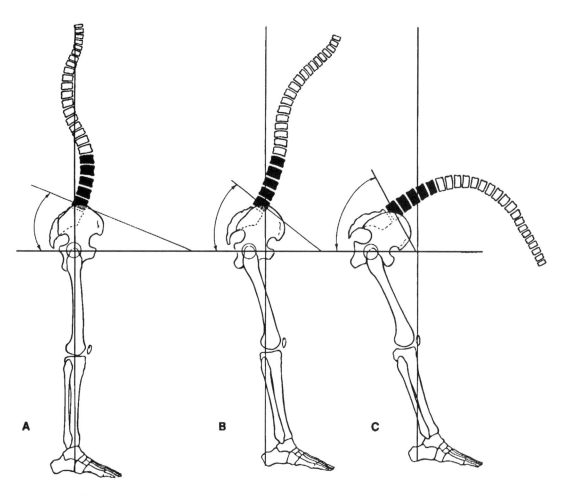

Figure 2-22. Lumbo-pelvic rhythm: A) Normal standing posture with lumbar concavity; body weight directly over hip joints; normal pelvic inclination angle with respect to horizontal. B) Flattening of the lumbar spine; pelvis begins to rotate anteriorly around the hips; hips and pelvis move posteriorly in the horizontal plane. C) Reversal of the lumbar spine into lumbar convexity; pelvis rotates anteriorly to the fullest extent; hips and pelvis are posteriorly displaced in the horizontal plane.

practitioners.[13] The symptoms associated with a variety of sacroiliac joint dysfunctions are similar; certain disease processes or mechanical problems will manifest themselves in localized sacroiliac pain. Diseases such as ankylosing spondylitis, Paget's disease, or tuberculosis all may give rise to sacroiliac pain as an initial complaint.[7,5] Therefore, differential diagnosis of the various sacroiliac joint problems depends upon a thorough understanding of sacroiliac joint biomechanics. Normal and dysfunctional motion about the principle sacroiliac joint axes is discussed in this section. Dysfunctional motion about the axes forms a basis for examination and a rationale for treatment. For simplicity, motion about each one of the axes is described individually. It must be remembered, however, that very few motions in the human body occur in a single plane about a single axis. So it is with the sacroiliac joint.

In the general population, acute strains with joint involvement are actually rare. This may not be true in certain populations such as athletes and the military.[18] Far more common in terms of mechanical dysfunction are structural and muscular imbalances and joint hypermobilities which give rise to sacroiliac complaints. Upslips of the ilium on the sacrum are fairly common, but downslips, inflares, and outflares are far less common. Cyriax considers SI joint problems to be more common in females than in males.[4]

Iliosacral Dysfunctions

The sacroiliac joint can be considered mechanically as two joints: the *iliosacral* and the *sacroiliac*. The term iliosacral implies the innominates moving on a fixed sacrum. The term sacroiliac implies the sacrum moving within fixed innominates.

Innominate Rotations

There are two principle rotatory dysfunctions of the innominates: anterior (forward) and posterior (backward) rotations. The axes through which these rotations occur are the Transverse Pelvic Axis and the Inferior Transverse Axis of the sacrum. Innominates found to be in dysfunction are described either as anterior or posterior according to the side of involvement (e.g., left posterior, right anterior innominate). By far the most common of these dysfunctional rotations is the left posterior innominate with the right anterior being the next most commonly occurring. These two dysfunctions make up the vast majority of dysfunctions of the sacroiliac joint.

Posterior innominate dysfunctions occur most frequently in the following situations: 1) Repeated unilateral standing; 2) A fall onto an ischial tuberosity; 3) A vertical thrust onto an extended leg; 4) Lifting in a forward bent position with the knees locked; 5) Intercourse positions in females (hyperflexion and abduction of hips).

Anterior innominates occur most frequently in the following situations: 1) Golf or baseball swing; 2) Horizontal thrust of the knee (dashboard injury); 3) Any forceful movement on a diagonal (ventral) PNF pattern such as chopping wood.

Pubic Shears

Pubic shears are, as the name implies, a sliding of one joint surface in relation to the other in a superior or an inferior direction. Pubic shears are probably the most commonly overlooked pelvic dysfunction, however, their recognition and proper treatment are mandatory for treating pelvic and sacroiliac dysfunctions successfully. Pubic shears are associated with innominate rotations and upslips/downslips.

Superior Innominate Shears (Upslips)

Innominate shears, particularly the superior, were once thought of as rather rare. However, Greenman[9] has indicated that their occurrence is much more common than previously thought. As the name suggests, a dysfunction here is a sliding of one entire innominate superiorly in relation to the other. These shears are usually traumatic in nature and result from a fall onto an ischial tuberosity or as an unexpected vertical thrust onto an extended leg.

Sacroiliac Dysfunctions

Sacral Torsions

Sacral torsions are perhaps the hardest dysfunctions to conceptualize. They occur as fixations on either of the oblique axes, usually during the gait cycle, and are held dysfunctionally by the piriformis muscle (right piriformis restricts the left oblique axis). Torsions do not occur purely on one of the two oblique axes but have a sidebending component as well as a flexion/extension component. Torsions are defined by the direction in which the face of the sacrum has turned and by the axis on which this motion has occurred. It must be remembered that anatomic referencing takes place from the standard anatomic model but clinically, patients with back problems are viewed from the posterior aspect. Confusion can arise if this is forgotten.

To help visualize the concept of sacral torsion, the reader is invited to take a matchbook cover to represent the sacrum in three-dimensional space. Hold the top left corner and the bottom right corner between the thumb and long finger. The diagonal axis between the fingers represents the left oblique axis. Push forward on the top right corner of the matchbook and allow the "sacrum" to rotate between the fingers. This action approximates that of a sacral torsion to the left occurring on the left oblique axis. Thus, this torsion is labeled a Left Forward Sacral Torsion on the Left Oblique Axis or Left-on-Left Forward Torsion (L-on-L).

By simply changing the finger holds on the matchbook to the opposite diagonal corners and pushing forward on the top left corner, the reader has now approximated a Right Forward Torsion on the Right Oblique Axis or a Right-on-Right Forward Torsion (R or R). *Note that forward torsions are only right-on-right or left-on-left.*

Backward sacral torsions positionally in space appear to be identical to forward torsions. They are, however, quite different. To visualize this concept, again take the matchbook and hold it on the left oblique axis (top left and bottom right corners). Now pull back on the top right corner. This approximates a Right Backward Torsion on the Left Oblique Axis or a Right-on-Left Backward Torsion (R-on-L). Grasping the opposite diagonal corners (top right and bottom left) and pulling the top left corner backward approximates a Left Backward Torsion on the Right Oblique Axis or a Left-on-Right Backward Torsion (L-on-R). *Note that backward torsions are only left-on-right or right-on-left.*

Unilateral Sacral Flexions

This dysfunction begins with the sacrum being fully nutated about the middle transverse axis. At this point, usually secondary to trauma, the sacrum is forced down the long arm of the joint where it becomes restricted. Thus, there is a large sidebending component in this dysfunction as well as a flexion component.

Because of this, the sacrum is unable to counternutate on that side.

Again using the matchbook cover, hold it about one-third the way down on each side. This simulates the middle transverse axis. Turning the cover forward between the fingertips simulates nutation. Now, by turning forward with one hand and turning backward with the other and adding a downward tilt to the side turning backward, the sacral flexion lesion is approximated.

REFERENCES

1. Beal M: The Sacroiliac Problems: Review of Anatomy, Mechanics and Diagnosis. JAOA 81(10):667-679, June 1982.

2. Caillet R: Low Back Pain Syndrome. 2nd edition. FA Davis, Philadelphia PA 1982.

3. Colachis S, Warden R, et al: Movement of the Sacroiliac Joint in the Adult Male. Arch Phys Med Rehab 44:490, 1963.

4. Cyriax J: Diagnosis of Soft Tissue Lesions. Textbook of Orthopædic Medicine, Vol 1, 8th edition. Bailliere-Tindall, London 1982.

5. DiAmbrosia R: Musculoskeletal Disorders, 258-260. JB Lippincott, Philadelphia PA 1977.

6. Farfan H: Mechanical Disorders of the Low Back. Lea and Febiger, Philadelphia PA 1973.

7. Frigerio N, Stowe R and Howe J: Movement of the Sacroiliac Joint. Clin Orthop and Rel Res 100:370, 1974.

8. Gray's Anatomy. R Warwick and P Williams, eds. 35th British edition. WB Saunders Philadelphia PA 1973.

9. Greenman P: Innominate Shear Dysfunction in the Sacroiliac Syndrome. Manual Med 2:114, 1986.

10. Gregerson G and Lucas D: An In Vivo Study of Axial Rotation of the Human Thoracolumbar Spine. JBJS 49A, 1967.

11. Grieve G: Common Vertebral Joint Problems. Churchill-Livingstone, New York NY 1981.

12. Kapandji I: The Physiology of the Joints. Vol 3 of The Trunk and the Vertebral Column, 2nd edition. Churchill-Livingstone, New York NY 1974.

13. Mitchell F, Moran P and Pruzzo N: An Evaluation and Treatment Manual of Osteopathic Muscle Energy Procedures. Mitchell, Moran and Pruzzo Associates, Valley Park MI 1979.

14. Mitchell F: Structural Pelvic Function. AAO Yearbook II: 178, 1965.

15. Nachemson A: The Lumbar Spine, An Orthopædic Challenge. Spine 1:50-71, 1976.

16. Shah J: Structure, Morphology and Mechanics of the Lumbar Spine. In The Lumbar Spine and Low Back Pain. M Jayson, ed. Pitman Medical, London 1980.

17. Solonen K: The Sacroiliac Joint in the light of Anatomical, Roentgenological and Clinical Studies. Acta Orthop Scand (Suppl 27):1-115, 1957.

18. Stratton S: Evaluation and Treatment of the Sacroiliac Joint. Course Notes and Personal Communication. Sept 1984.

19. Travell J, and Simons D: Myofascial Pain and Dysfunction. Vol 2 of The Trigger Point Manual. Williams and Wilkins, Baltimore MD 1992.

20. Weisel H: Movements of the Sacro-Iliac Joint. Acta Anat 23:80-91, 1955.

CHAPTER 3

PRINCIPLES OF SPINAL EVALUATION AND TREATMENT

INTRODUCTION

The role of the physical therapist in evaluation and treatment of musculoskeletal disorders is broadening to assume a position of greater responsibility in the medical field. More and more evidence is pointing to the importance of patient education, exercise and other rehabilitation methods as the only effective ways to achieve long term success with low back pain patients.[3, 8, 9, 16, 12, 18, 22, 24, 25, 26] No longer can a physical therapist responsibly practice without a proper knowledge base from which to plan the treatment of a musculoskeletal problem. The physician, due to the immense proliferation of information, can no longer encompass the totality of medical knowledge. Except in a few cases, physicians are not skilled in musculoskeletal evaluation, assessment and treatment planning. The high level of activity of their practices has forced some to turn to nurse clinicians, physician assistants and other ancillary personnel to screen and treat their patients.

Since the physical therapist already possesses many of the skills necessary to carry out musculoskeletal evaluation, assessment and treatment, it seems obvious that he or she should seek this role since it is the physical therapist who continues to see the patient as the treatment plan is carried out. Therefore, it is paramount that the training of physical therapists be expanded so they become experts in the area of problem assessment and conservative management of disorders that affect the musculoskeletal system.

A void presently exists in this area described by James Cyriax, MD, as the "vacuum in orthopædic medicine."[7] His reference was to the gap between prescription of a drug for a particular problem on the one extreme and surgical intervention on the other. It is from this "vacuum" that the orthopædic physical therapy specialization has emerged. When the physician and the physical therapist who specializes in orthopædics develop a complementary working relationship, the patient truly receives effective and efficient management of the problem. For this management to be effective, the treatment planning must involve the physical therapist because it is the physical therapist who has the most thorough knowledge of the indications for, the contraindications to and the effects of physical therapy techniques and modalities at his or her disposal.

Today, most patients treated by a physical therapist soon realize that physical therapy is not just the application of modalities and exercises, but the application of a comprehensive, systematic approach to the patient's problem. This approach involves the areas of patient evaluation, problem assessment, treatment planning, application of treatment techniques, reassessment, modification of the treatment program, rehabilitation, education and prevention.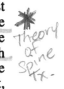

Theory of spine Tx.

When weighing the relative importance of each of the above components in this systematic approach, we must recognize that the evaluation is a vital part. Evaluation, through a series of pointed questions and objective tests, provides a knowledge base from which assessment of the problem can occur.

The assessment of the patient's problem should be based upon correlation of comparable signs and symptoms arising from the objective and subjective components of the evaluation. The assessment is a continual process during the evaluation and leads the physical therapist to a working diagnosis. Well-organized, meaningful evaluation and assessment build the patient's confidence in the physical therapist; the time it takes to perform a complete evaluation is time well spent. The patient will have confidence in the subsequent treatment regimen, recognizing that it is based on a thorough understanding of his or her particular problem. It should be noted that all pieces of the puzzle may not fall into place or be apparent during the initial evaluation and assessment process. A written record of the patient's signs and symptoms is imperative to the successful management of the problem.

Following the initial evaluation and assessment, treatment is instituted based on the assessment. After all, selection of modalities and techniques, no matter how skillfully applied, will be ineffective if applied inappropriately to a particular problem. Thus, treatment, in relation to evaluation and assessment, is of lesser importance, lying in the psychomotor domain more than in the cognitive.

Reassessment begins during and following the initial treatment according to patient response. Reassessment takes place prior to any subsequent treatment, for as the patient's condition changes, the signs and symptoms may alter dramatically, sometimes implicating a totally different area or structure than first assessed. Thus, treatment may have to be modified according to these noted changes in the data base. The therapist's experience, skill, judgment and knowledge all come into play during these phases with reassessment and treatment modification ongoing as the patient's condition resolves. Also, as the condition is resolving, the therapist is educating the patient in management and preventative measures, helping the patient assume responsibility for the ultimate management of his or her own condition to the greatest extent possible.

In the past, we have been far too concerned with doing things for the patient to "make him or her better." Now we must realize that our task is to teach the patient to bring about his or her own cure. The difficult insurance reimbursement issues of the 1990's are forcing us to justify our treatments better than ever before. If we cause a patient to become dependent on passive treatment, we are not only interfering with that patient's inherent ability to help him- or herself, but we will probably not get paid for our services.

Most back disorders are not the result of a single traumatic injury.[4,5,20,19,21] Rather, they are the result of the cumulative effects of poor posture, faulty body mechanics, stressful living and working habits, loss of strength and flexibility and a general decline in the level of physical fitness (Fig 3-1). Months or years

may pass before these factors result in an actual disorder. Recognition of this fact changes the overall management concept for the back pain patient dramatically, shifting emphasis from the acute phase to the long term rehabilitation/education/prevention stage. While attention must be given to the disorder when it is in an acute or subacute stage, the primary focus should be directed toward teaching the patient what he or she can do to effect a lasting "cure."

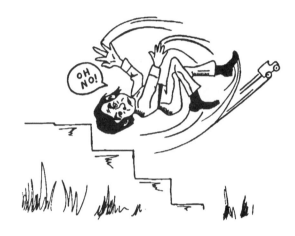

Figure 3-1. Contrary to popular belief, most back disorders are not the result of a single traumatic incident.

Back pain is common. Current estimates are that approximately 80% of the adult population will have low back pain significant enough to miss work and/or see a doctor during their lifetimes.[3] But at the same time we tell our patients not to worry, since most episodes of back pain are minor in nature and go away in a few days or weeks. We unintentionally reinforce this attitude by performing passive treatments designed to make the pain "go away."

But do these patients really recover? Industrial studies show that 25-50% of injured workers with low back pain who return to work for full, unrestricted duty will have another episode of low back pain again in the following year.[1,2,3,8] So the conclusion must be that although the patient becomes pain free and is able to return to work, he or she has not, in fact, fully recovered from his or her back problem. One reason for our treatment failure is that we have traditionally relied on pain as the criterion for assessing improvement. If we used function (strength, flexibility, fitness and the ability to perform work activities) as our criterion for assessing improvement, we would find that many of our patients still have problems even after the pain of the acute episode has subsided.

This is the single most important factor to remember when treating patients with back pain. We must treat function and judge improvement by function

- not pain. If we do this, our patients will truly recover. If we teach them what they can do to prevent reoccurrence of the problem, they will not necessarily become another disability statistic.

The Quebec Task Force Study[22] gives us important information concerning the treatment of workers with low back pain. Its findings must be analyzed carefully, however, to avoid misinterpretation. For example, of all Quebec workers who were disabled with back pain in 1981, 76% were off work less than one month and accounted for only 7.6% of total workers' compensation expenses. On the other hand, 7.4% were off work longer than six months and accounted for 76% of all costs. With this in mind, one might assume that we should concentrate our efforts on the small percentage of low back pain patients who have the complicated, chronic problems. After all, these few patients are the most costly to the system.

Before we subscribe to this philosophy, however, we should ask the question, "Do the patients with complicated, chronic, costly back problems start out with minor, simple back problems?" Could we prevent a minor back problem from becoming a chronic problem through early, effective treatment? We can if we direct our attention to patient education, exercise programs and other rehabilitation techniques instead of concentrating only on the acutely painful episode.

Therefore, most of a physical therapist's back pain patients need long-term rehabilitation in the form of aggressive exercise, body mechanics training and education. This is not to imply that we must continue treating patients for months and months until the goals of maximal strength, flexibility and fitness are met. The physical therapist must closely examine his or her professional involvement with the patient to determine when his or her services are no longer medically necessary. The question we must ask ourselves every day, with every patient is, "Does this patient continue to require the skilled services of a physical therapist?" If we realize that our goal is to be "the profession that teaches patients to help themselves,"[17] then we will appropriately discharge the patient from our care when he or she is able to continue the task of rehabilitation independently.

Increased emphasis must also be placed on prevention. One must recognize that there are limitations as to what can be done in the presence of certain degenerative processes, especially if in advanced stages. Since most back disorders tend to "come and go" as intermittent episodes of back pain, treatment of most back disorders should concentrate on prevention of the next episode. Thus, prevention and rehabilitation are really one and the same. Only three cents of every medical dollar spent in America

is for preventative measures.[6] While there seems to be unlimited resources to treat many apparently hopeless disorders, there is often no financial support for preventative diagnostic procedures and educational programs. It is often a frustrating fact that while insurance companies are willing to pay up to $30-40 for a hot pack, they will not pay for preventive education or a postural device such as a lumbar roll. These tendencies seem to be slowly reversing, but much more needs to be accomplished to put into effect the many advances which have been made in preventive physical therapy during the past few years. This trend is beginning and physical therapy is truly the profession that can lead the way.

VARIED APPROACHES TO EVALUATION AND TREATMENT

Several different approaches can be taken in the evaluation and treatment of spinal pain. The first approach bases the treatment plan on a specific pathological diagnosis. The idea is that every pathological entity presents a unique clinical picture and that a particular treatment regime will effectively resolve the pathology. This approach is ideal, but some health care professionals believe that an accurate pathological diagnosis often cannot be made.[22] Others believe that an accurate diagnosis can be made in most patients.[11]

The second approach to evaluation and treatment attempts to identify the patient's problems such as pain, decreased soft tissue or joint mobility, abnormal posture and muscle weakness. Treatment is then directed toward resolution of these problems, with the assumption that improved function will occur as a result.

These two approaches, "Treatment by Diagnosis" and "Treatment by Problem," are discussed in detail in Chapters 5 and 6. Two other factors to consider in evaluation and treatment of spinal disorders are the location of the symptoms and the chronicity of the condition.

When considering the location of symptoms, one uses the principles of centralization and peripheralization. The assumption is that any increase in peripheral symptoms usually indicates the condition is worsening, and any decrease in peripheral symptoms usually means the condition is improving. The physical therapist can therefore provide treatment and assess its effect by using these principles. The therapist should note, however, that some conditions exist in which effective treatment does cause some peripheralization of symptoms. Examples of these conditions include adhered nerve roots and restricted neural structures (see Chapter 7, Evaluation and Diagnosis of Pelvic Girdle Dysfunctions).

When treating any condition, we must always consider its chronicity. One must realize that chronically painful tissue is physiologically different from acutely painful tissue. In the case of chronic pain patients, many of the problems facing them have to do with the stiffness, weakness, deconditioning, fear and other factors that have developed since the original injury. Most of the treatment effort must focus on these problems in the chronic phase if a successful outcome is to be expected. Therefore, the physical therapist is making a mistake if he or she treats acute and chronic conditions the same.

THE EVALUATION PROCESS

In physical therapy, evaluation is an ongoing process. Thus, even though it may be possible to complete a full and thorough evaluation during the patient's first examination, signs and symptoms must be rechecked during the course of treatment to determine the patient's progress or lack of progress. This ongoing evaluation and assessment forms the basis for treatment modification.

The need to continue the evaluative process is also a key factor in total patient management. The initial examination, no matter how thorough, cannot provide all the answers. A trial treatment should be administered and its effects assessed to determine whether a more definitive treatment program is necessary.

EXAMINATION

The examination is the foundation on which effective treatment rests. The examination findings guide the therapist to select appropriate treatments. Because many different tests, measurements and sequences can be used to collect the required data, the format chosen largely depends on individual preference. To succeed, however, the therapist must internalize a methodical and complete examination process.

When performing a musculoskeletal examination, the therapist should adhere to one method. This will allow full development of the therapist's intuitive skills. Several recognized methods of evaluation are taught in orthopædic physical therapy settings. While there are some differences in the order of questioning and emphasis, the essentials of the examination differ little. The emphasis, of course, should always be on thoroughness and accuracy.

The only exception to the rule of performing a complete examination and assessment of the patient's status on the initial visit is in the case of acute, severe pain or pain which is by history highly irritable (see definitions on page 37). In this case, the practitioner must determine if the problem is of a musculoskeletal nature, ruling out such things as fractures or dislocations if trauma is involved. A complete history should be taken and, if the history does not contraindicate the objective information available, the therapist can proceed with treatment of the symptoms both to relieve pain and to expose its underlying cause. However, when the symptoms of acute pain have subsided sufficiently, the therapist must carry out a complete evaluation.

COLLECTING DATA

During an evaluation, the physical therapist must collect data that are relevant, accurate and measurable. It is most desirable to measure and record data as objectively as possible. For example, it is essential to measure and record a positive straight leg raise test in degrees, to take actual circumferential measurements and to state restrictions of movement in degrees or inches. The advent of the electronic inclinometer has made the objective measurement of spinal range of motion an easier task. It is important to record objective data accurately since changes in these data will be used later to assess the effects of treatment.

Any subjective information must be collected and recorded in an objective manner also. This seemingly contradictory task can be accomplished by recording some objectively measurable factors which correlate with the subjectively described symptoms. Examples of this include the length of time the symptoms persist after a certain activity, or the distance the patient can walk before the onset of symptoms.

The subjective questioning protocol and objective tests must be individualized by the therapist to maximize the information obtained. The therapist should ask the patient only purposeful questions that are directed at determining the patient's problem. In addition, objective tests should be used that are geared to the therapist's individual size, dexterity, physique and experience. Similarly, certain questions and tests will have more or less meaning with individual patients. For example, the result of an individual test or the answer to a question can lead to further questioning and testing to determine the relevance of the item to the present signs and symptoms. Correlation of comparable signs and symptoms is the key.

The tendency to jump to conclusions during the data collection phase of the evaluation process must be resisted. Only careful, accurate, thorough collection coupled with proper interpretation will ensure correct assessment and treatment.

We must be cautious about overuse of laboratory and radiological tests that are not only expensive, but may prove to be misleading. While there are definite circumstances when these tests are indicated, clinicians in the United States tend to use them far too often as a part of a routine examination. Laboratory and radiological tests are indicated when the patient has a previous history of cancer or other serious illness, has suffered trauma or in the case when the patient does not respond to routine conservative treatment. When these tests are overused, they may distract the clinician from finding the real cause of the patient's problem. For example, when one sees degenerative changes, spondylolisthesis, a sacralized lumbar vertebra or a bulging disc on the radiological exam, it is easy to implicate these "objective findings" as the cause of the patient's problem. Sources have suggested, however, that there is often little or no correlation between the radiological findings and the patient's symptoms.[10, 13, 14, 15, 22, 23]

Similarly, we must use caution when describing these findings to the patient. Using medical terminology without adequate explanation may be frightening to patients and may convince them they have no control over their problems. The clinician is not always aware that he or she is inadvertently causing this fear and confusion. The clinician should beware of telling patients they have "degenerative arthritis," a "birth defect," a "slipped disc," a "joint out of place" or other dreaded problems. Since patients know that exercise cannot cure a birth defect, they will be less likely to take self-responsibility for their disorder. Even when patients have such conditions, they should be described in terms of those factors on which the patient can have an effect, such as stiffness, weakness or postural faults.

RECORDING DATA

During an examination, it is important to record data in a format that physicians and other health professionals can interpret easily. The recommended format is the S-O-A-P note. S-O-A-P stands for the elements of Subjective, Objective, Assessment and Plan. This format can be used for all patients seen in a physical therapy clinic. The subjective portion contains the patient's pertinent past medical history and present complaint. The objective portion is a summary of all the clinical tests which the therapist performs and has available to evaluate the problem. The assessment portion lists the problems determined in the subjective and objective sections and gives a working diagnosis. The planning section consists of an outline of the treatment plan, goals and prognosis.

Progress notes and the discharge summary should also follow the S-O-A-P format. In combination with the initial examination, assessment and treatment plan, they become the complete physical therapy record for most patients. Special tests that require an additional form, such as a complete muscle test or a nerve conduction study, can be attached to the initial evaluation.

The use of dictation equipment and a word processor aids efficiency and clarity in record keeping. The evaluation report can be an effective communication instrument, but to achieve this, it must be concise and clear. A handwritten evaluation report is seldom as neat, easy to read, concise and complete as one that is typewritten. In addition, physicians and other health care personnel are less likely to read an evaluation if it is much more than one page in length, particularly if it is handwritten. However, thoroughness should not be sacrificed to keep the written evaluation brief. Material should always be arranged in the same order so frequent

PHYSICAL THERAPY WORKSHEET

SUBJECTIVE:
   Complaint:
   Nature:
   Location:
   Onset:
   Behavior:
   Course and Duration:
   Previous Treatment:
   Occupation/Hobbies
   Other Medical Problems:

OBJECTIVE:
   Structural:
   Mobility:
   Strength:
   Neurological:
   Palpation:
   Special Tests:
   Doctor's Report, Lab, X-ray:

ASSESSMENT:
   Problem List:
   Goals:

PLAN:
   Treatment/Education:
   Timeframes (Frequency, Duration):
   Return to Work Plan:

Figure 3-2. Evaluation worksheet used to record the results of the examination.

referral sources will know where to find certain information, and reference must be made to negative as well as to positive findings. For example, if the therapist should note that, "The neurological exam was within normal limits," he or she has said very little that is meaningful to a physician, for what constitutes a normal neurological exam to the therapist may not constitute a normal exam to the physician. If, however, the therapist records all tests done as positive or negative, this will assure the physician that the patient was well evaluated and managed.

To assure that all important parts of the evaluation are performed and recorded, a worksheet should be used (Fig 3-2). Even the most experienced practitioner may not recall all of the pertinent questions and tests that are necessary for a complete and thorough examination. Therefore, a worksheet is used to record all findings during the examination and as an outline for the formal written examination. The worksheet in Figure 3-2 helps the therapist organize his or her thoughts better for dictating. The actual written report looks much like the worksheet, except that all of the pertinent details are included. For most spinal evaluations, the final report is about one to one and a half pages long.

SEQUENCE OF EXAMINATION

When conducting an examination, the therapist should follow a sequential list of tests and questions to avoid unnecessary movement of the patient (Fig 3-3). The therapist should perform all tests which can be done with the patient in one position before asking the patient to change positions. This assures that nothing is overlooked or forgotten and it keeps the physical therapist moving along in an organized and efficient manner. This sequencing should be applied to examination of all major musculoskeletal areas, and data gathering sheets should be developed for use as a reference to assure thoroughness in testing.

A SEQUENCE OF SPINAL EVALUATION LUMBAR, MID AND LOWER THORACIC SPINE		**B** SEQUENCE OF SPINAL EVALUATION CERVICAL & UPPER THORACIC SPINE	
STANDING POSITION	**SUPINE**	**STANDING**	**SUPINE**
Gait	Passive (gross) FB (knees to chest)	Posture	Passive (gross) cervical ROM
Posture	Passive (gross) rotation	Sacral base (structural symmetry)	Cervical segmental mobility tests
Sacral base (structural symmetry)	Abdominal muscle testing	Aids and assistive devices	Upper limb tension test
Palpate soft tissue and bone	SLR and variations		Babinski's test
Correct lateral shift	Hip flexion, rotation tightness	**SITTING**	Distraction/Compression tests
Correct leg length	SI tests	Posture	Sensation testing
Standing flexion test	Palpate soft tissue and bone	Upper thoracic segmental flex/ext	1st rib mobility test
Active (gross) FB and BB	Sensation testing	Vertebral artery test	
Active (gross) SB	Resisted hip flexion	Active (gross) cervical ROM	**PRONE**
Heel-toe raises	Clear hip	Resisted cervical muscle tests	Upper thoracic segmental rotation
Weight shift test	Babinski's test	Resisted shoulder elevation	1st rib mobility test
Aids and assistive devices		Resisted shoulder abduction	Interscapular muscle strength
	SIDELYING	Clear shoulder	
SITTING POSITION	Segmental flexion and rotation	Resisted elbow flexion	
Posture	Palpate soft tissue and bone	Resisted elbow extension	
Sitting flexion test	Tensor fasciae latae tightness	Clear elbow	
Active (gross) rotation	SI tests	Resisted wrist extension	
Segmental mobility - flexion		Resisted wrist flexion	
Reflex testing	**PRONE**	Resisted thumb extension	
Resisted knee extension	P/A segmental mobility	Resisted finger abduction	
Clear knee	Passive BB (gross and segmental)	Distraction/compression test	
Resisted great toe extension	Palpate soft tissue and bone	Palpate soft tissue and bone	
Resisted ankle DF	Prone knee bend	Adson's test	
Clear ankle	Hip extension tightness	Costoclavicular test	
Distraction test	Paraspinal muscle strength	Hyperabduction test	
Slump test		Roo's test	

Figure 3-3. Sequence of spinal evaluation. A) Lumbar, mid and lower thoracic spine; B) Cervical and upper thoracic spine.

REFERENCES

1. Abenhaim L, Sulsa M, Rossignol M: Risk of Recurrence of Occupational Low Back Pain Over Three Year Follow Up. British Journal of Industrial Medicine 45:829-833, 1988.

2. Bergquist-Ullman M and Larsson U: Acute Low Back Pain in Industry: A Controlled Prospective Study With Special Reference to Therapy and Confounding Factors. Acta Orthop Scand 170: 1-117, 1977.

3. Bigos S and Battie M: Acute Care to Prevent Back Disability: Ten Years of Progress. Clin Orthop and Rel Res 221:121-130, Aug 1987.

4. Cady L et al: Strength and Fitness and Subsequent Back Injuries in Firefighters. Joul of Occ Med 21:269-272, 1979.

5. Chaffin D: Manual Materials Handling. Joul of Environmental Pathology and Toxicology 2:31-66, 1978.

6. Cooper H: The Aerobics Way. Bantam Books, New York NY 1977.

7. Cyriax J: Treatment by Manipulation. Massage and Injection. Textbook of Orthopædic Medicine, Vol 2, 10th edition. Bailliere-Tindall, London 1980.

8. Dimaggio A and Mooney V: The McKenzie Program: Exercise Effective Against Back Pain. The Journal of Musculoskeletal Medicine, Dec 1987.

9. Fitzler S and Berger R: Chelsea Back Program: One Year Later. Occupational Health and Safety 52:52-54, 1983.

10. Gall E: Lumbar Spine X-rays - What Can They Reveal? Occ Health and Safety 48:32-35, 1979.

11. Kirkaldy-Willis W: Managing Low Back Pain, 2nd edition. Churchill Livingstone, New York NY 1988.

12. Klaber Moffett J, et al: A Controlled Prospective Study to Evaluate the Effectiveness of a Back School in the Relief of Chronic Low Back Pain. Spine 11:120-122, 1986.

13. Magora A and Schwartz A: Relation Between Low Back Pain and X-ray Changes IV: Lysis and Olisthesis. Scand J Rehabil Med 12:47-52, 1980.

14. Magora A and Schwartz A: Relation Between Low Back Pain and X-ray Findings I: Degenerative Findings. Scand J Rehabil Med 8:115-126, 1976.

15. Magora A and Schwartz A: Relation Between Low Back Pain and X-ray Findings II: Transitional Vertebra (Mainly Sacralization). Scand J Rehabil Med 10:135-145, 1978.

16. Mayer T, et al: A Prospective Two Year Study of Functional Restoration in Industrial Back Injury. JAMA 258:1763-1767, Oct 2, 1987.

17. McKenzie R: The Lumbar Spine. Spinal Publications, Waikanae New Zealand 1981.

18. Nachemson A: Exercise, Fitness and Back Pain. In Exercise, Fitness and Health: A Consensus of Current Knowledge. C Bouchard, et al, eds. Human Kinetics Books, Champaign IL 1990.

19. Nachemson A: Low Back Pain, Its Etiology and Treatment. Clinical Medicine 18-24, 1971.

20. Nachemson A: Toward a Better Understanding of Low Back Pain: A Review of the Mechanics of the Lumbar Disc. Rheumatology and Rehabilitation 14:129-143, 1975.

21. Nordby E: Epidemiology and Diagnosis in Low Back Injury. Occupational Health and Safety. 50:38-42, Jan 1981.

22. Quebec Task Force Study: Scientific Approach to the Assessment and Management of Activity Related Spinal Disorders. Spine 12:7S, 1987.

23. Quinet R and Hadler H: Diagnosis and Treatment of Backache. Sem in Arth and Rheu 8:261-287, 1979.

24. Saal JA and Saal JS: Nonoperative Treatment of Herniated Lumbar Intervertebral Disc with Radiculopathy-An Outcome Study. Spine 14:431-437, 1989.

25. Tramposh A: Musculoskeletal Injuries Demand New Treatment Model. Occupational Health and Safety (Apr 1989) 20-25.

26. Waddell G: A New Clinical Model for the Treatment of Low Back Pain. Spine 12:632-644, July 1987.

SECTION 2
Evaluation and Treatment

CHAPTER 4

EVALUATION OF THE SPINE

SECTION ONE: GENERAL EVALUATION TECHNIQUES

INTRODUCTION

Chapter Four contains the general sequence and important principles to consider when conducting the subjective and objective portions of a spinal evaluation. The principles discussed in Section One are general and apply to all areas of the spine, from cervical spine to pelvis. Section One provides the framework for a solid, well-planned evaluation. The evaluation is organized according to the S-O-A-P format and follows the worksheet described in Chapter 3 (refer to Fig 3-2). A suggested evaluation sequence was also discussed in Chapter 3, and should be reviewed (Fig 3-3). The examiner will find that with practice, the examination can be conducted smoothly and efficiently if the sequence is followed. The clinician unfamiliar with the evaluation worksheet or the sequence should use a clipboard and paste a copy of the evaluation sequence onto the clipboard for easy reference. With time, the evaluation sequence will become quite natural and the "cheat sheet" will rarely be needed.

After the reader has developed a thorough understanding of the general thought processes necessary to complete a good spinal evaluation, he or she should refer to Sections Two and Three for a more detailed discussion of the evaluation techniques that pertain to specific anatomical areas. Section Two discusses cervical and upper thoracic techniques and Section Three discusses mid and lower thoracic and lumbar techniques.

SUBJECTIVE EXAMINATION OF THE SPINE

During the initial subjective examination (history), the clinician should always be in control of the situation. Some questions, particularly those directed to the chronic pain patient, lend themselves to long discourses by the patient. The clinician must develop the fine art of not appearing to be rushed, yet must be able to direct the interview so that time is not wasted by superfluous information volunteered by some patients.

Each musculoskeletal disorder presents a unique history. The physical therapist must possess a thorough understanding of musculoskeletal pathology and the clinical picture that each disorder presents. Even with this in mind, it is a mistake to consider treating a pathological disorder such as degenerative disc disease with a routine or "cookbook" approach. The signs and symptoms of a specific disorder in one patient may differ significantly from those in another, or signs and symptoms may alter from treatment to treatment in the same patient.

It is essential to good practice to sit down with the patient in the examination room and obtain a detailed history of the condition and events that led to the onset of symptoms. It is a mistake to accept sketchy or inadequate information blindly, even if it came from a physician. Based on knowledge of mechanics, posture and activities of daily living, the therapist very often asks an entirely different set of questions than the physician does. With the history completed, the clinician may sometimes wish to leave the room to finish recording the history, review the notes from the subjective examination and plan the objective examination. Although one cannot always assign more importance to the subjective examination than the objective examination, often much of the information needed to make a correct assessment can be elicited from the patient during the subjective examination.

The following is a step-by-step description of some common areas of questioning that should be included in the subjective examination to obtain an adequate patient history.

Patient Complaint

When taking the history, the first question to ask is simply, "What is your complaint?" This gives the patient a chance to tell in his own words anything that he believes is important. This first question facilitates the rest of the interview by placing both the clinician and the patient at ease. It is useful to ask the patient to rate his symptoms on a 1-10 scale. It is also important to know if today is a good day, bad day or medium day, as the patient's complaints may be different from day to day.

Nature

The clinician often has to ask more detailed questions about the patient's complaint. Pain, weakness, numbness, stiffness and hypersensitivity are common symptoms. The clinician should ask for a specific description of the symptoms such as a "constant deep ache," "intermittent pain" or "sharp stab of pain," but should not lead the patient by suggesting descriptions.

It is important to differentiate carefully between "pins and needles" and/or "tingling" or "numbness" descriptions. The patient should be asked if there is an area of skin that can be pinched or pricked with a pin and not be felt. If this is the case, nerve root impingement or peripheral nerve entrapment is a probability. "Pins and needles" and/or "tingling" are often non-specific descriptions that many patients use regardless of the disorder involved.

Weakness that is present without pain suggests a neurological deficit or disease process or may be associated with prolonged disuse. Painless weakness associated with a peripheral nerve entrapment or spinal nerve root compression often follows a specific dermatome or myotome distribution. Weakness associated with a neurological disease or disuse will typically be more generalized. If weakness is present with pain, it is sometimes difficult to determine if the pain alone is causing the weakness or if there is also an underlying neurological deficit.

Often the patient will describe a slipping, popping or clicking sensation that is associated with certain movements. It is important to determine if this sensation occurs every time the particular movement is repeated. Many joint noises are the result of carbon dioxide gas forming because of the decreased pressure that occurs when the joint surfaces are suddenly separated. When this type of pop occurs, it cannot be repeated for a certain period of time. This is a normal phenomenon. If a joint cannot be popped it is an indication that it is hypomobile and if a joint seems to pop easily it may be an indication that the joint is hypermobile.

If the patient describes a joint noise that can be repeated over and over it is an indication of: 1) an unstable joint that may be subluxing or partially subluxing with certain movements, 2) a mechanical roughness or abnormality of the joint surfaces such as a meniscus tear or osteophytosis or 3) thickening and scarring of the soft tissue (ligament and capsule) that surrounds the joint.

Location

The patient should be asked to identify the location of the symptoms, but the clinician should remember that the location that the patient describes is not necessarily a reliable indicator of the actual site of pathology.[9] Most disc syndromes cause bilateral pain in the spine, while most spinal facet joint problems are unilateral. Pain limited to one spinal segment suggests a joint or nerve root disorder, whereas pain over several spinal segments usually describes a muscular inflammation or systemic disorder.

Ralph Cloward, MD, has described areas in the interscapular region that, when painful, may correspond to anterior disc pathology in the cervical spine.[8] He found these areas when performing cervical discography in the 1950's. When stimulating the anterior surface of cervical discs with a needle, he found that patients complained of an immediate deep, dull ache in a predictable pattern. Conversely, when the same area was injected with Novocain, the symptoms immediately disappeared. The so-called "Cloward's areas" are depicted in Figure 4-1. Cloward also found that stimulation of the posterior surface of the discs caused pain, but in a less predictable pattern. When a patient complains of interscapular symptoms, the clinician should consider cervical disc pathology as one of several possible causes. Correlating signs

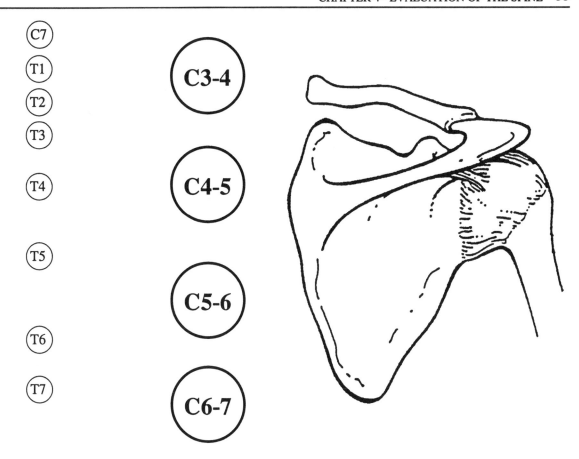

Figure 4-1. Cloward's areas. The small circles represent spinous processes. The large circles are Cloward's areas. Pain in these general areas corresponds to possible disc pathology at the level indicated inside the large circles.

and symptoms for differential diagnosis is important, as many other pathological conditions can cause interscapular pain.

Pain and other symptoms are often referred distally and are rarely referred proximally. For example, cervical pain is often felt in the rhomboid muscle area, shoulder pain in the upper arm, and lower back pain in the buttocks and posterior thigh.

Pain that migrates from one joint to another suggests a systemic disease rather than a musculoskeletal disorder. Pain that spreads from the original site to the surrounding tissues is usually caused by inflammation and/or muscle spasm, both of which are often secondary reactions to the primary disorder.

The use of a body diagram to document the patients complaints, nature and location aids the clinician in two ways: First, it helps keep the clinician organized during the evaluation and decreases the likelihood that the clinician will forget to ask important questions. Secondly, it allows the clinician to remember details of the patient's original complaint, so that the patient can be specifically questioned about his or her

status during future reassessments. The body diagram is kept as a part of the patient's permanent medical record (Fig 4-2).

Onset of Symptoms

The original onset of symptoms and the onset of the most recent episode should be considered. Knowing the exact mechanism of injury can be helpful. For example, joint locking is often caused by a sudden, unguarded movement, whereas sprains and strains involve aggravation or trauma. Inflammatory and systemic disorders present a more subtle onset. Disc disorders usually have an insidious onset caused by repeated activities related to slumped sitting, forward bending and lifting, but the patient may perceive the onset as a sudden event related to one particular activity in which he was engaged when the pain was first noticed.

It is important to realize that the patient will always try to remember some incident that caused the problem. This may not be reliable and it is often misleading to place too great an emphasis on the onset as described by the patient. The patient also may

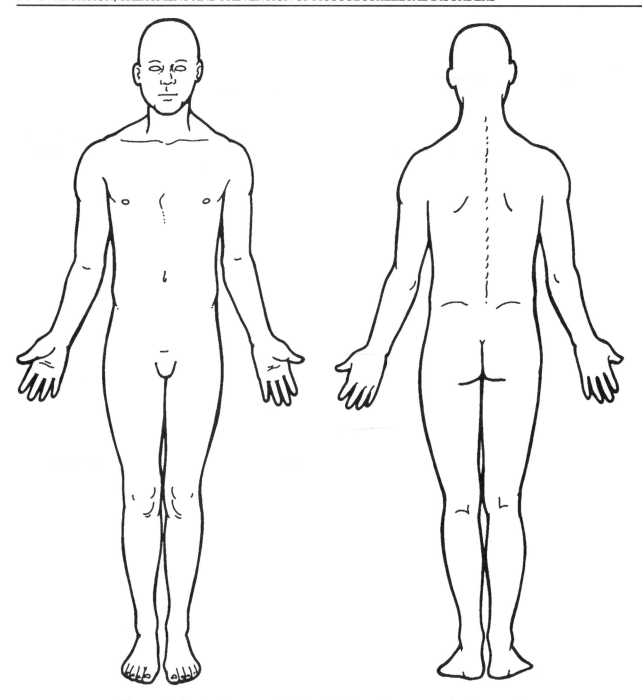

Figure 4-2. Body diagram used by the clinician to document patient's symptoms.

attempt to relate present complaints to old injuries. This can be very misleading.

Since many musculoskeletal disorders are caused by the cumulative effects of poor posture, faulty body mechanics, stressful working and living habits, loss of flexibility and strength and a general state of poor physical condition, one should be certain that these areas are discussed in detail with the patient. Often the answers to both the cause and the cure of the problem are found in this area of questioning. In fact, when considering a corrective or preventive exercise program, it is usually more helpful to understand the patient's occupation, lifestyle and hobbies than it is to know about the incident that led to the current episode of symptoms.

Behavior of Symptoms

What movements, positions or activities irritate the symptoms? What movements, positions or activities ease the symptoms? Does the patient wake up with the pain in the morning? Does the weakness appear only after activity? Is there a pattern to the symptoms over a 24-hour period? The answers to these questions will help the clinician plan the objective portion of the evaluation. The effect of position can be an important clue to the cause of pain. For example, spinal pain arising from the disc is aggravated by sitting and forward bending, whereas walking tends to give relief. Pain arising from the facet joints will often be irritated by walking and relieved by sitting and forward bending. Pain associated with movement in any direction is often related to acute injury and/or inflammation, whereas pain that is aggravated by movements in only one or two directions is often due to joint or soft tissue dysfunction or disc pathology. Pain while resting suggests the presence of an inflammatory process. Night pain suggests a possible tumor, infection or systemic disease process.

It is important for the clinician to identify and distinguish between an irritable and a severe condition. The information gained will help the clinician decide how vigorous and/or complete the objective part of the exam should be. If a condition is highly irritable or severe by history, the clinician's initial physical exam may have to be modified. If a position or activity causes pain, does the pain last after the position is changed or the activity is ceased? Once irritated, does the pain last for hours or days? Lingering pain indicates an irritable condition. If the condition is highly irritable, the clinician may choose to perform a fewer number of tests to avoid causing an increase in symptoms that may last for several hours or days after the initial evaluation. If a position causes pain, is it so intense that the patient cannot maintain the position? Inability to maintain the position indicates a severe condition. If the patient's symptoms are severe but not highly irritable the clinician may be able to perform a relatively thorough evaluation by simply avoiding the end range of positions that are known by history to be problematic.

Musculoskeletal symptoms are usually irritated by certain movements and positions and are generally relieved with rest. If the symptoms do not seem related to movement or position and are not relieved with rest, and the clinician cannot elicit a change in symptoms during the movement exam, one should suspect a systemic disease or visceral disorder and should consult with a physician.

Course and Duration of Symptoms

It is important for the clinician to consider the length of time since the onset of the symptoms to figure out whether the condition is in an acute, subacute or chronic state. The degree of acuteness or chronicity will influence treatment.

The natural progression of the condition should be considered, too. Was the pain greatest when the injury first occurred, or did it worsen on subsequent days? Overall, is the condition getting worse, getting better or staying the same? Has the patient continued to work since the onset of the symptoms? Is this the patient's first back or neck injury, or have there been previous episodes? In the case of multiple episodes, how does this episode differ from previous ones?

Effect of Previous Treatment

It is important to know the effect of any previous treatment. If the patient has been to a chiropractor or other medical practitioner, did the treatment affect the condition? If the patient has had a previous episode of this condition and a certain treatment helped, such treatment should be considered again as a possible means of treatment. Has the patient been instructed in any home treatment or exercises? Which exercises? Is the patient still doing the exercises? What medication has been prescribed? The clinician should ask if and how often the patient is taking the medication.

Other Related Medical Problems

Special questions involving other medical problems such as general health, bowel and bladder problems, any recent unexplained weight loss or any recent illnesses also must be considered. Previous surgery should be noted. If the patient has had a history of malignancy, the possibility of a metastatic spinal lesion should be ruled out. Hypertension or heart disease should be noted, as well as any conditions that would interfere with the patient's ability to exercise. The patient's physician should be consulted as needed.

Occupation/Hobbies

The patient's occupation and hobbies are very important to note, even in a non-work related injury. For instance, a computer programmer whose hobbies are gardening and bowling has a lifestyle that involves many flexion activities. The exercises chosen for this individual may need to be extension-oriented to balance his lifestyle.

For a work related injury, the clinician needs to know any current work restrictions that have been set by the physician. The patient also should be asked to describe current duties at work if he or she is on light or modified duty. Often, a patient may not be working at the level allowed by the physician because there is no work available at that level. For example, the post office normally handles a variety of packages that can weigh up to 70 pounds. A mail handler who is on a 30 pound weight restriction may be temporarily sorting letters instead of handling packages, however. An astute clinician will supplement the patient's work activities and prevent deconditioning by having the patient practice lifting packages as a part of the rehabilitation. As the patient improves, the clinician will add more weight to his functional activities, and thus can give the physician input regarding appropriate changes in the patient's work restrictions.

Furthermore, the clinician needs to understand the patient's regular job duties, to set functional goals. For example, if the above patient needs to lift 20 pounds frequently and up to 70 pounds occasionally to return to the mail handler job, the clinician will identify this as a specific goal in the assessment portion of the initial evaluation report. The exercises and functional activities chosen for treatment will be oriented in part toward achieving this goal. For more details on functional rehabilitation, see Chapter 13, Spinal Rehabilitation.

Doctor's Report, Lab and X-ray

The patient should be asked about the results of tests performed and the physician's diagnosis. This gives the clinician information about the patient's understanding of his or her condition. The clinician may need to explain the diagnosis further or clarify misconceptions about the patient's condition. The clinician should always confirm the patient's verbal report of the diagnosis and any tests performed with the physician's office.

OBJECTIVE EXAMINATION OF THE SPINE

General Comments

The objective portion of the spinal evaluation consists of seven main categories: The Screening exam, the Structural exam, the Mobility exam, the Strength exam, the Neurological exam, the Palpation exam and Special Tests. The rest of this section will be devoted to describing the purpose for each of these exams, and the main points the evaluator should consider when completing each exam. For techniques that relate to specific areas of the spine, the reader should refer to Sections Two and Three of this chapter.

Screening Examination

When a patient presents with extremity symptoms, the exact location of the disorder is sometimes unclear. The patient complaining of arm symptoms may have a cervical disorder. Leg symptoms may be referred from the lumbar spine or the hip joint. The screening examination should be a quick overview of several areas to provide the physical therapist with enough information to decide what specific areas must be examined in detail. If the screening examination proves negative, it must be repeated since there is the possibility that something was missed. If no abnormalities are found and symptoms persist, the clinician should consult with a physician and further medical diagnosis should be pursued.

Screening exams are performed when the patient's primary complaint is extremity symptoms. One must always consider that extremity symptoms may be related to spinal pathology, even in the absence of spinal symptoms. The neck should always be examined if the patient is complaining of an upper extremity symptom. Similarly, the lower back should always be examined if the patient is complaining of a lower extremity symptom. The screening exams are ideally suited for these cases. If, on the other hand, the patient's original complaint is in the spine, the screening exam is not necessary as the clinician will perform a thorough evaluation of the spine anyway.

The screening exam begins with the clinician's initial observations of how the patient carries himself, his posture, gait and balance even prior to entering the examination room. The patient is unaware that he is being evaluated and may show inconsistent patterns, which may indicate symptom magnification.

Structural Examination

Areas of specific complaint or areas that have shown some questionable signs during the screening examination should be examined in detail. The detailed objective examination of a specific area begins with general observation of the patient. The way the patient responds to the clinician's questions should be noted. What kind of attitude does the patient seem to have toward his condition - apprehensive, resentful or depressed? Since the behavioral attitude of the patient often has a bearing on the success of the treatment, the clinician should take time to think about this important aspect of the patient's condition.

How does the patient walk and sit? Does the patient seem to be in excruciating pain? Are there any obvious abnormalities in the way he or she moves about? Such observations are important for the clinician to note, as they may later tell more about the patient's progress than direct questioning does.

The structural exam involves a closer, more specific inspection of the area of complaint. Inspection involves the observation of bony, joint and muscular structures in the areas involved. It is essential that the parts to be examined be adequately free of clothing. Gym shorts and halter tops (females) are essential because they allow adequate observation, yet avoid embarrassment.

Posture

Postural assessment should be made considering the entire spine even if the patient's complaint concerns only one area of the spine. Any asymmetries found may be significant if correlated with other subjective and objective findings. Three types of asymmetries are discussed: Anterior/Posterior, Lateral, and Cephalocaudal.

Anterior/Posterior Symmetry

There should be a gentle continuation of anterior/posterior curves the entire length of the spine. An excessive curve in one area will usually cause an abnormal curve in an adjacent area. For example, excessive lumbar or cervical lordosis may be accompanied by increased thoracic kyphosis. Suboccipital muscle and/or joint tightness will cause extension of the occiput and upper cervical spine, which causes a compensatory flattening of the lower cervical and upper thoracic spine to achieve a level head position. The flattened cervical lordosis is a problem that needs to be addressed in this type of patient, as it can lead to more serious problems including cervical disc herniation and TMJ dysfunction.[33] A characteristic feature seen with this syndrome is the forward head position and rounded upper thoracic spine. The forward head posture is often seen following cervical strains and can become the major cause of symptoms in the chronic stages of these injuries. Forward head posture is also often seen because of certain working positions and habits.

The lumbar and cervical spine should show a mild lordotic curve and the thoracic spine should have a mild kyphotic curve. Absence of any of the curves may indicate restriction of mobility or a disc disorder, whereas excessive lordotic curves may suggest the presence of any of a variety of structural and postural problems including joint hypermobility. "A straight spine is stiff and a curved spine is flexible" is usually a good rule of thumb. Many pathological processes present certain predictable changes in lordosis and kyphosis and can be important clues to aid in diagnosis.

It is also very important to observe the patient's sitting posture. Often the slumped lumbar flexion (flat back) posture contributes to loss of lumbar extension and to the development of a posterolateral lumbar disc protrusion. Additionally, patients with slumped lumbar sitting postures usually have forward head posture and abducted scapulæ. These problems contribute to cervical and upper thoracic disorders that cannot be resolved unless the lumbar sitting posture is addressed. Indeed, sometimes the most important aid used to correct a cervical posture problem is a lumbar roll or cushion.

Lateral Symmetry

Scoliotic curves in the spine are abnormal and are classified as either functional or structural or as caused by a specific pathological process. A structural scoliosis is caused by a defect in the bony structure of the spine such as wedging of the vertebral bodies. A functional scoliosis can be caused by a nonspinal defect such as unequal leg length, muscle imbalance or poor postural habits.

Cephalocaudal Symmetry

The clinician should observe for any cephalocaudal asymmetries, including asymmetries in the ribs or skin folds. Close attention is also paid to the sacral base during the structural examination. The sacral base should be checked closely, even in patients with complaints in the cervical spine. Compensatory scoliotic curves are often present in the cervical spine and may need to be treated by correcting the sacral base.

Assistive Devices and Supports

Any special assistive devices or supports used by the patient should be noted. Care should be taken to assess whether the device has been properly fitted and if it is being used correctly.

Mobility Examination

The mobility exam consists of posture correction and active, passive, and segmental mobility tests. The mobility exam helps determine what structures are involved (muscle, joint or neural tissue) and to what extent they are involved. It is important for the physical therapist to understand the reason mobility testing is performed. When performing any type of mobility test – active, passive or segmental – the clinician should ask two main questions:

1. What does the test do to the patient's symptoms?

2. Is the amount of movement normal, hypermobile or hypomobile?

The findings of the mobility exam are significant if the test changes the patient's symptoms or if the amount of movement seen or felt is abnormal. To perform a thorough mobility examination, the clinician must include in the examination all tissues from which the patient's symptoms might arise, including the joints, discs, connective tissues and muscular tissues.

Since posture often plays an important role in both the cause and treatment of many musculoskeletal disorders, an important part of the mobility exam involves observing the effects of correcting postural abnormalities. Posture correction is done to figure out if return to normal posture is possible and if the patient's symptoms are altered when posture is corrected. This may help find which structures are at fault and also will help the clinician decide to what extent the postural deformity is involved with the patient's current complaint.

Clinical observation shows that many spinal musculoskeletal disorders start as local pain in the neck or lower back but as the condition worsens, the pain and other symptoms begin to spread toward the periphery (arm or leg). Therefore, as a rule, a neck or lower back movement or position that increases arm or leg pain is harmful, whereas a neck or lower back movement or position that increases local pain only may not be causing harm.

The tissues may be divided into two groups - non contractile and contractile. The non contractile tissue group includes capsules, ligaments, bursæ, nerves and their sheaths, cartilage, intervertebral discs and dura mater. The contractile tissue group includes muscles and tendons with their attachments. To differentiate between contractile and non contractile tissue as the cause of the patient's symptoms, the clinician considers the results of mobility and strength testing.

Active mobility testing gives the clinician a general assessment of available range of motion and the patient's willingness to move. Active movements involve both contractile and non contractile elements but may occur in certain predictable patterns that help determine the origin of the patient's symptoms. For example, a painful recovery from forward bending often implicates a disorder of muscular origin, since the patient is using the muscles most when the pain is

the greatest. Pain only at the end of range of motion in the absence of severe muscle shortening or spasm is more indicative of a non contractile problem because the joint is the main structure being stressed at end range. The specific level of hyper- or hypomobility cannot be determined, but a general impression of problem areas can be gained.

Passive range of motion is tested to differentiate between contractile and non contractile structures. These tests determine if the joint range is reduced (hypomobile), increased (hypermobile) or normal. If passive range of motion is greater than active range of motion, this implies that contractile tissue is at least in part responsible for the patient's symptoms. If active range of motion is greater than passive range of motion, the patient is probably not able to relax well enough to allow the clinician to complete the passive range of motion testing.

The *passive* mobility tests give the clinician a general picture of the patient's joint mobility, while the *segmental* mobility tests help to find exactly where the abnormal motion is originating. Even if the patient has normal passive range of motion, the segmental mobility tests can still be useful because abnormal joint mechanics may still be present. For example, one joint may be extremely stiff, but the clinician may not be able to detect it in the passive mobility exam because other joints are mobile enough to compensate for one stiff joint, giving the appearance of normal mobility. Another reason for performing segmental mobility tests is to determine if the structure being tested (stressed) is painful, suggesting a potentially pathological process.

Segmental mobility testing is the most difficult part of the objective examination for many clinicians. Developing the skill of detecting subtle differences in motion from one joint to the next requires experience. Initially, the clinician should not be concerned about detecting these very subtle differences. It is enough to perform the segmental mobility testing procedures on every patient one encounters. Very soon, the clinician will begin to recognize that a certain segment "feels abnormal" or "is definitely stiff" when compared to the hundreds of other segments examined in the past. Eventually, that clinician will be able to detect very subtle differences. The most serious mistake the inexperienced clinician can make is to avoid testing segmental mobility for fear of not understanding the results.

A very good method to use when performing segmental mobility tests is to find the tender segment(s) first through palpation. The tender segments can be identified through palpation of the soft tissues surrounding them, the interspinous spaces, or central or unilateral posterior/anterior pressures on the spinous processes or transverse processes of each segment. The clinician then performs specific segmental mobility tests to identify any differences in mobility between the tender and the adjacent non tender segments. If the tender segments move more than the non tender ones, hypermobility is present. If, on the other hand, the tender segments move less, hypomobility is present.

Many clinicians use the following scale to grade segmental mobility:[26]

1. Ankylosed

2. Considerable restriction

3. Slight restriction

4. Normal

5. Slight increase

6. Considerable increase

7. Unstable

The use of the above scale is not universal, however, and it is usually sufficient and perhaps even more desirable to use the descriptive words rather than the numerals when describing segmental mobility in one's report.

If range of motion is full and painless in all planes, it should be repeated with overpressures to try to reproduce symptoms. Segmental mobility testing should be performed in an attempt to find a joint that, when moved, reproduces the patient's symptoms. If none of the mobility tests and the strength tests described below reproduce the patient's symptoms, the area is considered free of musculoskeletal pathology, and the complaint is unlikely to stem from a problem that can be helped by a physical therapist.

Strength Examination

The strength exam is performed to rule out muscular involvement as the source of symptoms, to decide if muscle imbalances are a source of the problem and to provide a baseline for any strengthening that will be performed as a part of the treatment. Strength tests are usually done in a comfortable neutral position within the available range of motion. The clinician attempts to elicit a strong muscle contraction with very little or no joint movement. If resisted muscular contraction of an extremity muscle produces pain, there is pathology within the muscle, tendon or its attachment. If no pain or weakness is observed, the muscle group (contractile) is ruled out as a source of the symptoms. Weak and painful muscle contractions do not necessarily indicate true weakness, since the pain may be interfering with the patient's ability to contract. A weak and painless contraction, on the other hand, suggests neurological involvement or weakness due to inactivity (see Neurological Examination).

While strength tests are very helpful in differential diagnosis of the extremity joints, they are of very little use in definitely implicating or ruling out muscular pathology in the lumbar and thoracic spine because of the difficulty in isolating muscle contraction without the occurrence of joint movement, especially compression, in these areas. Resisted muscle tests may be somewhat helpful in ruling out muscular involvement in the cervical spine.

Strength tests of the lumbar spine are most useful because of the relationship between trunk weakness and lumbar injury.[3, 12, 17, 20, 32] The lumbar paraspinals and the abdominal muscles are tested for weakness. The weakness is usually treated through exercise, whether or not the muscles are the source of the patient's symptoms.

Neurological Examination

The neurological portion of a musculoskeletal evaluation consists of a series of tests to determine if there is impingement or encroachment upon a spinal nerve root, entrapment of a peripheral nerve or central nervous system involvement.

Resisted Muscle Tests

Resisted (isometric) muscle tests as described above are done to decide whether muscular pathology or weakness is present. They are also useful for determining neurological involvement. When weakness is present with a painful contraction the clinician cannot be certain if the muscle is weak because of a neurological deficit or because of the pain itself. If pain, inactivity and/or immobilization has been present for a long time, the muscle also can be weak because of disuse. Specific muscular weakness that is not associated with pain or disuse is considered a positive neurological finding if it follows a nerve root distribution and correlates with other objective findings. Resisted muscle tests are done bilaterally simultaneously, when possible. This makes it easier to find slight differences in strength. It also makes it more difficult for the patient to exaggerate a weakness. A true weakness will be smooth and present throughout the range of motion, whereas an exaggerated weakness or weakness caused by pain will often be jerky or intermittent through the range of motion.

Muscle Stretch Reflexes

Muscle stretch reflexes are often helpful in finding neurological deficits. As a rule, hyperactive reflexes suggest upper motor nerve pathology and hypoactive reflexes suggest impingement, entrapment or injury of a lower motor nerve (spinal nerve root or peripheral nerve). Normal reflexes vary a great deal from person to person. Occasionally, reflexes appear hypoactive or hyperactive, but are symmetrical. These findings are probably normal for those patients. When a reflex appears hypo or hyperactive when compared to the corresponding reflex on the opposite side, the finding is significant.

It is important to remember that referred pain can facilitate motor activity in the area of referral. This increased muscular activity can inhibit the antagonistic muscle group. For example, pain arising from pathology in any pain producing structure in the lower lumbar spine can be felt as pain down the posterior aspect of the thigh. This referred pain may cause increased muscular activity in the hamstring muscles, which may inhibit the quadriceps group. This inhibitory influence on the quadriceps may cause a hypoactive muscle stretch reflex. The implication is that some muscle stretch reflex changes can be caused by referred pain in addition to spinal nerve root impingement or peripheral nerve entrapment.[31]

Sensation Testing

The patient is questioned closely during the subjective examination concerning aberration of sensation. The clinician should remember that patients will confuse paresthesias with anesthesias. Paresthesias are of subjective value and can suggest a certain nerve root level if they follow a given pattern but they are not considered positive neurological signs. Anesthesia of the skin, however, is a positive neurological finding. If the patient has indicated there is a sensory deficit, the clinician should find with pin prick testing the extent and exact location of involvement. An area of numbness that follows a dermatomal pattern or the distribution of a peripheral nerve suggests nerve root impingement or nerve entrapment or injury. If the area of numbness involves the entire circumference of an extremity (glove or stocking effect), a sensory nerve deficit due to a vascular insufficiency or other medical disorder is suspected rather than musculoskeletal pathology.

Pain that follows a dermatomal, sclerotomal or myotomal pattern does not necessarily indicate nerve root impingement or peripheral nerve entrapment. Pain may be referred from muscles, joints and/or other structures that are innervated by the same spinal nerve level or peripheral nerve. Pain producing structures in the spine are: 1) Paraspinal musculature; 2) Facet joints: 3) Dura mater; 4) Outer layers of the annulus fibrosis 5) Intervertebral disc; and 6) Spinal ligaments.[15, 18, 34, 35]

Nerve root pain is often felt as a deep burning pain specific to one nerve root segment, whereas referred pain is felt as a diffuse aching pain. Since the sensory nerves supplying pain producing structures of the spine are not specific to one level, referred pain is usually felt in more than one dermatome. Both referred pain and nerve root symptoms are usually felt first in the proximal ends of the involved dermatomes and spread toward the periphery as the symptoms intensify.

Neural Tension Tests

Physical therapy clinicians are familiar with performing neural tension tests to implicate the neural tissues for potential pathology. Examples of the most common tests performed include passive neck flexion, the straight leg raise and the prone knee bend. More recently, however, researchers have expanded the role that adverse mechanical neural tension (AMNT) may play in a patient's symptoms or dysfunction.

Because the human nervous system is a continuous tissue tract,[5] any peripheral limb movement will have a mechanical consequence on the peripheral and possibly central nerve tissues. For example, the ulnar nerve is stretched when the elbow is flexed, while the median and radial nerves are shortened. Apparently the human body normally provides for built-in anatomical protection of the neural tissues during movement to ensure continued chemical and electrical neural conduction. It seems appropriate, then, that an examination of the response of the neural tissues to mechanical stresses should be included in a complete examination of the spine or extremities.

Symptoms related to mechanical deformation of the nervous system can result from any of three processes:[5]

1. *Interruption of blood supply to neural tissues*

2. *Interruption of axonal transport systems*

3. *Irritation of the connective tissues of the nervous system*

Also, there are many potential mechanical tissue interfaces where mobility of the neural tissues may be affected. These may be myofascial, bony or ligamentous. For example, the posterior interosseus branch of the radial nerve pierces the supinator muscle (myofascial), the ulnar nerve rests in the ulnar groove (bony), and the median nerve lies under the transverse carpal ligament (ligamentous). Thus, the clinician could consider these interfaces as possible causes of decreased neural tissue mobility and possibly related to symptom provocation in the peripheral limbs.

Researchers are starting to implicate the role of AMNT in many disorders of the neuromusculoskeletal system. Recent clinical studies have linked positive neural tension tests to various peripheral limb symptoms.[5]

For this reason, the possibility of AMNT should be examined in any patient presenting with non-irritable symptoms where there may be a potential neural tension component. This would include any patient complaining of central or peripheral symptoms where the symptoms cannot be definitively traced to a non-AMNT source.

David S. Butler's Mobilization of the Nervous System[5] is the definitive resource on this subject. The neural tension tests are documented well in Butler's text. Most physical therapists are already familiar with the three traditional tests (passive neck flexion, straight leg raise and prone knee bend). Recently developed tests include the upper limb tension tests (ULTT's) and the Slump tests. The ULTT tests are generally indicated for the upper limbs and the Slump tests are indicated for lower limbs and trunk. They are described in detail later in this chapter in Sections Two and Three.

Neural tissue is by nature highly irritable. Therefore, neural tension testing is usually not indicated for severe, irritable, inflammatory or pathological disorders. The reader should review the definitions of severity and irritability found earlier in this chapter. Care should be taken when performing the tests. The testing or treatment of neural tension disorders should only be considered as a contributing factor to the patient's complete clinical picture.

In summary, testing for potential AMNT is a new concept to most physical therapy clinicians. It is included in this text because it is an exciting area of clinical research and a potential contributing component to the evaluation of many clinical disorders that are seen by the physical therapist. The body of knowledge in this area is continuing to evolve; scientifically designed clinical and anatomical studies should lend continued valuable information to the clinician. Mobilization of the Nervous System by Butler[5] is strongly recommended reading for further information on this subject.

Palpation Examination

The palpation portion of the evaluation procedure can give valuable information to the examiner about the condition of the structures and tissues in question. During the palpation exam, an inexperienced examiner uses a single palpation procedure to gain information concerning tenderness, muscle tone and position of the bone. A better approach is to study each element of the palpation exam as a separate procedure. The elements considered are the skin, subcutaneous tissue, muscle, ligament and bone.

The skin is palpated and examined for tenderness, color, temperature, moisture and texture. Because pain can be referred from a proximal site, the area where the patient describes the symptoms may not be the site of the primary disorder.[9] For example, a patient may complain of posterior thigh pain, but the pain may be coming from the lumbar spine. Tenderness to palpation can be a reliable indication about the location of the primary pathology, but prolonged muscle guarding and spasm in response to referred pain can fool the inexperienced examiner. Temperature changes help find areas of pathology. A warm area may suggest acute inflammation or a cool area may mean chronic pathology such as soft tissue hypomobility. Dry, smooth, shiny skin indicates a chronic condition, whereas a slight rise in moisture may mean an acute condition.

The subcutaneous tissue is palpated for abnormal amounts of fat, tissue fluid, tension, localized swelling and nodules. Normally the skin can be rolled over the underlying muscle and bone freely and painlessly. If there are pathological changes at a segmental level, the subcutaneous tissue may be tight and painful when the skin rolling test is done (Fig 4-3). Any moles on the skin are examined to find whether they are superficial or deep.

Muscle tenderness is examined and careful interpretation is given to any positive findings. Muscle guarding and/or spasm is noted. When documenting muscle changes, the clinician must take care to avoid indiscriminate use of the word "spasm." True muscle spasm is somewhat rare, especially in chronic cases. Unless the soft tissue changes found show true muscle spasm (where the muscle is in a contracted state and is unable to relax), other word choices that are more descriptive should be used.

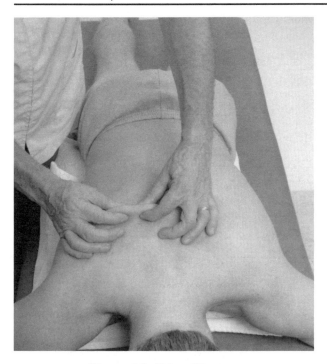

Figure 4-3. Skin rolling test.

Next, the condition of the palpable ligaments is noted. They may be tender if the joint is sprained or inflamed. They may be thickened and coarse if joint hypomobility is present.

The position of the bone is felt to rule out dislocation, subluxation or positional changes such as seen with facet joint impingement. The examiner must not assume that all bony abnormalities are pathological. Some may be congenital and may be unrelated to the patient's present complaint.

Special Tests

The special tests section is included in the objective evaluation because certain areas of the spine have tests that are unique for that area. The tests that are unique to the cervical spine and the lumbar spine are described in their respective sections that follow.

It should be noted that physical therapists as a group, perhaps because of their innate desire to help and make their patients feel better, sometimes fall victim to manipulative patients who have secondary gain, conversion syndromes or other psychophysiological reasons for their complaints. While no one can deny that psychological and emotional factors can significantly influence a patient's perception of pain and actually increase muscular tension, one needs to be attuned to the possibility of these factors for the patient's total management picture.

Sections Two and Three contain specific tests that help decide whether a non-organic component to the patient's pain is present. In addition, the following mnemonic "M-A-D-I-S-O-N" is provided as a guide for psychophysiological factors being present:

M Multiplicity. When one symptom goes, another one comes. The patient presents a history of bizarre or non-organic symptoms in multiplicity.

A Authenticity. The patient seems more concerned with convincing the clinician that the symptoms are real than with the symptoms themselves.

D Denial. The patient refuses to consider the possibility that the symptoms may be psychogenic.

I Interpersonal variation. Symptoms get better when the patient is enjoying him- or herself and worse when a professional is around.

S Strangeness. No one else has ever had anything exactly like this patient has.

O Only you can help! Patients are setting the clinician up for a fall. "All those other doc's before you were incompetent, but you'll figure out what it is."

N Never varies. Symptoms are always terrible and are theatrically described with superlatives.

When psychophysiological factors are suspected, or when the patient is suspected of having secondary gain issues, treatment should still be initiated if the patient has objective physical findings that correlate with his or her complaints. But the clinician should beware of a prolonged course of passive treatments with such a patient, especially when the patient's condition is not improving. Treatment which emphasizes self-responsibility and rehabilitation is most appropriate.

Correlation with Other Reports and Tests

Upon completion of the evaluation, the clinician correlates his findings with other information that is available such as medical diagnosis, physician's reports, x-rays, lab and other tests. So that the evaluation is done without bias, this correlation should be done at the conclusion of the evaluation instead of at the beginning. Knowledge of any severe or serious pathology is, of course, important and should be considered immediately.

SECTION TWO: EVALUATION OF THE CERVICAL AND UPPER THORACIC SPINE

INTRODUCTION

The subjective and objective examination of a patient with spinal pain was discussed in Section One. Section Two takes a closer look at the objective examination of the cervical and upper thoracic spine. The reader should become familiar with the concepts found in Section One before proceeding.

Section Two is organized according to the seven components of the objective evaluation: the Screening exam, the Structural exam, the Mobility exam, the Strength exam, the Neurological exam, the Palpation exam and Special Tests. The order follows the evaluation worksheet found in Figure 3-2. Organizing the evaluation in this way helps the examiner record and report the evaluation results in a clear, concise manner. When performing the objective evaluation, however, the examiner should attempt to perform all tests that can be done in one position at once. This becomes even more important when evaluating the lumbar spine and pelvis, but is still a consideration in the cervical and upper thoracic spine evaluation (see Sequence of Evaluation, Figure 3-3).

After completing the subjective portion of the evaluation, the physical therapist often has an idea of where to concentrate his or her objective examination. It is important, however, to perform a thorough objective evaluation to avoid missing any non-obvious clues because of the clinician's preconceived biases.

OBJECTIVE EXAMINATION

Upper Quarter Screening Examination

The upper quarter screening examination consists of a series of mobility and neurological tests to identify problem areas in the cervical and upper thoracic spine, shoulder, elbow, wrist and hand (Fig 4-4). It is most valuable when performed on a patient complaining of upper extremity symptoms and little or no neck pain. With such a patient it is important to clear the cervical spine as a source of the upper extremity symptoms. The screening examination is redundant if the patient is already complaining of cervical symptoms, and the clinician should skip to the rest of the objective evaluation.

A good screening examination performed by a skilled evaluator can make the rest of the evaluation more concise and efficient. The purpose of the screening examination is to identify what anatomical areas deserve a detailed evaluation. After the screening examination, the clinician will know which anatomical areas have been cleared and which ones need a closer look. The testing is done with the patient sitting in a straight backed chair or on the edge of a treatment table.

First, a postural assessment should be made, then the cervical spine is taken through the active ranges of motion as the clinician watches for signs of pain, muscle spasm and/or limited range of motion. If no signs or symptoms are observed with active range of motion, passive overpressure is performed. If still no signs or symptoms are observed, the joints of the cervical spine are considered "clear" and are not the causal structures involved.

The quadrant test is a useful screening test for cervical spine involvement. The quadrant test can be performed in a sitting or supine position. The cervical spine is passively taken to end range of extension, rotation and sidebending in one direction. Overpressure is applied. This places the facet joints on the ipsilateral side in a maximally closed position and rules out or implicates the cervical spine as a source of peripheral symptoms. *The clinician should perform the vertebral artery test prior to performing the quadrant test* (Fig 4-6).

1. Postural assessment
2. Active range of motion of cervical spine
3. Passive overpressures if symptom free
4. Vertebral artery test
5. Quadrant test
6. Resisted muscle tests cervical spine (rotation C-1)
7. Resisted shoulder elevation (C-2, 3, 4)
8. Resisted shoulder abduction (C-5)
9. Active shoulder flexion and rotations
10. Resisted elbow flexion (C-6)
11. Resisted elbow extension (C-7)
12. Active range of motion of elbow
13. Resisted wrist flexion (C-7)
14. Resisted wrist extension (C-6)
15. Resisted thumb extension (C-8)
16. Resisted finger abduction (T-1)
17. Babinski's reflex test (UMN)

Figure 4-4. Upper quarter screening exam.

Next, resisted pressures are exerted to the cervical spine in all planes of motion with the head in a neutral mid-range position. If these isometric resisted muscle tests produce no pain and no weakness is observed, the musculature of the cervical spine is considered "clear." Resisted rotation of the cervical spine is also a neurological test of spinal level C1. Resisted shoulder elevation is a test for a disorder in the upper trapezius, levator scapulæ and rhomboid muscles and neurological involvement of the spinal levels C2 through C4.

The patient is then asked to hold the arms abducted to 90° with the elbows flexed while downward resistance is applied, testing the deltoid and supraspinatus musculature and spinal level C5. This is followed by active shoulder flexion and external and internal rotation with overpressure to clear the shoulder joint. The clinician should look closely for asymmetries or problems with scapulohumeral rhythm while active shoulder flexion and abduction are being performed. Abnormalities in scapulohumeral rhythm are clues to abnormal muscular forces in the shoulder girdle and upper back. Resisted elbow flexion and extension test the musculature of the upper arm and spinal levels C6 and C7. Active range of motion completes clearing of the elbow. The wrist and hand and spinal nerve roots C6 through T1 are cleared by testing resisted wrist extension (C6), wrist flexion (C7), thumb extension (C8) and finger abduction (T1). The upper quarter screening is completed by doing a Babinski reflex test for upper motor neuron involvement.

Structural Exam

The evaluator should review Section One for general comments relating to structural examinations. This section will concentrate on details used for the structural examination of the cervical spine and upper extremities.

Posture

The evaluator should remember that postural assessment should include the entire spine even if the patient's complaint concerns only one area of the spine. Any asymmetries found may be significant if correlated with other subjective and objective findings. We will discuss three types of asymmetries: Anterior/ Posterior, Lateral, and Cephalocaudal.

Anterior/Posterior Symmetry

There should be a gentle continuation of anterior/ posterior curves the entire length of the spine.

Abnormal posturing often involves extension of the occiput and upper cervical spine, which causes a compensatory flattening of the lower cervical and upper thoracic spine to achieve a level head position. Scapular abduction/protraction and humeral internal rotation is usually seen as well. This posture is often called the forward head, rounded shoulder position (Fig 4-5). It is often caused by repetitive working positions or habits related to a sedentary lifestyle. When the patient habitually holds the occiput in extension, the suboccipital muscles adaptively shorten. This can be a source of headaches that originate in the suboccipital area. The flattened lower cervical lordosis that accompanies this habitual posture can lead to more serious disorders including cervical disc herniation and TMJ dysfunction.[33] The forward head posture is also often seen following acute cervical strains and can become the major cause of symptoms in the chronic stages of these injuries.

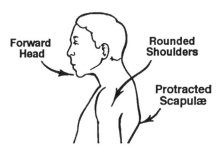

Figure 4-5. Forward head posture.

It is important to observe the patient's posture in a variety of positions. For example, patients with slumped lumbar sitting postures usually have forward head posture and protracted scapulæ. These problems contribute to cervical and upper thoracic disorders that will not resolve unless the lumbar sitting posture is addressed. Indeed, sometimes the most important aid used to correct a cervical posture problem is a lumbar roll.

Lateral Symmetry

The patient should be observed closely from the front and back. Is the head slightly tipped to one side or the other? Lateral asymmetries can be the result of functional or structural abnormalities. Facet joint impingement may cause an acute functional scoliosis in the cervical spine. This disorder involves the entrapment of soft tissue within the facet joint. If this happens, the patient may tip the head toward the opposite side of impingement to take the weight off the painful structure.

Often, a lumbar or thoracic scoliosis will cause adaptive positional changes of the head and neck.

These can be thought of as functional if they are still reversible, and structural if they are long-term enough to cause permanent structural changes.

Cephalocaudal Symmetry

Cephalocaudal asymmetries can often cause lateral asymmetries. Therefore, these two conditions are closely related. When the patient is observed from the front, are the eyes and ears level? The height of the shoulders and the inferior angle of the scapulæ also should be examined to decide whether they are level. Often, however, the shoulder and scapula on the dominant side are positioned lower. This is considered normal and care should be taken to avoid drawing conclusions from shoulder and scapula height asymmetries. Asymmetrical scapulohumeral rhythm during shoulder flexion and abduction is a more significant finding. Scapulohumeral rhythm should be checked in all patients with cervical and thoracic symptoms, as asymmetries or general weakness of the interscapular musculature can contribute to problems in these areas. For example, weak interscapular musculature is often associated with protracted scapulæ, forward head posturing, dysfunction of the levator scapulæ and trapezius muscles, and tightness of the suboccipital muscles.

The clinician should look for any asymmetries in the ribs or skin folds, sacral base and lower extremities. The sacral base should be checked closely even in patients with complaints in the cervical spine because compensatory scoliotic curves are often present in the cervical spine and may need to be treated by correcting the sacral base. The method for checking the sacral base is discussed in Section Three of this chapter. Occasionally, significant abnormalities in the lower extremities (for example, unilateral genu recurvatum or subtalar pronation) also can be problematic. The clinician must use common sense and must correlate objective findings carefully when deciding if a long standing lower quarter postural defect is related to upper quarter complaints.

Assistive Devices and Supports

Any special assistive devices or supports that the patient uses, such as a cervical collar or lumbar roll, should be noted at this time. Care should be taken to assess if the device has been properly fitted and if it is being used correctly. Cervical collars are typically sold in three to five inch heights. If the patient is in acute discomfort, the taller heights are sometimes less comfortable. But if the collar is too short, it allows the patient to slump into a forward head posture. The patient must be educated about proper posture while

using the collar, or it can cause more harm than good. This is especially true if the collar is used for more than a few days. Long term use should be discouraged because of the collar's detrimental effects on the strength, range of motion and function of the cervical spine. When fitting the collar, the clinician should make sure that the collar is most comfortable when the patient is assuming proper posture. If the collar is uncomfortable when the patient slumps into undesirable posture, this is acceptable because the collar then serves as a reminder to use good posture.

Mobility Exam

General Comments

As mentioned in Section One, it is important for the physical therapist to understand the reason mobility testing is performed. When performing any type of mobility test, whether it is active, passive or segmental, the clinician should ask two main questions:

1. How does the test affect the patient's symptoms?

2. Is the amount of movement normal, hypermobile or hypomobile?

The findings of the mobility exam are significant if the test changes the patient's symptoms or if the amount of movement seen or felt is abnormal.

Vertebral Artery Testing

The vertebral artery test is a well-known screening procedure performed to ensure that the movements performed during cervical mobility testing or treatment will not compromise the circulation of the vertebral artery. Most clinicians are taught to perform the test during the initial examination. However, the integrity of the vertebral artery should be reassessed any time the clinician plans to perform testing or treatment that will increase the available range of motion of the cervical spine. For example, if a patient lacks significant extension and rotation mobility, the vertebral artery test probably will be negative initially. The test should be repeated as the patient gains range of motion, since it is possible that the newly gained motion could cause a compromise in vertebral artery circulation.

The test is traditionally performed passively with the patient in a supine position. It also can be performed actively with the patient sitting. The clinician instructs the patient to keep the eyes open throughout the procedure. The patient fully extends and rotates the neck to one side, holding the position for a minimum of 10 seconds (Fig 4-6). The patient should report on any symptoms of tinnitus, dizziness, nausea, throbbing, confusion or unusual sensation. The clinician observes for pupillary constriction/dilation or confusion both during and a few seconds after the test. The opposite side is tested as well. If the test is performed actively, the clinician should make sure that the patient is fully extending and rotating the upper cervical spine. If unsure, the clinician should perform the test passively until the patient becomes familiar with the test movements.

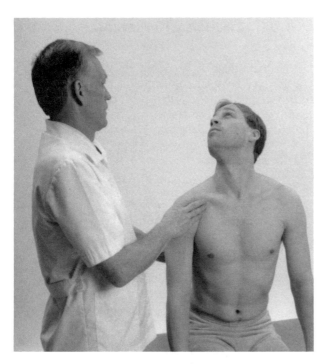

Figure 4-6. Vertebral artery test.

Wendy Aspinall[2] describes a gradual progression of vertebral artery tests. When patients complain of dizziness or other symptoms that are suspicious of vertebral artery occlusion, a gradual progression may be advisable. Since vertebral artery tests themselves can compromise the artery, the progression Aspinall proposes produces minimal stress because the least potentially provocative tests are applied first. The details of the progression are not described in this text. Clinicians desiring more information about her tests should consult the article referenced herein.

If the vertebral artery test is positive, the clinician must avoid mobilization and cervical spine movements that cause extension and rotation into the ranges of motion that produced the symptoms. The patient's physician also should be alerted to the positive finding.

Posture Correction

Postural correction for the cervical and upper thoracic spine often involves the forward head, slumped sitting, abducted/protracted scapula posture that is seen in many patients who complain of a variety of musculoskeletal disorders. If correction of the poor posture can be accomplished, it should be done. If correction of posture results in some increased neck pain, it is usually acceptable. However, if posture correction causes increased pain or other symptoms in the upper extremity, attempts to correct the poor posture should be ceased.

The "head back, chin in" position has long been a favorite of clinicians who are trying to correct their patient's posture. Yet care must be taken when prescribing it. If a patient already has a flattened mid cervical lordosis, improper technique when performing head back, chin in can make it worse (Fig 4-7). The clinician should instruct the patient as follows. First, the patient must be sitting upright with an adequate lumbar lordosis. The scapula should be retracted and the sternum elevated. This should not be done forcefully, but gently and naturally. Care should be taken to avoid elevating the shoulders. Often, this position alone is enough to effect the head back, chin in posture (Fig 4-8). If suboccipital muscle tightness is present, the patient should be instructed to gently nod the occiput, without flexing the cervical spine. If scapular muscle weakness or anterior shoulder tightness is present, these areas also should be addressed.

Active Mobility Testing

Atlanto/Occipital Joint

For active motion, the joint can be tested with the patient seated or supine by simply asking the patient to nod his head slightly. The cervical spine should be in neutral for this test. A neutral position is most easily achieved by asking the patient to sit up straight with a normal lumbar lordosis, and elevate the sternum. The clinician may then use the nose and the midline of the face for reference and observe for any lateral deviations of the head during the nodding movement. Deviation to one side suggests a restriction in movement of the A/O joint on that side. Palpation of the suboccipital area during active motion helps the clinician to feel the quality of movement and to make sure that the movement is only taking place at the A/O joint.

Atlanto/Axial Joint

When testing active mobility of the atlanto/axial joint, one should remember that this joint is oriented

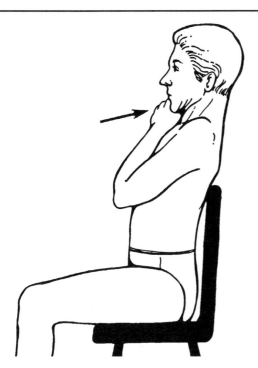

Figure 4-7. Improper correction of forward head posture, decreasing the normal cervical lordosis.

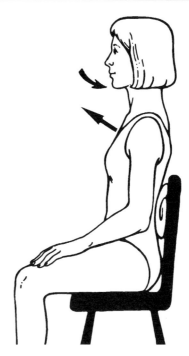

Figure 4-8. Proper correction of the forward head posture, maintaining normal cervical lordosis.

in the horizontal plane. Rotation is the main motion of the A/A joint. It has only small excursions of flexion, extension and sidebending. If a rotatory restriction of the cervical spine is present, the A/A joint should be considered as a probable factor. Rotation of the A/A joint can be effectively tested actively in a sitting position by asking the patient first to fully flex the cervical spine, then rotate. This technique isolates rotation of the A/A joint by "locking" the rest of the cervical spine into flexion (Fig 4-9).

Mid and Lower Cervical and Upper Thoracic Spine

Active range of motion of the mid-lower cervical and upper thoracic spine is examined with the patient sitting. Gross range of motion is observed when the clinician asks the patient to actively forward and backward bend, sidebend and rotate in each direction. Any movements that are limited or that change the patient's symptoms are noted.

Next, the clinician palpates between the spinous processes while the patient performs active flexion, extension and rotation of the upper thoracic spine. This is actually a segmental mobility palpation technique, but is included in the active mobility section for simplicity because it is performed during the active mobility exam. Flexion and extension movement can be felt by placing the finger between the spinous processes as the patient forward and backward bends. Active rotation can be assessed by placing the thumbs

on the spinous processes or pinching the spinous processes at two levels and watching and feeling the movement between the levels. This test also can be done with the patient lying prone, rotating the head from one side to the other (Fig 4-10). Palpating segmental mobility during active motion of the cervical spine is not as effective, as it is easier to palpate

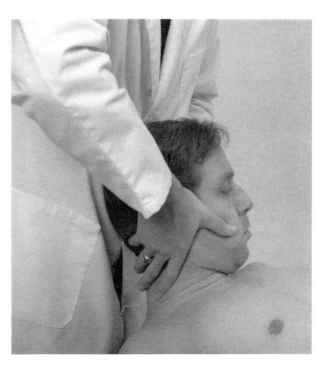

Figure 4-9. Testing rotation mobility at the A/A joint.

cervical motion using the prone and supine segmental mobility tests described later.

If all active range of motion is within normal limits and is symptom free, the movements are repeated and passive overpressures are given at the end of range of each movement. If no pain or other symptoms arise, even when overpressures are applied, the area is clear of musculoskeletal pathology.

Passive Mobility Testing

Passive range of motion is tested to differentiate between contractile and non contractile structures. These tests determine if the joint range is reduced (hypomobile), increased (hypermobile) or normal. In a supine position, the cervical spine is moved through each plane of motion passively by the clinician, with

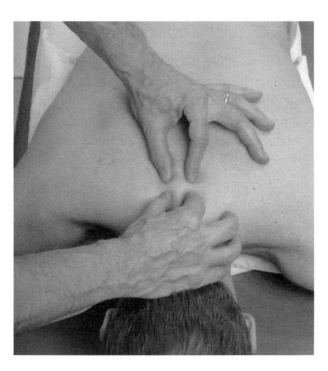
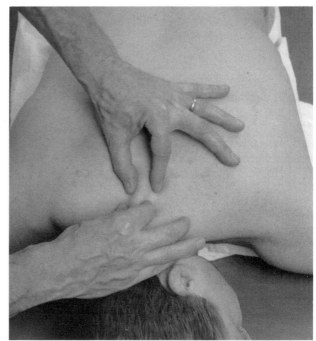
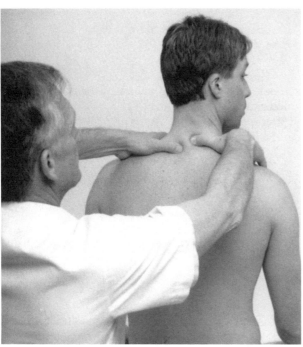
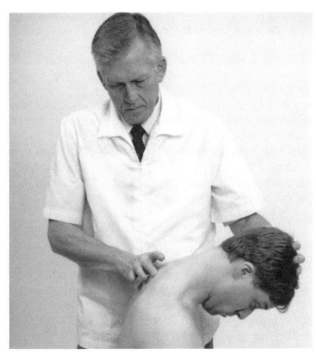

Figure 4-10. Palpating segmental mobility during active mobility testing - lower cervical and upper thoracic spine.

care being taken to ensure the patient is relaxed and not voluntarily contracting his or her musculature. If active range of motion is less than passive range of motion, this implies that contractile tissue is at least in part responsible for the patient's symptoms. If active range of motion is greater than passive range of motion, the patient probably cannot relax well enough to allow the clinician to complete the passive range of motion testing. This is common in cases where the patient is extremely painful or anxious. In such cases, the passive range of motion testing should be repeated later when the patient is more comfortable and at ease.

Segmental Mobility Testing

Atlanto/Occipital Joint

To palpate segmental mobility of the A/O joint, the clinician stands at the head of the table with the patient lying supine. The head is fully supported under the occiput by both hands while contact is made with the transverse processes of the atlas by the index or middle fingertips. This contact is indirectly made through soft tissue between the mastoid and the ramus of the mandible. This hand support and palpation technique can be used by the clinician for forward/ backward bending, sidebending and rotational movements (Fig 4-11).

Forward/Backward Bending - The clinician passively moves the head in a nodding movement.

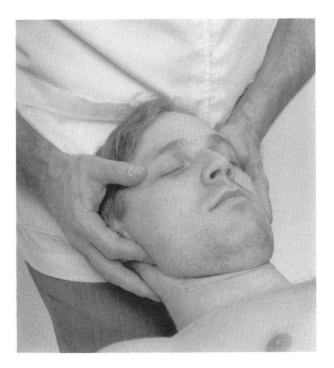

Figure 4-11. Palpating segmental mobility - A/O joint.

Care should be taken to avoid flexing the entire cervical spine. The transverse processes should move symmetrically or not at all.

Sidebending - The clinician passively sidebends the head on the neck. Care should be taken to avoid sidebending the entire cervical spine. The transverse process of the atlas will become more prominent on the side opposite the direction of sidebending.

Rotation - The transverse process keeps a constant relationship between the mastoid and ramus during the first few degrees of rotation. At the end of rotation range, the transverse process can be felt to approximate or even disappear behind the mastoid or the ramus depending which way the head is turned. For example, if the clinician turns the head to the left, the right transverse process will approximate/disappear behind the right mastoid. In right rotation, the opposite should occur. The two sides are compared for symmetry of movement.

Atlanto/Axial Joint

The clinician stands at the head of the table with the patient lying supine, using the same hand placement that was used in the A/O evaluation. The clinician then fully flexes the cervical spine, to "lock" the cervical spine from any other motions. The clinician then tests the A/A joint for a restriction in its ability to rotate by rotating the head each direction, taking care to maintain full flexion during the movement. No other segmental mobility tests of the A/A joint are performed, since rotation is its main movement.

Mid and Lower Cervical and Upper Thoracic Spine

The segmental mobility tests for the cervical spine are forward bending, backward bending, rotation, sidebending and side glide. They enable the clinician to feel specific areas of hyper- or hypomobility in the cervical spine.

The patient is positioned supine with his or her head extending over the end of the treatment plinth. It is important for the clinician to support the patient's head in such a way that the patient can relax completely, having confidence that the clinician has full control of the movements. The treatment plinth must be adjusted to the correct height for the individual clinician. The patient's head is rested against the anterior aspect of the clinician's hip (Fig 4-12). The clinician must observe the neck musculature (scalenes and sternocleidomastoids) to be certain that the patient is relaxed. The hands are cradled to hold the patient's head and neck. The index fingers support the articular pillar superior to the segment to be tested (Fig 4-13).

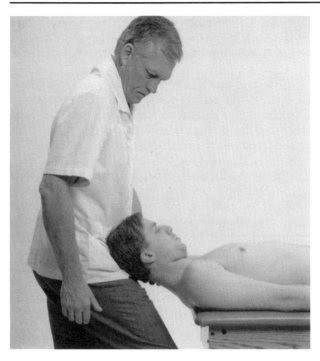

Figure 4-12. Position of the patient for cervical spine segmental mobility testing.

Cervical Forward Bending

Forward bending in the cervical spine involves superior and anterior glide of the superior articulating surface on the inferior articulating surface bilaterally. The patient's head and neck are held in 30° of forward bending. This aligns the plane of the cervical facet joints perpendicular to the floor. Forward bending is done by lifting straight upward with both hands. To start, the clinician's knees should be slightly bent. The clinician extends his or her knees slightly to keep the patient's head in the correct position (Fig 4-14). Most of the force is directed through the index fingers, but contact is maintained with all of the neck and head so that it is carried along with the movement.

Cervical Backward Bending

Backward bending is performed in the same manner, except that the head and neck are not carried along with the movement and the test is begun with the head and neck in a neutral position. Only force through the index fingers is applied. This causes backward bending to occur at the segments adjacent to the contact point. In effect, the index fingers act as a fulcrum with the weight of the patient's trunk on one end and the head on the other end stabilizing inferiorly and superiorly (Fig 4-15).

Cervical Rotation

Cervical rotation involves superior and anterior glide of the superior articulating facet on the inferior articulating facet on one side and slight inferior and posterior glide on the opposite side. Therefore, rotation is tested in the same manner as forward bending, except to only one side at a time, and it is done from the neutral position. For example, to do left rotation, the right hand lifts upward to perform the movement, while the left hand supports (Fig 4-16).

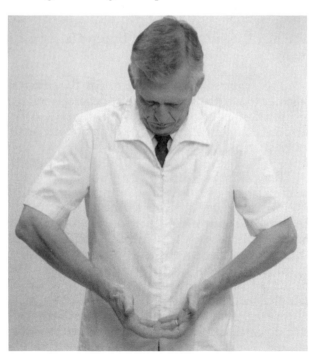

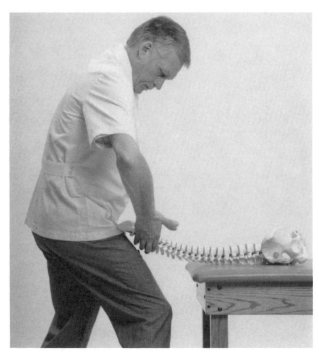

Figure 4-13. Position of the therapist's hands for cervical spine segmental mobility testing.

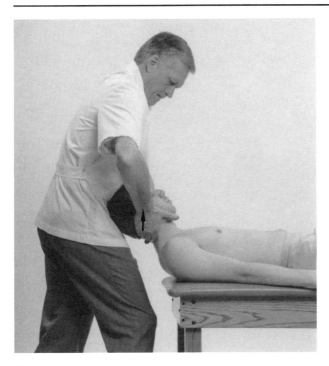

Figure 4-14. Segmental mobility testing - cervical forward bending.

Cervical Sidebending

The same positioning is used for cervical sidebending. Force is applied in a medial and slightly inferior direction through the base of the index finger as it contacts the lateral aspect of the articular pillar. The point of contact on the index finger is lateral and slightly toward the palmar surface of the metacarpophalangeal joint. This force causes the segment adjacent to the contact to sidebend to the same side as the mobilizing force. In effect, the index fingers act as a fulcrum as the spine is stabilized by the trunk inferiorly and by the opposite hand against the side of the head superiorly (Fig 4-17).

Cervical Side Gliding

The same basic position is used for cervical side gliding. Force is applied in a medial direction through the index finger as it contacts the lateral aspect of the articular pillar, causing movement to occur at the segment below the contact. The point of contact on the index finger is on the palmar surface of the metacarpophalangeal joint. The patient's head is carried to the side with this movement. To do this, the clinician must shift his or her hips in the direction of the movement (Fig 4-18).

Upper Thoracic Flexion, Extension and Rotation

Segmental mobility of the upper thoracic spine can be palpated during active mobility testing as

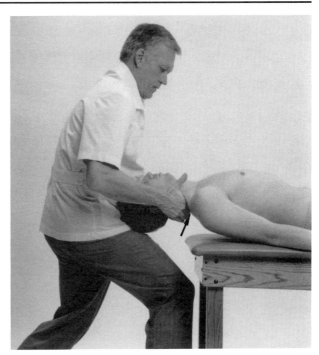

Figure 4-15. Segmental mobility testing - cervical backward bending.

described earlier. The clinician palpates between the spinous processes when the patient is performing active flexion, extension and rotation of the upper thoracic spine so that active and segmental mobility testing is performed simultaneously. Flexion and extension movement can be felt by placing the finger between the spinous processes as the patient forward and backward bends. Rotation can be assessed with

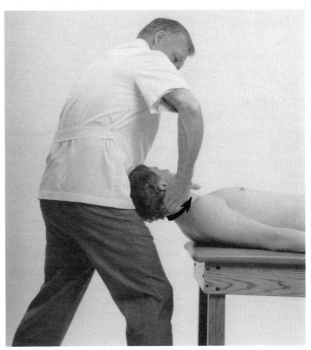

Figure 4-16. Segmental mobility testing - cervical rotation.

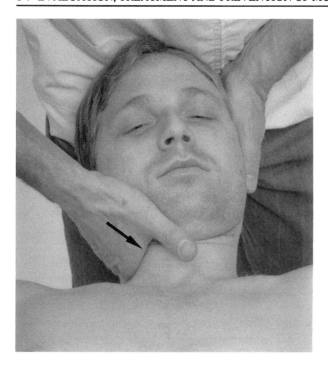

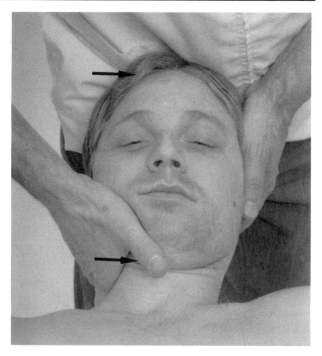

Figure 4-17. Segmental mobility testing - cervical sidebending.

Figure 4-18. Segmental mobility testing - cervical side gliding.

the patient sitting or lying prone by placing the thumbs on the spinous processes or pinching the spinous processes at two levels and watching and feeling the movement between the levels as the patient rotates the head from side to side (Fig 4-10).

Posterior/Anterior Palpation Techniques for Cervical and Upper Thoracic Spine

With the patient lying prone, central posterior/anterior pressure can be applied to the spinous processes of the cervical and upper thoracic spine. Unilateral P/A pressures applied to the transverse processes are also very helpful in assessing general mobility and symptom response. These techniques assess general mobility and symptom response and are not specific tests for flexion, extension or rotation mobility. A positive response to these P/A pressures should be correlated with other mobility tests (Fig 4-19).

Special Mobility Tests for the 1st Rib

The cervical-thoracic junction represents the transition of cervical segments into the thoracic spine and the rib cage. Because of its soft tissue attachments and its attachment to T1, 1st rib mobility is important to assess in a complete cervical and upper thoracic mobility examination.

The patient is supine on the examination table. While supporting the head under the occiput, the clinician induces passive sidebending to the left. At the same time, the clinician's right thumb is palpating the 1st rib lateral to the C7 transverse process. The clinician notes the point in sidebending range of motion when the 1st rib starts to move cephalically into the palpating thumb (Fig 4-20). This is compared to the contralateral side. Asymmetries should be noted. Early 1st rib movement when the cervical spine is sidebent may be indicative of scalene muscle tightness on the same side being palpated. Joint dysfunction of the 1st rib can be confirmed or ruled out by the segmental mobility test described below.

Segmental mobility of the 1st rib is tested with the patient lying prone. The clinician palpates the 1st rib by placing the thumbs underneath (anterior to) the muscle belly of the upper trapezius right next to the cervical spine. A caudally-directed pressure is applied (Fig 4-21). The first firm resistance felt caudally will be the 1st rib. The clinician then applies pressure onto the 1st rib to detect differences in mobility from one side to another, and to determine whether the patient's symptoms are provoked.

Use of an Inclinometer in Range of Motion Testing

The AMA Guides to the Evaluation of Permanent Impairment, 1990 state that standard goniometric techniques for measuring spinal movement can be highly inaccurate and that measurement techniques

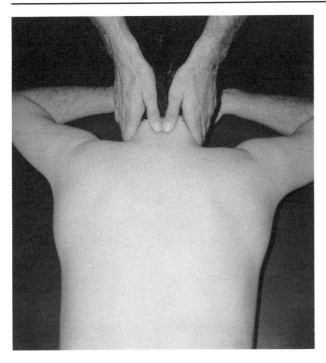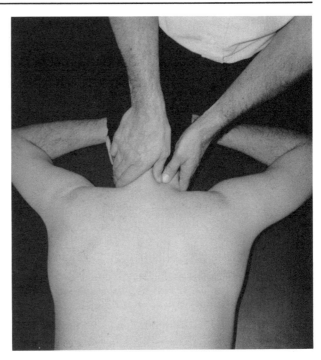

Figure 4-19. Palpating segmental mobility. A) Central P/A pressure on a cervical spinous process; B) Unilateral P/A pressure on a cervical transverse process.

using inclinometers are necessary to obtain reliable spinal mobility measurements.[1] For this reason, many clinicians are using inclinometers to measure and report spinal range of motion (Fig 4-22). Inclinometers are also useful because improvements during treatment can be measured objectively.

Another issue related to use of an inclinometer for measuring spinal range of motion is the lack of agreement on norms and protocols. Limited information is available in the medical literature and much research is needed to establish norms for varying sex and age groups. Normal ranges of spinal mobility are presented in this section to provide some broad,

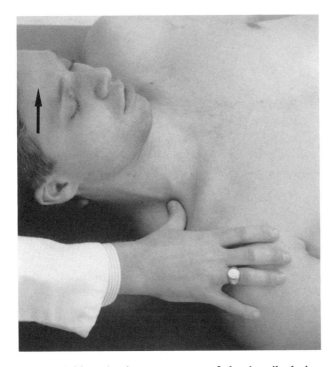

Figure 4-20. Palpating movement of the 1st rib during contralateral sidebending of the cervical spine.

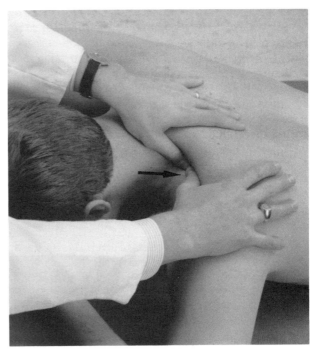

Figure 4-21. Palpating segmental mobility - 1st rib.

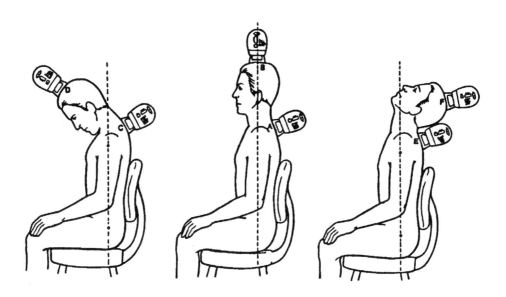

Figure 4-22. Inclinometer used for cervical range of motion testing.

general guidelines (Fig 4-23). These are based on these authors' interpretations of the limited information available.[1, 4, 12, 21, 22, 23, 28, 39] For further discussion on inclinometer usage, see Section Three.

While we must recognize that we have not established adequate norms for range of motion of the spine, we also must recognize that the inclinometer does provide us with a much more accurate and objective method of measuring range of motion than we have previously had available. Exact instructions for measuring spinal range of motion using an inclinometer are not included in this section, as inclinometers do vary and protocols are usually included with the inclinometer when purchased.

Strength Exam

The resisted movement tests to determine muscular involvement in the cervical and upper thoracic spine are done with the patient sitting. The head is held well supported in a neutral, mid range position as the patient is asked to hold against resistance in each range of motion direction (Fig 4-24). Shoulder elevation is tested with the patient sitting to figure out if the upper trapezius and/or rhomboid muscles are involved (Fig 4-25). The middle and lower trapezius

CERVICAL		
Flexion	40°	
Extension	75°	
Sidebending	35° - 45°	
Rotation	80° - 90°	
THORACIC		
Flexion	20° - 30°	
Extension	25° - 35°	
Sidebending	20° - 25°	
Rotation	5° - 10°	
Posture	30° - 40°	Kyphosis
LUMBAR		
Lumbosacral Angle	15° - 30°	
Standing Posture	30° - 40°	Lordosis
Standing Hip Flexion	45° - 65°	
Flexion	40° - 60°	
Extension	20° - 30°	
End Range of Flexion	0° - 20°	Kyphosis
End Range of Extension	60° - 75°	Lordosis
Sidebending	20° - 30°	
Rotation	5° - 10°	

Figure 4-23. Normal ranges of spinal mobility (authors' compilation from many sources.[1, 4, 12, 21, 22, 23, 28, 39])

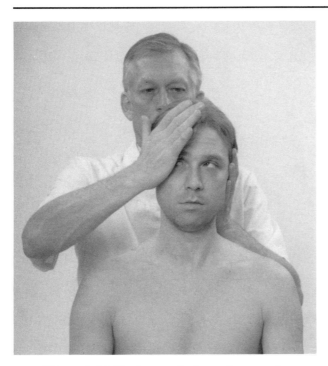

Figure 4-24. Testing cervical muscle strength.

muscles are tested with the patient prone (Fig 4-26). A strong muscle contraction is elicited with very little or no joint movement. A weak and painless contraction suggests neurological involvement or weakness due to prolonged disuse (see Neurological Exam).

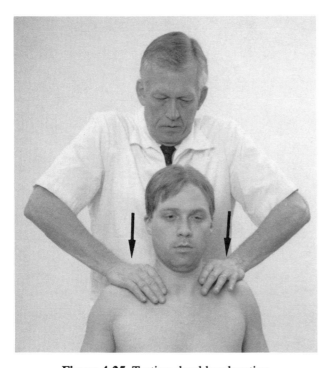

Figure 4-25. Testing shoulder elevation.

Neurological Exam

As a rule, neurological involvement of levels C4 through C7 is more indicative of a cervical nerve root disorder such as a herniated disc or encroachment of the nerve root within the intervertebral foramen. The C7 nerve root is the most common root affected.[19] If neurological involvement of C8 or T1 is seen, it is often suggestive of thoracic outlet syndrome or another disorder and not cervical spine pathology.

Resisted Muscle Tests

As noted earlier, if resisted muscle tests are painful or painful and weak, muscular pathology may be involved. If they are painless and weak, however, and disuse atrophy is ruled out, a neurological disorder is suggested. All resisted muscle tests for the cervical spine are done with the patient sitting.

The tests for the cervical spine involve the following muscle groups:

- Cervical rotation (C1) is tested with the head and neck held in a neutral, mid-range position. The patient is asked to hold as a rotational force is applied (Fig 4-27).

- To test shoulder elevation (C2,3,4), the shoulders are elevated and the patient is asked to hold against resistance (Fig 4-25).

- To test shoulder abduction (C5), the shoulders are abducted to 90° and the patient is asked to hold against resistance (Fig 4-28).

- Elbow flexion (C6) is tested with the elbows flexed to 90°. The patient is asked to hold against resistance (Fig 4-29).

- Elbow extension (C7) is tested with the elbows flexed to 45°. The patient is asked to hold against resistance (Fig 4-30).

- Wrist extension (C6) is tested with the wrists held in extension as resistance is applied (Fig 4-31).

- Wrist flexion (C7) is tested with the wrists held in flexion as resistance is applied (Fig 4-32).

- Thumb extension (C8) is tested with the thumbs held in extension as resistance is applied (Fig 4-33).

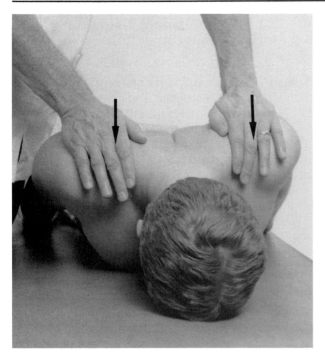

Figure 4-26. Testing the interscapular muscles.

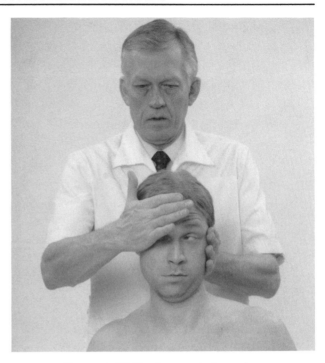

Figure 4-27. Testing cervical rotation.

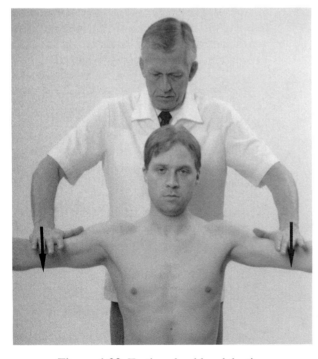

Figure 4-28. Testing shoulder abduction.

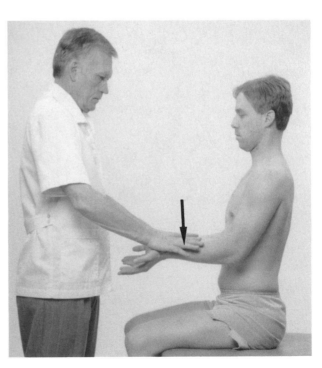

Figure 4-29. Testing elbow flexion.

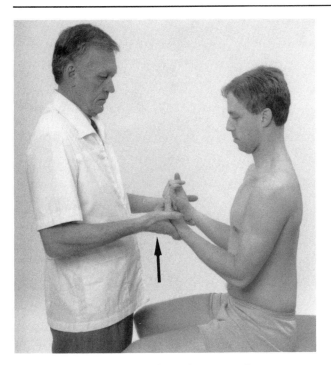

Figure 4-30. Testing elbow extension.

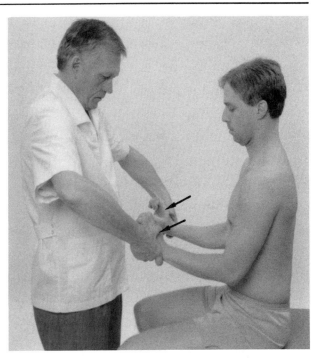

Figure 4-31. Testing wrist extension.

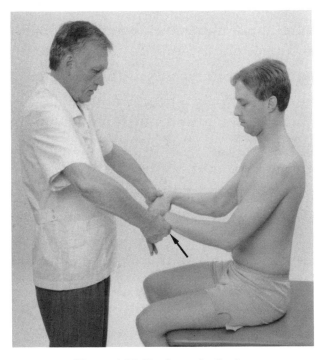

Figure 4-32. Testing wrist flexion.

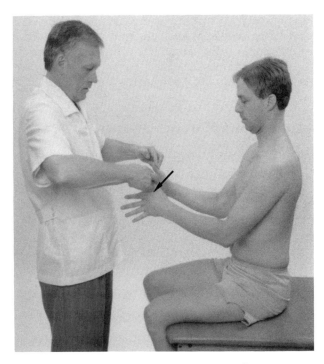

Figure 4-33. Testing thumb extension.

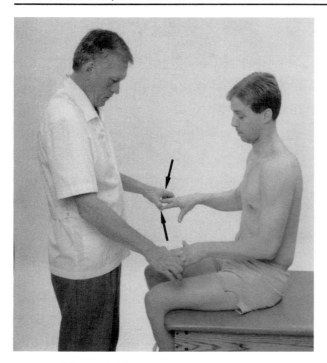

Figure 4-34. Testing finger abduction.

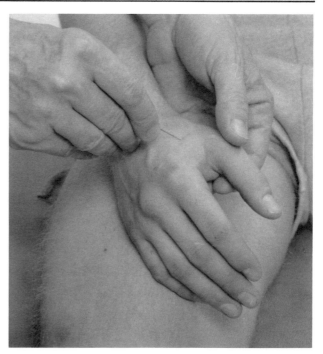

Figure 4-35. Testing sensation.

- Finger abduction (T1) is tested with the fingers held in abduction as resistance is applied (Fig 4-34).

Sensation Testing

Specific sensation testing is carried out with the patient sitting. The clinician carefully maps out areas of numbness by using the pin prick method (Fig 4-35). The C5 neurological level supplies sensation to the lateral arm from the shoulder to the elbow. The purest patch (autonomous zone) of C5 innervation lies over the lateral portion of the middle deltoid muscle. C6 supplies sensation to the lateral forearm, the thumb, the index finger and one-half of the middle finger, with the purest patch being on the lateral portion of the web space between the thumb and index finger. C7 supplies sensation to the middle finger. Since middle finger sensation is also occasionally supplied by C6 or C8, there is no autonomous zone for C7. C8 supplies sensation to the ring and little finger of the hand and the distal one-half of the ulnar forearm. The ulnar side of the little finger is the purest area for C8 testing. T1 supplies sensation to the upper one-half of the medial forearm and the medial portion of the arm. T2 supplies the axilla (Fig 4-36).

Muscle Stretch Reflexes

The biceps (C5-6), brachioradialis (C6) and triceps (C7) muscle stretch reflexes are tested in the sitting

position (Fig 4-37). A decreased response when compared to the contralateral limb suggests pathology at the corresponding nerve root level.

Neural Tension Tests

Many clinicians consider the neural tissue tract as a potential contributing source of symptomatic complaints and limited mobility.[5, 13, 24, 26] Thus, a complete examination should evaluate the effects of applying functional stresses to the neural tissues and their supporting connective tissue interfaces to assess the effect on the patient's clinical signs and symptoms.

The tests for neural tension in the upper limb are almost exclusively used by physical therapists at this writing. Continued research should encourage other disciplines to use them as a part of a complete orthopedic and neurological evaluation.

Previously described as the "brachial plexus tension test" or the "test of Elvey," the current accepted term is the Upper Limb Tension Test (ULTT). Kenneally, et. al.,[24] have called the ULTT the "straight leg raise of the arm." This analogy describes the potential usefulness of the ULTT when examining upper limb and cervical spine disorders just as the straight leg raise is useful when examining lower limb and lumbar spine disorders.

The ULTT is generally recommended for all patients presenting with non-irritable conditions of

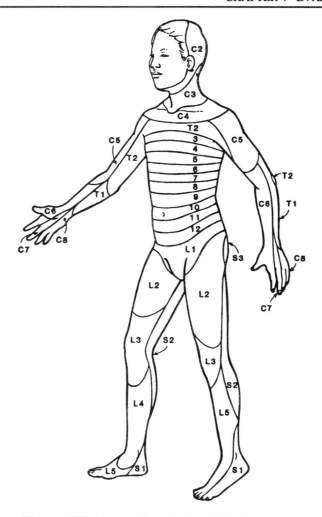

Figure 4-36. An anterolateral view of the dermatomes.

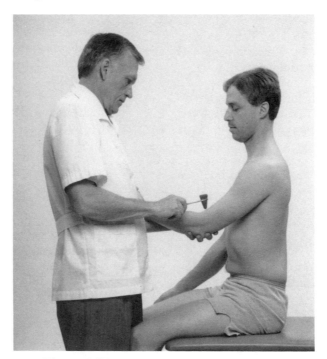

Figure 4-37. Testing upper extremity reflexes

the head, cervical spine, thoracic spine and upper extremities. The basic ULTT is particularly important if symptoms are in the distribution of the median nerve.[13] Variations of the basic ULTT can be performed, but these are not described in this text. Interested clinicians can find more information in Butler's text.[5]

Contraindications to neural tension testing and treatment include the following:

1. Irritable conditions

2. Inflammatory conditions

3. Spinal cord signs

4. Malignancy

5. Nerve root compression signs

6. Severe, unremitting night pain

7. Neurological signs (includes true numbness, weakness or reflex changes)

8. Recent paresthesia/anesthesia

9. Active spinal motions easily provoke distal symptoms, paresthesia, or anesthesia

10. Reflex sympathetic dystrophy

Normal responses for the ULTT have been identified in a recent study by Kenneally of 400 subjects without pathology or complaints.[24]

• Deep ache or stretch in the cubital fossa (99% of subjects) extending down the anterior and radial forearm into the radial hand (80% of subjects)

• A definite tingling in the thumb and 1st three fingers

• A stretch feeling in the anterior shoulder area (small percentage of subjects)

• Increased responses with cervical sidebending away from the tested side (90% of subjects)

• Decreased responses with cervical sidebending toward the tested side (70% of subjects)

Therefore, the clinician must be careful when deciding whether the results of the ULTT are positive or whether they are a normal response to placing neural tissues on stretch.

A tension test can be considered positive in the following circumstances:

• If it reproduces the patient's symptoms

• If the test response can be altered by moving distant body parts that alter tension on neural tissues alone. For example, when the patient is in the test position, the symptoms are changed by isolated movement of the wrist or cervical spine.

• If the test response differs from side to side and from a normal response described above

Any symptoms or decreased mobility found should fit with other clinical findings. It should be noted that any pathological process that causes less space for neural tissue to slide freely will produce an earlier onset of symptoms with the ULTT.[13]

The basic ULTT is performed in the following manner:[5]

1. Cervical Spine Neutral - The patient lies in neutral, supine on the treatment table, close to the edge of the side being tested. The clinician faces the patient, one leg in front of the other, supporting the upper extremity at the wrist. Prior to the exam, the patient is instructed how to sidebend the cervical spine away from and toward the upper extremity to be tested, to avoid substitution or a rotatory component in later steps.

2. Shoulder Girdle Depression - The clinician depresses the shoulder girdle by reaching under the scapula and pulling it caudally. This position is sustained throughout the rest of the procedure. Any change or onset in symptoms should be noted (Fig 4-38).

3. Glenohumeral Abduction - The clinician grasps the patient's elbow while supporting the upper arm with the thigh. This allows mild horizontal extension of the humerus. Approximately 110° of abduction should be attained (Fig 4-39).

4. Wrist/Finger Extension, Forearm Supination - While maintaining Step 3, the wrist and all

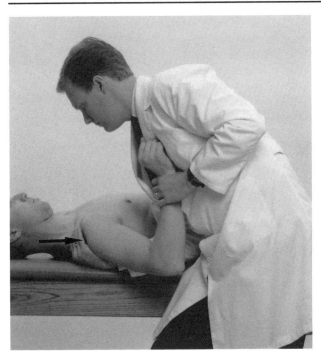

Figure 4-38. Upper limb tension testing. Shoulder girdle depression.

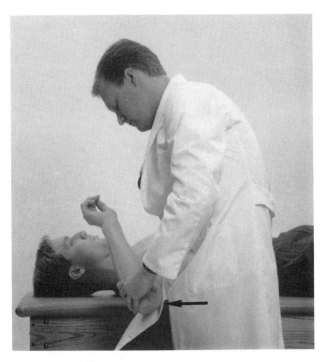

Figure 4-39. Upper limb tension testing. Glenohumeral abduction.

fingers are extended, while the forearm is supinated (Fig 4-40).

5. <u>Glenohumeral External Rotation</u> - The clinician externally rotates the glenohumeral joint to approximately 60° while Steps 1-4 are maintained (Fig 4-41).

6. <u>Elbow Extension</u> - The clinician extends the patient's elbow to the point of symptom onset or resistance (Fig 4-42).

7. <u>Cervical Sidebending</u> - The patient is then instructed to sidebend the cervical spine away from the limb being examined. This is followed by sidebending to the ipsilateral side. Symptom response is noted.

Each individual step must be maintained during the test, especially when the next step is added. The onset or change of symptoms or resistance should be identified and recorded after each step. Examination should include both upper limbs.

In any tension testing, it is important to consider the following:

- Before beginning, carefully identify all the patient's symptoms and complaints.

- Note which symptoms are present in the starting position.

- Carefully note any change in symptoms or onset of new symptoms during each step of the test.

- Move the patient's limb in each step to the point of <u>onset or change</u> in symptom complaints.

- Compare the findings of the test to the contralateral limb and what is considered normal.

As with any musculoskeletal test, reassessment of the test at later intervals will help the clinician decide whether treatment is effective. To compare later findings, the clinician must document the following thoroughly:

- The range of motion at which the symptoms first appear

- The nature and location of the symptoms

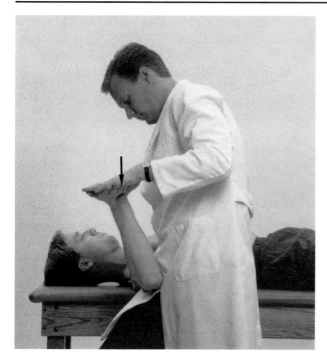

Figure 4-40. Upper limb tension testing. Wrist and finger extension, forearm supination.

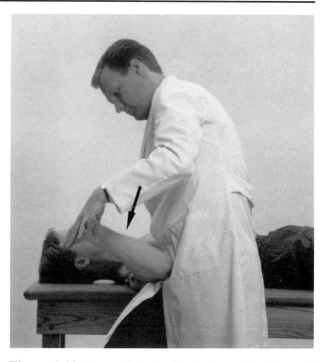

Figure 4-41. Upper limb tension testing. Glenohumeral external rotation.

• Any abnormal resistance felt by the clinician during the test

Babinski's Test

The neurological exam is completed by doing a Babinski test. The test is done by quickly drawing a blunt instrument across the sole of the foot, starting at the heel, moving along the lateral aspect and crossing the ball of the foot. A positive reaction consists of extension of the great toe, usually associated with fanning (abduction and slight flexion) of the other toes. A positive Babinski test suggests an upper motor neuron disorder (Fig 4-43).

Thoracic Outlet Syndrome Tests

A discussion of thoracic outlet syndrome is included in this text because of its close association to the cervical spine and because differential diagnosis of cervical involvement and thoracic outlet compression is often difficult. Thoracic outlet compression syndrome can involve compression or stretching of the subclavian artery, subclavian vein and/or the brachial plexus as they pass through the thoracic outlet. The syndrome can cause symptoms that are primarily vascular or neurological or both.

Diagnosis of arterial compression is accomplished by the techniques described below and other objective tests not readily available to physical therapists such as arteriography and plethysmography. Diagnosis for brachial plexus compression in the thoracic outlet is primarily done through ruling out other pathology in

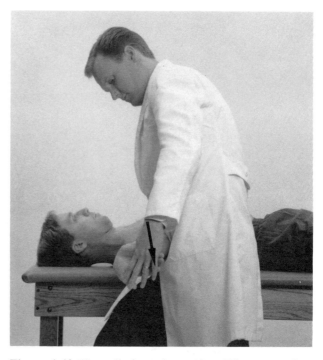

Figure 4-42. Upper limb tension testing. Elbow extension.

the cervical spine and upper extremities that could cause similar symptoms.[25] If the tests described below reproduce neurological symptoms, and if other pathology is ruled out, thoracic outlet syndrome is a likely cause of the patient's neurological symptoms.

Neurological compression accounts for 90-97% of all thoracic outlet syndrome cases, venous compression is responsible for 2% of cases, and arterial compression is responsible for 1%.[25, 38] Arterial compression is potentially the most serious, particularly if arterial embolism occurs. The clinician should be aware of the signs and symptoms that may be present with arterial, venous or nerve compression.

With arterial compression, the patient will report pain and fatigue during activity that goes away with rest. Often, symptoms will start distally and proceed proximally. In later stages, cold sensitivity may be present. Any signs of possible emboli, such as cyanosis in one or more fingers, are considered serious and require immediate medical attention.[25]

Venous compression may lead to edema, skin tightness, cyanosis, pain and fatigue. After activity, venous distention may be seen in the extremity. The edema should decrease after a change in the precipitous activity. If the edema does not diminish, it is a sign of a possible venous thrombosis, and requires the attention of a physician for further evaluation.

Nerve compression causes various symptoms including pain, tingling or numbness that usually follows the nerve trunk. Ulnar nerve symptoms are more common than median nerve symptoms.[25] Night pain is common.[25, 30]

Adson's Test

Adson's test helps decide whether the neurovascular bundle is being compressed as it passes between the scalenus anticus and medius. Occasionally, a congenital defect in the scaleni may cause the bundle to pass through the muscle mass, rather than between the two muscles. A review of the literature reveals that there is no clear consensus on the exact method for performing Adson's test.[7, 14, 16, 30] The test as described here combines many elements of the test as described by the various authors, to place the neurovascular bundle and scaleni on maximum stretch.

The clinician should palpate the patient's radial pulse at the wrist as the patient takes a deep breath and holds it. The patient's arm is abducted and extended and the patient extends and rotates the cervical spine toward the arm being tested (Fig 4-44). If a marked decrease or obliteration of the radial pulse is felt, and the patient's symptoms are reproduced, the test is positive. The test is repeated with cervical extension and rotation away from the arm being tested.

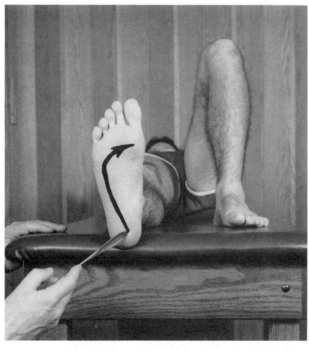
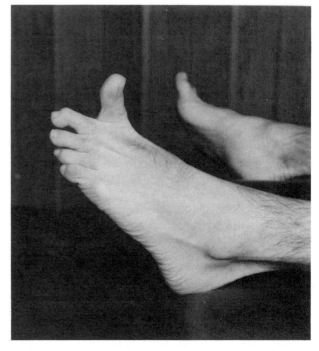

Figure 4-43. Babinski's test. A positive result is great toe extension, with fanning (abduction and slight flexion) of the other toes.

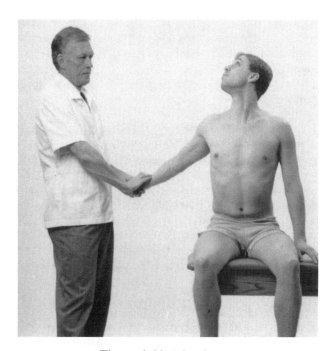

Figure 4-44. Adson's test.

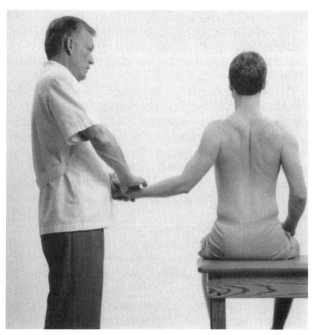

Figure 4-45. Costoclavicular (military bracing) test.

Costoclavicular (Military Bracing) Test

The costoclavicular test checks for the possible compression of the neurovascular bundle as it passes between the clavicle and 1st rib by approximating the two structures.

Again, the clinician palpates the radial pulse at the wrist. The patient is asked to assume an exaggerated military position by drawing the scapulæ backward and downward (Fig 4-45). Again, the test is positive if a marked decrease or obliteration of the radial pulse is felt, and the patient's symptoms are reproduced.

Hyperabduction Test

The hyperabduction test helps to determine whether the neurovascular bundle is being compressed between the pectoralis minor muscle and the ribs.

The clinician palpates the radial pulse at the wrist while abducting the shoulder as far as possible (Fig 4-46). The clinician should concentrate on performing true abduction, without flexion.[25] As with the other pulse palpation tests, the test is positive if a marked decrease or obliteration of the radial pulse is felt, and the patient's symptoms are reproduced.

Roo's Test (EAST Test)

Named for Dr. David Roo, this test involves full shoulder external rotation and abduction to 90°. It is also called the Elevated Arm Stress Test (EAST). The patient holds this position bilaterally for three minutes while repeatedly opening and closing the fists (Fig 4-47). After completing the test, the clinician quickly looks for objective changes and the patient's subjective response. If increased pallor, cyanosis, swelling, vein distention, tingling, numbness or pain is felt, the test is positive. The clinician should compare the affected limb to the unaffected limb.

Bilateral Brachial Blood Pressure Comparison

Cherry Koontz reports that a comparison of bilateral brachial blood pressures can give useful information about arterial compression syndromes. A difference of more than 20-30 mm Hg may be suspicious for subclavian artery stenosis.[25]

Neural Tension Tests for Thoracic Outlet Syndrome

All of the pulse palpation techniques described above are more definitive for thoracic outlet syndrome involving arterial compression. If neurological symptoms are reproduced with the tests, they are helpful at pointing toward neurological compression as well. Since neurological compression accounts for 90-97% of all thoracic outlet syndromes,[25,38] the neural tension tests described in the previous section are extremely useful. When performing the neural tension test for the upper limb (ULTT), the clinician can look for symptoms reproduction and can also appreciate any tissue resistance felt during the test. When symptoms reproduction or tissue resistance is encountered, the clinician must consider both local sources of compression (the 1st rib, lower cervical and upper thoracic vertebral segments and the scaleni) and remote contributing factors such as tight acromioclavicular and glenohumeral joints, or imbalanced trapezius, levator scapulæ, pectoral and cervical musculature. Butler describes variations of the basic ULTT that can be more specific for the lower trunks of the brachial plexus, and his text should be consulted for further investigation of the use of neural tension testing for thoracic outlet syndrome.[5]

Palpation Exam

The palpation exam of the cervical and upper thoracic spine involves inspection of the skin and subcutaneous tissue as described above. When palpating the muscles, the examiner must pay close attention to the suboccipital, upper trapezius and rhomboid muscles. Muscle guarding and spasm in these muscles is often associated with various syndromes in the cervical spine. Painful trigger areas are often found in the levator scapulæ insertion. It is often necessary to treat muscle guarding and spasm in these muscles even though they are not the primary disorders. Injury or prolonged muscle guarding of the rhomboid muscles often causes a coarseness or crepitus that can be palpated. Muscle guarding and spasm of the suboccipital muscles are often associated with

headaches. Trigger points can often be palpated along the occipital line and in the belly of the upper trapezius muscles. The clinician should rule out 1st rib involvement when a painful response to palpating the upper trapezius muscles is found, as the 1st rib lies directly beneath the upper trapezius and can be painful to palpation.

The supraspinous ligament and spinous processes of the lower cervical and upper thoracic spine can be palpated. In the mid and upper cervical spine, the spinous processes usually cannot be palpated. The facet joint lines of the mid-cervical spine (articular pillar) can be palpated for tenderness during segmental range of motion testing.

Special Tests

Distraction Test

The distraction test is a neurological test and a mobility test. The clinician stands behind the patient if he or she is seated or at the head of the patient if he or she is lying supine and applies long axis distraction to the cervical spine through the occiput. This maneuver opens the foramina and stretches the joint capsules. If it relieves the patient's symptoms it may show that a spinal nerve root is impinged. It should be noted that facet joint or disc pain also may be relieved with this test and it is, therefore, not a completely reliable test for spinal nerve root impingement. The test is most

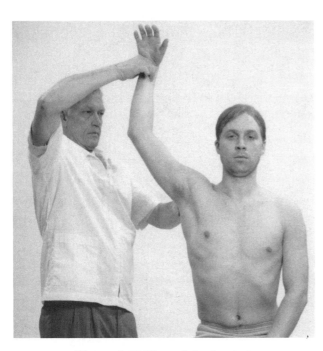

Figure 4-46. Hyperabduction test.

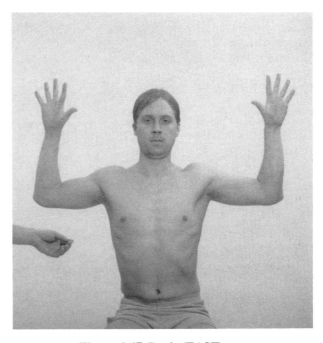

Figure 4-47. Roo's (EAST) test.

valuable because it is a good test for whether traction or a cervical support to decrease vertical loading will be beneficial during treatment (Fig 4-48 A & B).

Compression Test

The clinician presses down on top of the patient's head either while he or she is seated or lying supine. The test is repeated with the neck in slight extension/

sidebending and with the neck in slight flexion. If symptoms increase when the head and neck are held in slight extension and sidebending, it is a good indication that foraminal encroachment or facet joint pressure may be the source of pain. Conversely, if symptoms are increased when the head and neck are held in slight flexion, a disc problem may be the source of the symptoms (Fig 4-48C).

Valsalva Test

The patient is asked to hold his or her breath and bear down as if having a bowel movement. If the patient notes an increase in pain or radiation, this may suggest the presence of a space-occupying lesion such as a herniated disc or tumor.

Dynamometer Grip Strength Test

Grip strength testing is done for two reasons. First, it provides very objective baseline data for cervical patients complaining of upper extremity pain. The test can be repeated during treatment to document improvement in the patient's condition.

Secondly, grip strength testing has been proposed as a method of detecting submaximal effort.[37] The Jamar Dynamometer is used. The patient is asked to perform grip strength testing in all five positions (three trials at each position are averaged). If the five values are plotted on a graph, the graph should follow a bell-shaped curve, with positions one and five weakest and position two or three strongest (Fig 4-49).

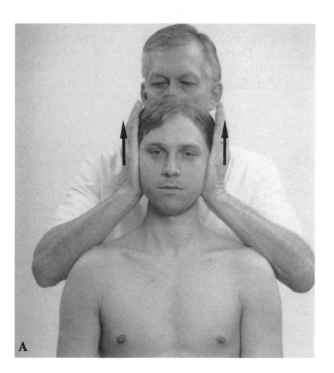

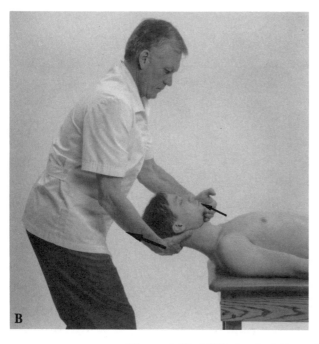

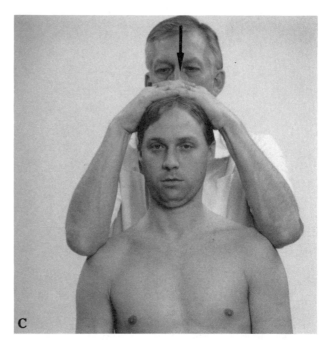

Figure 4-48. A&B) Cervical distraction tests; C) Cervical compression test.

The bell-shaped curve should be present even with true pathology. Therefore, if a bell-shaped curve is not found, or if there is less than a five pound variance between each value, it is probable that the patient is not exerting maximal effort.

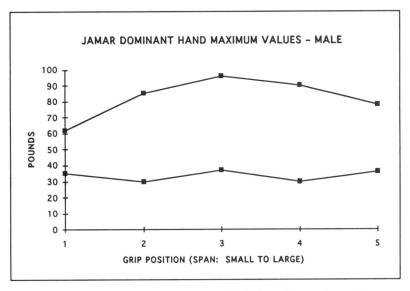

Figure 4-49. Dynamometer grip strength testing results. A normal bell-shaped curve (upper) is expected. A flat or irregular curve (lower) may indicate submaximal effort.

SECTION THREE: EVALUATION OF THE MID AND LOWER THORACIC AND LUMBAR SPINE

INTRODUCTION

Subjective evaluation of the spine was covered in detail in Section One. The general components of an objective evaluation of the spine were also discussed in Section One. Section Three contains a more detailed discussion of those components that are specific to the mid and lower thoracic and lumbar spine. The reader should become familiar with the ideas found in Section One before proceeding.

Section Three is organized according to the seven components of the objective evaluation: the Screening exam, the Structural exam, the Mobility exam, the Strength exam, the Neurological exam, the Palpation exam and Special Tests. The order follows the evaluation worksheet found in Figure 3-2. Organizing the evaluation in this way helps the examiner record and report the evaluation results in a clear, concise manner. When performing the objective evaluation, however, the examiner should attempt to perform all tests which can be done in one position at once (see Sequence of Evaluation, Figure 3-3). This avoids unnecessary movement of the patient, which will certainly be appreciated.

After completing the subjective portion of the evaluation, the physical therapist often has an idea of where to concentrate his or her objective examination. But it is still important to perform a complete objective evaluation to avoid missing any non-obvious clues because of the clinician's preconceived biases.

OBJECTIVE EXAMINATION

Lower Quarter Screening Exam

The lower quarter screening examination consists of a series of mobility and neurological tests to identify problem areas in the lumbar spine, sacroiliac area, hip, knee, ankle and foot (Fig 4-50). It is most valuable when performed on a patient complaining of lower extremity symptoms and little or no back pain. With such a patient it is important to clear the lumbar spine as a source of the lower extremity symptoms. The screening examination is redundant if the patient is already complaining of lumbar symptoms, and the clinician should skip to the rest of the objective evaluation. A good screening examination performed by a skilled evaluator can make the rest of the evaluation more concise and efficient. The purpose of the screening examination is to identify which anatomical areas deserve a detailed evaluation. After the screening examination, the clinician will know which anatomical areas have been cleared and which ones need a closer look.

---

1. Postural assessment
2. Active forward, backward and lateral bending of lumbar spine
3. Standing flexion test/Gillet's test
4. Toe raises (S-1)
5. Heel walking (L-4, 5)
6. Sitting flexion test
7. Active rotation of lumbar spine
8. Overpressures if symptom free
9. Straight leg raise (L-4, 5; S-1)
10. Resisted hip flexion (L-1, 2)
11. Passive range of motion to hip
12. Resisted knee extension (L-3, 4)
13. Knee flexion, extension, medial and lateral tilt
14. Femoral nerve stretch
15. Babinski's reflex test (UMN)

Figure 4-50. Lower quarter screening exam (adopted from Cyriax[9]).

The lower quarter screening examination begins with the patient standing so posture can be observed. Any postural abnormalities should be noted and investigated more thoroughly if they correlate with the patient's complaint or with other objective findings. The lumbar spine is then taken through active forward, backward and lateral bending as the clinician watches for signs of pain, muscle spasm and/or limited movement. The standing flexion test for iliosacral (p164) involvement is also performed (See Chapter 7, Evaluation and Treatment of Pelvic Girdle Dysfunctions). Heel and toe walking, which is a neurological test for L4 and L5 (heel) and S1 (toe), is then completed. Heel and toe walking also clears the ankle and foot when no pain or limitation of movement is observed. A quick technique to clear all joints of the lower extremity is to ask the patient to squat and then stand.

(p166) Next, the patient sits and the sitting flexion test for sacroiliac involvement is performed. The standing and sitting flexion tests are described thoroughly in Chapter 7 (Figures 7-6 and 7-10). Active lumbar rotation is also checked with the patient sitting. The patient is asked to extend the arms directly in front with the hands held together and then to twist to the right and left as far as possible. If no signs or symptoms are observed with active range of motion, passive overpressures are applied. If forward and backward bending, lateral bending and rotation produce no signs

or symptoms even with passive overpressure, the joints and muscles of the lumbar spine are considered clear for those movements.

Next, the patient is positioned supine for straight leg raising, which is a neurological test of spinal levels L4 through S1. Differentiation between tightness of hamstrings and sciatic pain is critical. Spring tests for sacroiliac involvement are also done at this time.

The hip is clear if passive flexion, internal and external rotation and resisted hip flexion do not produce any signs or symptoms. Resisted hip flexion is also a neurological test of spinal levels L1 and L2.

Resisted knee extension is a neurological test of spinal levels L3 and L4. Clearing of the knee is completed by passively testing flexion and extension and applying varus and valgus stresses.

A femoral nerve stretch in the prone position may be indicated if the patient has described symptoms in the anterior hip and thigh and/or groin area. The lower quarter screening is completed by doing a Babinski reflex test for upper motor neuron involvement.

Structural Exam

Areas of specific complaint or areas that have shown some questionable signs during the screening examination should be examined in detail. The detailed objective examination of a specific area begins with general observation of the patient. The evaluator should review Section One for general comments relating to structural examinations. This section will concentrate on details about the structural examination of the lumbar spine and lower extremities.

Posture

The evaluator should remember that postural assessment should include the entire spine even if the patient's complaint concerns only one area of the spine. Any asymmetries found may be significant if correlated with other subjective and objective findings. The three types of asymmetries, Anterior/Posterior, Lateral, and Cephalocaudal, will be discussed.

Anterior/Posterior Symmetry

There should be a gentle continuation of anterior/posterior curves the entire length of the spine. Lumbar and thoracic A/P curves can be objectively measured using an inclinometer (Fig 4-51). Objective measurements are useful for patient education and documenting changes as treatment progresses.

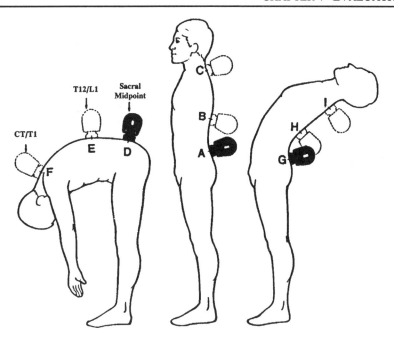

Figure 4-51. Using an inclinometer to objectively assess lumbar curvatures.

The lumbar and cervical spine should show a mild lordotic curve and the thoracic spine should have a mild kyphotic curve. Absence of any of the curves may suggest restriction of mobility, whereas excessive lordotic curves may suggest the presence of any of a variety of structural and postural problems. Increased lumbar lordosis may be associated with joint hypermobility, anterior pelvic rotation, weak abdominal muscles and tight hip flexor muscles. If this is the case, the patient may have a chronic postural strain and should be treated with a corrective exercise program. Absence or decrease of lumbar lordosis should be noted as it may be an indication of a disc disorder or may be the result of living and working in the sitting or forward bending posture over a long period. The patient with flat back posture often has very little lumbar extension mobility and often has tight hamstring muscles. The pelvis is posteriorly rotated.

The sway-back posture is often mistaken for the hyperlordotic posture, but it is actually quite different. The sway-back posture is characterized by forward displacement of the hip joint, posterior rotation of the pelvis, a flat lower lumbar spine, a slight lordotic curve in the upper lumbar spine and a slightly increased thoracic kyphosis[23] (Fig 4-52).

It is also very important to observe the patient's sitting posture in the waiting room and in the examination room. Slumped lumbar flexion posture often contributes to loss of lumbar extension and to development of a posterolateral lumbar disc protrusion.

Lateral Symmetry

Scoliotic curves in the spine are abnormal and are classified as either functional or structural or as caused by a specific pathological process. A structural scoliosis is caused by a defect in the bony structure of the spine such as wedging of the vertebral bodies. A structural scoliosis does not straighten during forward bending or sidebending away from the direction of the curve. Because lateral bending is always accompanied by rotation, the patient will have a "lumbar bulge" and/or "rib hump" when he forward bends if a structural scoliosis is present (Fig 4-53). A functional scoliosis can be caused by a nonspinal defect such as unequal leg length, muscle imbalance or poor postural habits. Generally, a functional scoliosis of this type will straighten during forward bending and sidebending away from the direction of the curve, but this may not be true if moderate to severe muscle spasm and guarding is present or if the soft tissue structures have shortened on the concave side of the curve. The patient should always be asked to hold his or her hands together when forward bending. This eliminates some chance of error in determining if a rib hump is a true structural scoliosis or just active rotation of the spine. If the patient has an uneven sacral base, it is important to "level" the sacral base by placing shims under the short leg before testing forward bending. This ensures that true spinal abnormalities (stiffness or structural scoliosis, for example) will be easier to identify.

Although consideration should be given to structural scoliosis, the clinician should remember that when seen in an adult, it will be a long-standing condition and may be only indirectly related to the patient's present complaint. Long-standing structural scoliosis may cause early degenerative joint/disc disease and may indirectly contribute to a variety of disorders. When seen in children and early adolescents, structural scoliosis has much more significance. It must be managed by someone knowledgeable and competent to give the special treatment required. Idiopathic scoliosis cannot be treated by physical therapy alone.

Facet joint impingement may cause an acute scoliosis in any area of the spine. This disorder involves the entrapment of soft tissue within the facet joint. If this happens, the patient may shift to the opposite side of impingement to take the weight off the painful structure.

A more common type of lateral curve seen with acute disorders in the lumbar spine is the "lateral shift" or "protective scoliosis" (Fig 4-54). According to McKenzie, a lateral shift will often occur as the nucleus pulposus moves posterolaterally. For example, if the nucleus moves posterolaterally to the right, the patient is likely to shift his body weight anteriorly and to the left. Thus, the patient would appear to have a flattened lumbar lordosis and a left lateral shift.[29] Finneson advances another explanation for an acute lateral curve in the lumbar spine, which he calls the "protective scoliosis."[10] If a protective scoliosis is present, he theorizes that it is caused by the patient moving the spinal nerve root away from the bulge of a disc herniation. If the bulge is lateral to the nerve root it is encroaching upon, the patient will shift to the opposite side (most common). If the bulge is medial to the nerve root it is encroaching upon, the patient will shift to the same side (uncommon) (Fig 4-55).

Cephalocaudal Symmetry

The height of the shoulders and the inferior angle of the scapulæ should be examined to decide whether they are level. Often, however, the shoulder and scapula on the dominant side are positioned lower. This is considered normal and care should be taken to avoid drawing conclusions from shoulder and scapula height asymmetries. The clinician also should look for any asymmetries in the ribs or skin folds. Close attention is paid to the sacral base during the structural examination. With the patient standing straight with the feet spread shoulder width apart and weight equally distributed, the height of the iliac crests, posterior/ superior iliac spines (PSIS), anterior/superior iliac

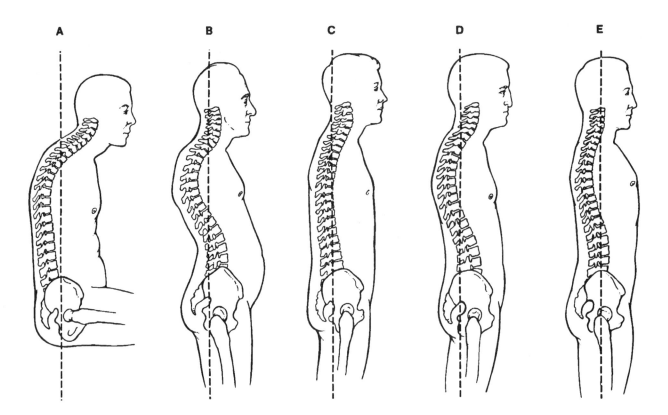

Figure 4-52. Common postural disorders. A) Forward head, rounded shoulders; B) Hyperlordosis, hyperkyphosis; C) Hypolordosis (flat back); D) Sway-back; E) Ideal posture.

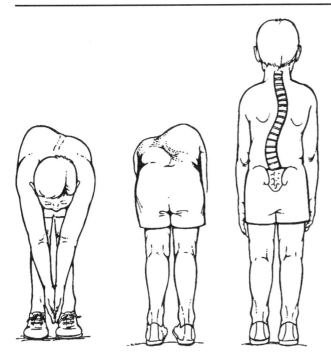

Figure 4-53. If structural scoliosis is present, a lumbar bulge or rib hump will be seen during forward bending.

spines (ASIS), trochanters, gluteal folds and fibular heads are checked to find if the sacral base is uneven and, if so, where the discrepancy lies (Fig 4-56). For example, if the PSIS's are uneven and the trochanters are even, the discrepancy lies between the two structures. The sacroiliac joint, the angulation of the femoral neck or the hip joint itself are possible areas of dysfunction.

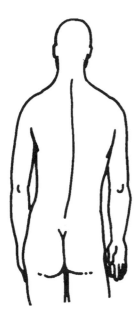

Figure 4-54. A lateral shift or protective scoliosis.

Leg length differences that cannot be corrected by treatment should be corrected with a shoe lift. If left uncorrected, an uneven sacral base will cause a lumbar scoliosis that will contribute to uneven weight distribution on the facet joints and the intervertebral disc. This may lead to early degenerative changes in the lumbar spine and hip and/or soft tissue shortening or imbalance.

The height of the iliac crests also should be checked in the sitting position because it is possible for one side of the pelvis to be larger than the other. This will cause an uneven sacral base and a lumbar scoliosis while sitting. It can be corrected by using a seat cushion that is thicker on one side.

It is important to make sure that any adaptive soft tissue changes such as unilateral paraspinal or hip muscle tightness or facet joint capsular tightness are addressed prior to and concurrent with leg length correction.

Assistive Devices and Supports

Any special assistive devices or supports, such as a lumbar corset, lumbar pillow or cane that the patient uses should be noted at this time. Care should be taken to assess if the device has been properly fitted and if it is being used correctly. Sometimes a patient will bring an assistive device to the appointment, even though it is not regularly used. Conversely, some patients have a device that is used regularly but is not mentioned during the subjective portion of the evaluation. The clinician should take care to note exactly if, when and how the assistive devices are used.

The use of a cane is rarely helpful with lumbar or lower extremity pain, and it can sometimes even be harmful. When a cane is used, the patient may lean on it, creating asymmetrical forces on the spine and pelvis. When true muscle weakness of a lower extremity exists, a cane could conceivably be useful for helping promote a safer, more even gait pattern.

Mobility Exam

Postural Correction

Postural correction in the lumbar spine involves either hypolordosis, hyperlordosis or a lateral scoliosis. Hypolordosis or hyperlordosis is evaluated during active forward and backward bending testing.

When an acute lateral lumbar scoliosis is seen during the examination an attempt should be made to correct it (Fig 4-57). If the lateral shift is caused by a mild to moderate disc protrusion as described by McKenzie, the correction procedure will often cause centralized pain in the lumbar spine but no increase of peripheral symptoms. An exception to this would involve a large bulge in which some of the disc material is being trapped outside the posterolateral edge of the vertebral bodies. In this case, attempted correction would cause increased pain or other symptoms in the lower extremity also.

If the scoliosis is a protective scoliosis as described by Finneson,[10] any attempt at correction will increase pain and other symptoms in the lower extremity. At this point in the examination, the following rule applies: If the acute lateral lumbar scoliosis can be corrected without increasing pain or other symptoms in the lower extremity, it should be done. If on the other hand, attempted correction increases the pain or other

symptoms in the lower extremity, attempts to correct the shift should be ceased (see discussion in Chapter 5, Treatment of the Spine by Diagnosis).

Active Mobility Testing

Active range of motion begins with the patient standing as he was for the sacral base test. If the sacral base is uneven, it should be leveled by placing the correct thickness of books or magazines under the short side. If this is not done during active range of motion testing, an accurate assessment of true range of motion in the lumbar spine cannot be made.

When examining active movements of the spine, the clinician is looking for two things.

1) Does the test recreate the patient's symptoms?

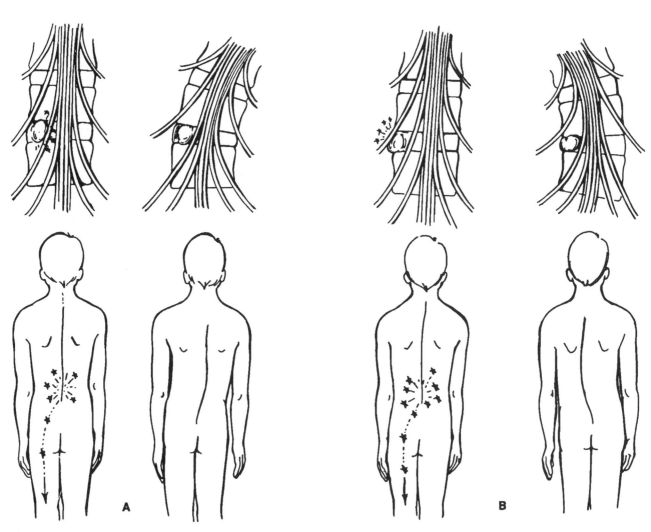

Figure 4-55. Protective scoliosis sometimes seen in patients with HNP-protrusion. A) Bulge lateral to the nerve root; B) Bulge medial to the nerve root (adapted from Finneson[10]).

2) Is the amount of movement normal?

The findings of the mobility exam are significant if the test changes the patient's symptoms or if the amount of movement seen or felt is abnormal.

Many patients may have mild to moderate movement dysfunctions without symptoms. To be significant, problems with movement often must be correlated with the patient's complaints. The clinician must use common sense and carefully analyze the results of the subjective and objective examinations to decide which areas need to be treated.

Forward Bending

Active forward bending is checked by having the patient bend forward as the clinician assesses the general and specific mobility of the spine (Fig 4-58). Does the normal lordosis in the lumbar spine flatten to neutral (normal) or does it round into considerable kyphosis (hypermobility) during forward bending? If the lordosis does not straighten completely, the spine is hypomobile. How much standing hip flexion is present? Does the thoracic spine show increased kyphosis? Is the movement smooth and is it uniform throughout the length of the spine? Does the patient experience pain, stiffness or any other symptoms? If so, is it central in the lower back or does it radiate into the lower extremity? Does the lower extremity pain linger after the patient returns to an upright posture? If the patient experiences increased pain when recovering from the forward bent position, he or she is said to have a "torturous recovery," which suggests an active lesion in the spinal muscles.[30] The patient with a torturous recovery will often "crawl" the hands up the thighs to regain the standing position. Does the patient drift to the left or right instead of bending straight forward? If so, it suggests unilateral hypomobility of the soft tissue, unilateral muscular tightness or posterolateral disc protrusion. It is often necessary to ask the patient to forward bend with eyes closed before this drift is seen because it is natural for the

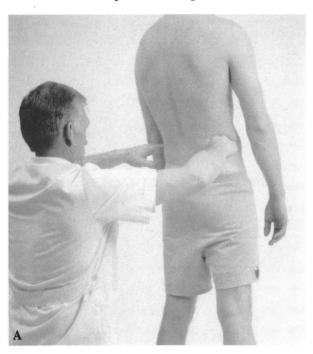

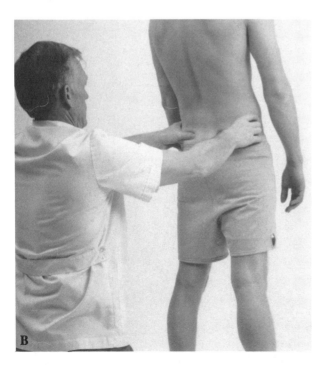

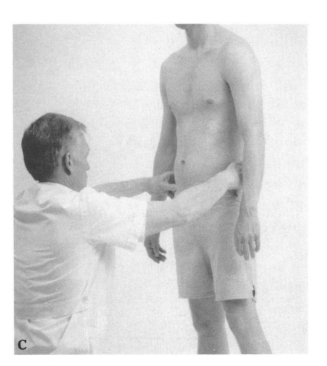

Figure 4-56. Sacral base and pelvic alignment testing. A) Iliac crest symmetry; B) PSIS symmetry; and C) ASIS symmetry.

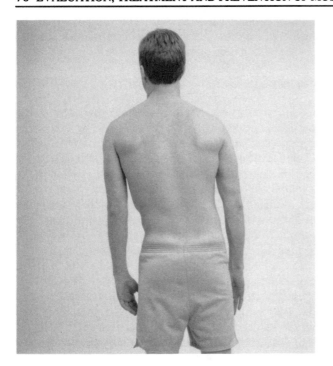
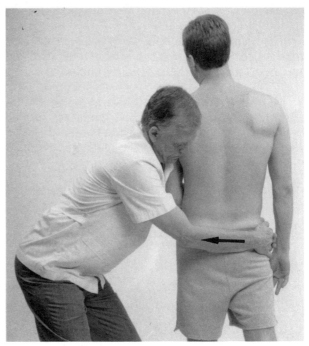

Figure 4-57. Correcting the patient's lateral shift.

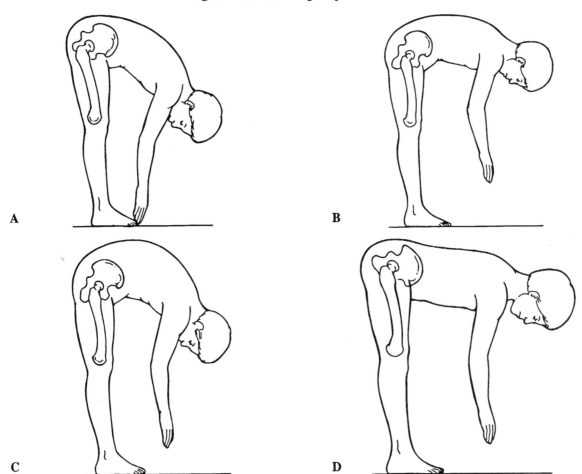

A

B

C

D

Figure 4-58. Active forward bending. A) Normal; B) Tight hamstrings but normal lumbar motion; C) Tight hamstrings and excessive lumbar flexion; D) Normal to loose hamstrings and decreased lumbar flexion.

patient to fix his or her eyes on the floor, thus overriding any tendency to drift laterally. Having the patient close the eyes will eliminate this chance of error.

Backward Bending

Active backward bending is also checked with the patient standing (Fig 4-59). Restrictions of backward bending are usually associated with disc protrusion, soft tissue hypomobility or facet joint pain.

During mobility testing, it is important to note what movements (changes in lordosis) cause the patient's pain to move centrally and what movements cause the pain to move peripherally. According to McKenzie,[29] for patients with lumbar disc protrusion, movements centralizing pain are helpful; ones peripheralizing pain are harmful. If the symptoms move peripherally when testing repeated lumbar forward and backward bending in standing, it indicates the movement is making the condition worse. For example, it may be causing further disc bulging. If movements centralize the pain, it is not necessarily an indication the condition is getting worse. When a stiff joint is moved, it will be painful but it must be moved to regain mobility. The most common example is that repeated forward bending will cause the pain to move away from the midline and into the buttock and thigh while repeated backward bending will cause increased pain in the center of the lumbar spine. When this is seen, it indicates the patient has a mild disc protrusion. Pain present at end of range when range is limited indicates soft tissue hypomobility. Pain throughout the range of motion is characteristic of acute inflammation, strain or sprain. A feeling of "slipping" or a moving sensation during range of motion testing is a sign of instability or hypermobility.

Even without a history of peripheral pain, increased central lumbar pain with backward bending must be analyzed carefully. The patient who has a flattened lumbar lordosis and who is not accustomed to backward bending will usually complain of increased lumbar pain with the backward bending testing. The clinician should ask if the movement reproduces the patient's exact symptoms. The clinician should also ask the patient to repeat it gently several times to see if it gets better, worse or stays the same. If the increased pain is not an exact reproduction of the patient's symptoms and if it does not increase significantly with repetition, it is probably due to stiffness. The patient with a decreased lumbar lordosis and decreased extension mobility will usually benefit from trying to increase it. To have the confidence to perform a corrective exercise program, he or she must be educated about the difference between soreness from stretching stiff soft tissue and a true reproduction of symptoms.

Sidebending

Active sidebending is examined by first having the patient bend to one side and then the other (Fig 4-60). Is the patient bending one way as far as the other? An easy way to assess this is to watch how far the patient's fingers reach on the side of his or her legs. One should see a gentle, smooth and continuous curve from the lumbosacral joint through the mid thoracic spine when the patient actively sidebends. Any straight areas suggest hypomobility and any areas of sharp bending suggest hypermobility (Fig 4-61). One must be careful to keep the patient from shifting the pelvis laterally when examining active sidebending. If the sacral base is uneven it is important that it is leveled before checking active sidebending.

Rotation

Active rotation is checked with the patient sitting on the edge of a treatment plinth with the arms held straight out in front and the hands together. A general assessment is made first, followed by a closer examination of the specific area of the patient's complaint (Fig 4-62). As rotation occurs in one direction, sidebending will occur in the opposite direction. The spinous processes also move in the opposite direction of the rotation. The physical therapist should observe the position of the spinous processes during rotation, looking for smoothness and symmetry in their positions (Fig 4-63).

Findings of Active Mobility Testing

The following discussion is included in this section to guide the clinician in appropriate clinical decision making. By considering carefully the "clues" that the results of active mobility testing provide, the clinician can begin to formulate an idea about what potential pathological entity or treatable problems the patient may have. The clinician must remember, however, that a correct conclusion cannot be made until the entire subjective and objective evaluation is completed.

Certain pathological entities present with specific findings during the active mobility tests. For example, inert soft tissue restrictions (facet joint capsule, ligaments, etc.) will generally be painful at the end of range of motion and will often tend to loosen up with repeated movement. Muscular restrictions will be most painful when the involved muscle is actively contracting, as in the torturous recovery described earlier. As a rule, unilateral restrictions are more noticeable during sidebending than in forward or backward bending. Conversely, bilateral restrictions will be proportionately more noticeable in forward bending.

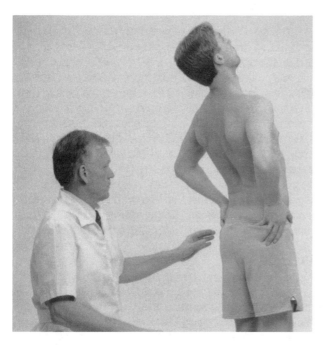

Figure 4-59. Active backward bending.

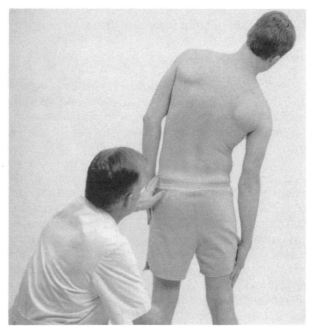

Figure 4-60. Active sidebending.

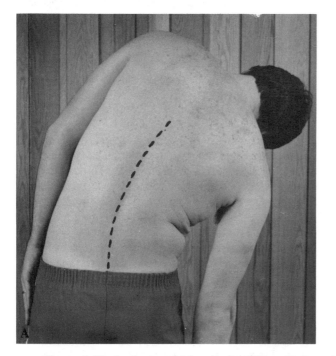

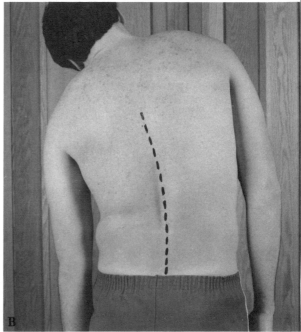

Figure 4-61. Analyzing sidebending mobility. A) Smooth curve; B) Straightened area indicating hypomobility.

Disc lesions tend to be irritated by certain repeated movements, especially forward bending, and the pain often lingers after the movement is stopped. For example, when using the standing forward bending test, if the patient has pain (mostly in the back) at the end of available range of motion and it is relieved when he starts to return to standing and if repeating the movement several times relieves the pain, one would suspect soft tissue hypomobility. If the pain felt at the end of range of motion worsens with repeated movements and lingers after the movement is stopped, one would suspect disc involvement. If the pain is felt mostly on returning from the forward bent position, one would suspect muscle involvement. A more detailed discussion on the objective findings of various conditions in found in Chapter 5, Treatment of the Spine by Diagnosis.

Passive Mobility Testing

The passive mobility tests that are most useful for the lumbar spine are the knees to chest (flexion) and the passive press up (extension). Passive overpressure in rotation is also very useful as a provocation test if no other mobility tests reproduce the patient's symptoms. Passive sidebending is more difficult to perform and does not provide much additional information. Passive range of motion of the hip joint must be tested thoroughly because of the possible involvement of hip musculature, particularly the iliotibial band, the iliopsoas and the piriformis.

Passive flexion is performed by having the patient hug both knees to chest when lying supine. He or she is then asked to repeat this movement several times, without letting go of the knees between repetitions. The clinician asks whether the pain increases, decreases or stays the same with repetition.

The results of passive flexion testing must be analyzed carefully. On one hand, passive flexion stretches the lumbar muscles, which may feel good to the patient. On the other hand, passive flexion compresses the disc which may be potentially harmful, causing increased peripheralization of the pain. When performing passive flexion repetitively, the patient

may initially have relief of back pain, but may later have increased symptoms.

Passive extension is performed by having the patient perform a prone press up. The starting position for the hands should be directly in front of the shoulders. The clinician makes sure the patient's lumbar musculature is relaxed, so that it is truly a passive movement. Again, the patient is asked to repeat the movement several times to determine whether a change with repetition occurs. The clinician also determines whether a normal lumbar curve exists. One should observe flattening of the mid and lower thoracic kyphosis and an increase in lumbar lordosis, especially in the lower lumbar area, with this test. The distance of the ASIS from the table should be measured (approximately 2 inches is considered within normal limits), although the quality of the curve is generally more important than the actual distance (Fig 4-64). Extreme obesity or thinness will interfere with interpretation of the measurement.

The prone press up position is a very convenient position for testing thoracic and lumbar extension with an inclinometer (Fig 4-65). Range of motion testing using an inclinometer is discussed later in this section.

Pain with hip motion or limitation of hip range of motion can be a clue to involvement of the piriformis or iliopsoas muscles. These muscles are commonly involved in the back pain patient and cannot be overlooked.

Internal rotation, external rotation and passive hip flexion are tested in supine with the hip and knee flexed to 90°. Hip internal rotation can also be tested in prone with the knees flexed to 90° and allowing the legs rotate laterally. Hip extension can be tested in prone. If the patient is positioned supine with the leg hanging over the edge of the plinth as in Figure 4-66, the length of the rectus femoris is tested as well. The clinician looks for symptom provocation or any range of motion differences from one side to the other.

Length of the tensor fascia latæ is assessed in sidelying. The patient's uppermost hip is extended then adducted (Fig 4-67). Restriction or symptom reproduction in extension and adduction (Ober's sign) is indicative of a tight tensor fascia lata .

Segmental Mobility Testing

Thoracic and Lumbar Spine

The segmental mobility tests for the lumbar and mid and lower thoracic spine are forward bending,

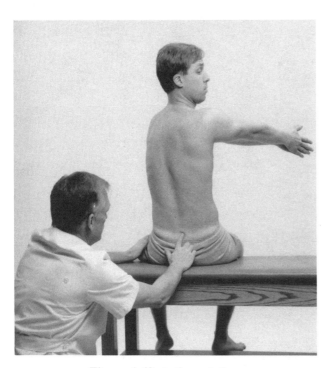

Figure 4-62. Active rotation.

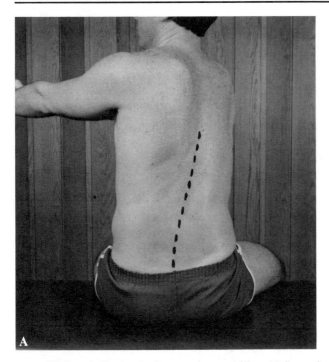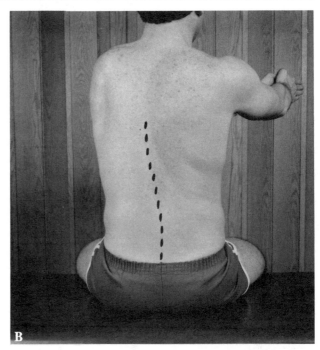

Figure 4-63. Analyzing rotation mobility. A) Smooth rotation; B) Straightened area indicating hypomobility.

backward bending and rotation. During segmental mobility testing it is often helpful to first identify the segments that are tender to palpation. Specific segmental tenderness is often a clue to a mobility problem at that segment. The tender segment(s) are then compared to the adjacent non tender segments. Using this method makes it easier to detect slight but often significant differences.

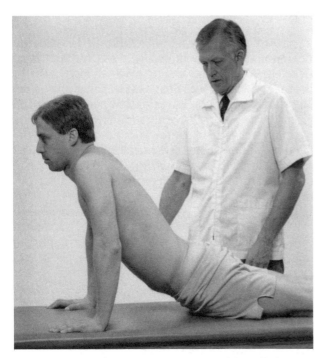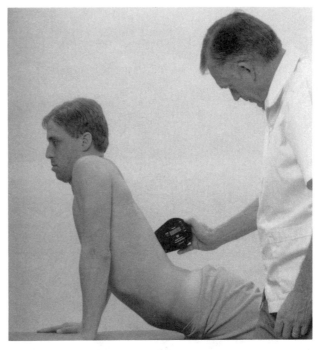

Figure 4-64. Passive backward bending with too little curve in the lumbar spine and ASIS far from the exam table.

Figure 4-65. Testing lumbar extension with an inclinometer in the press-up position.

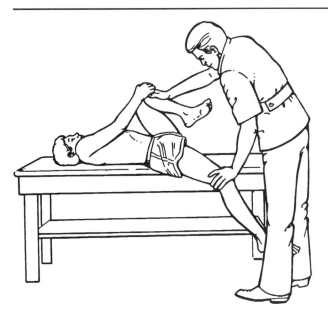

Figure 4-66. Testing rectus femoris length, hip extension and contralateral hip flexion simultaneously.

During normal forward bending, the spinous processes separate slightly. While feeling between two spinous processes with his or her finger, the clinician asks the patient to forward bend the spine. If the clinician feels the spinous processes separate slightly and the supraspinous ligament become taut under the finger, there is movement present at that segmental level. This amount of movement is compared to other levels and the clinician determines if the movement at the involved (painful) segment is hyper- or hypomobile, or if it is normal. This test is done with the patient sidelying (Fig 4-68 A & B) or in the "prayer" position for the lumbar and lower thoracic spine (Fig 4-68C), and sitting for the mid thoracic spine (Fig 4-69).

During normal backward bending, the spinous processes approximate. While feeling between two spinous processes with his or her finger, the clinician asks the patient to perform a prone press up. If the clinician feels the spinous processes come together and the supraspinous ligament become slack under the finger, there is movement present at that segmental level. This amount of movement is compared to other levels and the clinician determines if the movement at the involved segment is hyper- or hypomobile, or if it is normal.

During normal spinal rotation, each spinous process moves laterally in relation to the spinous process of the vertebræ below. For example, during right rotation, each spinous process moves to the left. During left rotation, each spinous process moves to the right. The clinician, with the patient positioned in

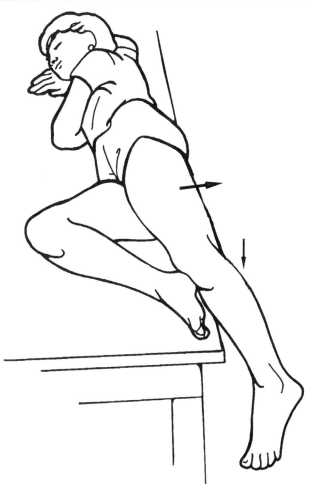

Figure 4-67. Ober's test for tensor fasciæ latæ length.

the sidelying position, stabilizes the inferior vertebra and passively rotates the spine superior to the segment being tested, while feeling between two spinous processes with his or her finger (Fig 4-70). If the clinician feels the superior spinous processes move laterally, as described above, there is movement at that level. This amount of movement is compared to other levels and is graded by the clinician. Right rotation should be tested with the patient lying on his left side, and the patient should lie on his right side to test left rotation. This technique is effective for the mid and lower thoracic and the entire lumbar spine. The clinician should begin testing superiorly and work his or her way inferiorly for ease of testing.

Segmental mobility in rotation also can be tested during the active mobility exam when the patient is sitting. The clinician palpates each interspinous space in the lumbar and lower thoracic spine as the patient actively rotates. The quality and quantity of motion between each segment should be roughly the same at adjacent levels and in right and left rotation at the same level. In the mid thoracic spine, the clinician can

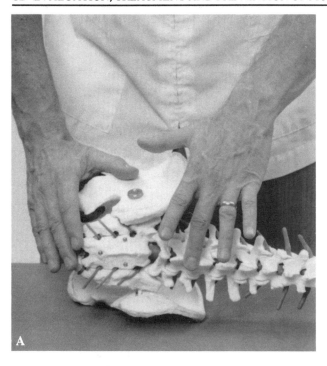

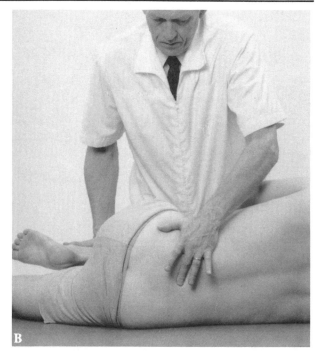

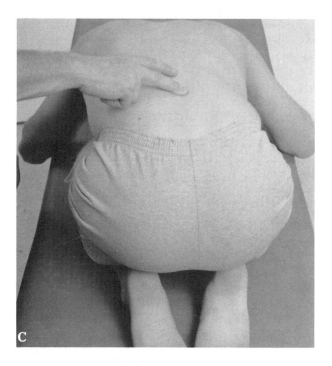

"pinch" two adjacent spinous processes to check for symmetrical motion (Fig 4-10).

The anterior spring test is a special mobility test that is done by contacting three spinous processes in a row with the thumbs (Fig 4-71). The patient is positioned prone. Downward (anterior) pressures are applied with both thumbs. This pressure is applied to the two spinous processes that are directly under each of the thumbs while the one spinous process between, which is being contacted by the tips of both thumbs, receives no direct pressure. If there is normal anterior/posterior movement, the two "outside" spinous processes are felt to move, while the one between is felt to stay in position.

A less specific but very useful spring test is performed with the heel of the clinician's hand placed over one or two segments. The clinician repeats a gentle but firm anterior spring up and down the length of the spine. This method is useful for determining the general mobility of an entire area of the spine (mid thoracic, for example) and can sometimes even be helpful for determining specific stiff or painful segments.

Figure 4-68. Segmental mobility testing - lumbar and lower thoracic flexion. A&B) In sidelying; C) In the prayer position.

Coccyx

The coccyx is palpated internally for segmental mobility and tenderness (Fig 4-72). The clinician grasps the coccyx with the index finger in the rectum, and the thumb on the coccyx externally. The position of the coccyx in neutral, flexion or extension can be felt, and PA glide can be assessed in this manner.

Tenderness and quality of the piriformis muscles can be palpated in the same position. The piriformis is assessed for tenderness or "ropiness." The internal contours of the anus should be smooth and relaxed. If ropiness or tenderness of the piriformis is found, pathology is indicated.

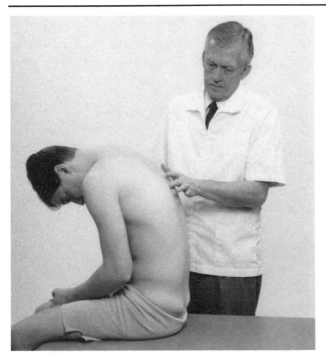

Figure 4-69. Segmental mobility testing - mid-thoracic flexion.

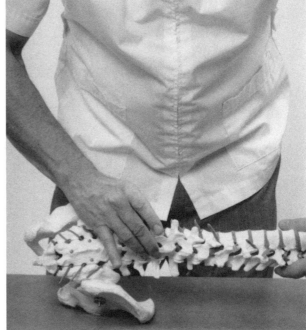

Use of an Inclinometer in Range of Motion Testing

The AMA Guides to the Evaluation of Permanent Impairment, 1990 state that standard goniometric techniques for measuring spinal movement can be highly inaccurate and that measurement techniques using inclinometers are necessary to obtain reliable spinal mobility measurements.[1] For this reason, many clinicians are using inclinometers to measure and report spinal range of motion and standing postural alignment (Fig 4-73). Inclinometers are also useful because improvements during treatment can be measured objectively.

More than one protocol exists for measuring spinal range of motion. One protocol for measuring spinal flexion/extension measures the curve angle at the end of range of motion[4, 12] (Fig 4-74A). Another protocol found in the literature, including the AMA Guides,[1] uses the standing position as the reference or zero point when measuring spinal flexion/extension. This protocol is seriously flawed if the subject does not have normal standing posture (Fig 4-75).

Since many, if not most, subjects do not have normal standing posture, we propose that measurement of the curve angle at the end of range of motion be used rather than the method the AMA Guides use for measurement of spinal flexion and extension.

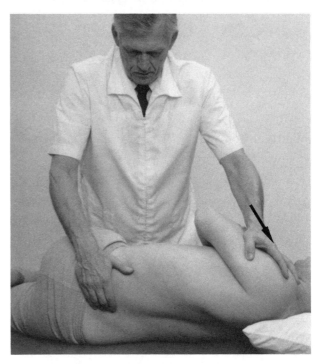

Figure 4-70. Segmental mobility testing - lumbar and lower thoracic rotation.

Assessment of the subject's standing and sitting posture is important and must be measure separately.

A typical example of how the AMA Guides provide us with incorrect and misleading information is shown in Figure 4-75. Here, because the AMA Guides Method shows that subject B has limited flexion range of motion, one might mistakenly assume the patient

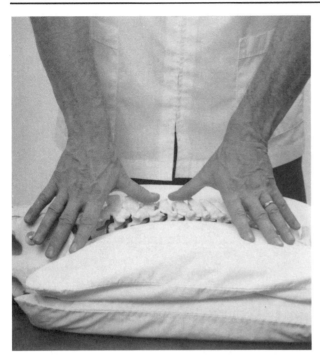 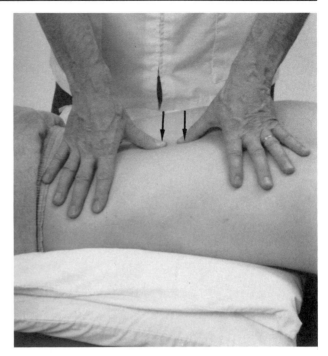

Figure 4-71. Spring test.

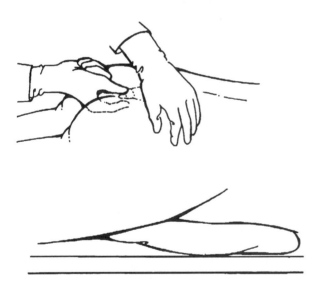

Figure 4-72. Coccyx palpation.

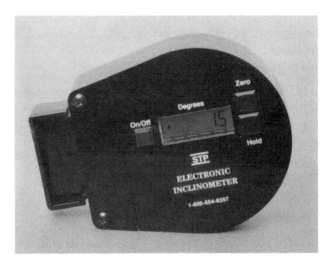

Figure 4-73. Inclinometer used for lumbar range of motion testing.

needs to work on flexion flexibility exercises, when in reality he or she probably needs to work on extension flexibility (because of the flat back posture).

Another issue related to use of an inclinometer for measuring spinal range of motion is the lack of agreement on norms. Limited information is available in the medical literature and much research is needed to establish norms for varying sex and age groups. Normal ranges of spinal mobility are presented in Figure 4-23 to provide some broad, general guidelines.

These are based on our interpretation of the limited information available.[1,4,12, 21, 22, 23, 28, 39]

In summary, while we must recognize that we have not established adequate norms for range of motion and posture of the spine and that protocols for measuring range of motion are not fully agreed upon, we also must recognize that the inclinometer does

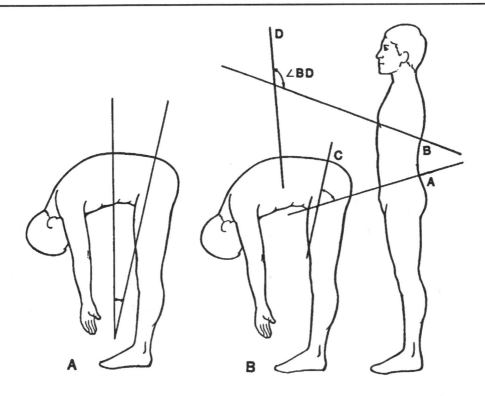

Figure 4-74. Two protocols for measuring lumbar flexion range of motion with an inclinometer. A) Measuring the curve angle at end range of motion; B) Using the AMA Guide's method. Angle AC is standing hip flexion, angle BD is gross flexion (BD - AC = lumbar flexion).

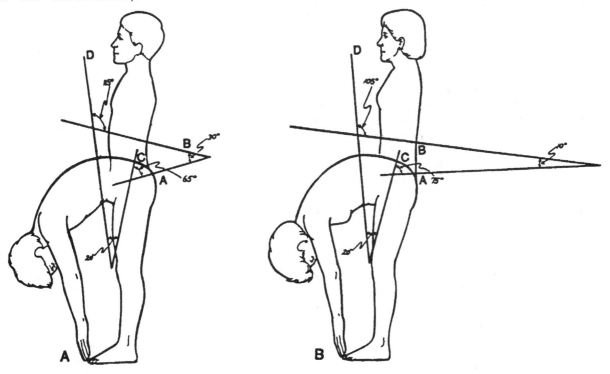

Figure 4-75. Figure showing a flaw in the AMA Guide's method of measuring lumbar flexion. Subjects A and B forward bend to the same point (20° using the curve angle at end range of motion method). However, subject A's gross flexion measures 115° and subject B's gross flexion measures 105°. The difference is due to the difference in the subject's standing posture (subject A = 30° and subject B = 10°), which the AMA Guide's method does not take into account. Using the formula BD - AC = lumbar flexion, subject A has 50° lumbar flexion and subject B has 30° lumbar flexion. Normal = 40° to 60°.

provide us with a much more accurate and objective method of measuring range of motion than we have previously had available. Exact instructions for measuring spinal range of motion using an inclinometer are not included in this section, as inclinometers do vary and protocols are usually included with the inclinometer when purchased. The clinician should make sure that the inclinometer he or she purchases makes use of the desired protocol, which is, in our opinion, measurement of the curve angle at the end range of motion.

Strength Exam

Although resisted muscle tests are very helpful in differential diagnosis of the extremity joints, their value in the lumbar and mid and lower thoracic spine is limited because of the difficulty of isolating the muscle contraction without at least some joint movement. Torturous recovery from the forward bent position, which was described under active movements, is probably the most valid mobility test for muscular involvement in the lumbar and mid and lower thoracic spine.

Strength tests of the lumbar spine are most useful because of the relationship between trunk weakness and lumbar injury.[3, 12, 17, 20, 32] The lumbar paraspinals and the abdominal muscles are tested for weakness, and weakness is usually treated through exercise, whether or not the muscles are the source of the patient's symptoms.

The lumbar paraspinals are tested with the patient lying prone, arms out in front. The patient is asked to extend both hips and raise the chest and arms off the table (Superman position). This position must be held effortlessly for at least 10 seconds (Fig 4-76). This test is preferred to unilateral hip extension against resistance, since the patient may brace with the opposite leg in the latter test .

If the patient is so stiff that the chest and legs cannot be raised from the floor simultaneously, the Superman position may not be optimal for testing paraspinal strength. Instead, the positions shown in Fig 4-77 can be used. These positions do not require as much flexibility as the Superman position does. The clinician can choose the position which works best for each particular patient.

The abdominal muscles are tested with the patient in the half sit-up position. The patient must be able to achieve the position shown in Figure 4-78, and must be able to hold it effortlessly for at least 10 seconds. If he or she cannot, the abdominal musculature should be strengthened.

Even when the patient has good trunk strength when tested as above, more aggressive trunk testing and strengthening exercises are often indicated in the treatment of patients with lower back pathology. The trunk musculature must have exceptionally good endurance to support the spine all day, especially in labor intensive occupations. Thus, common sense would tell us that the more conditioned the trunk, the less likely the patient is to experience a re-injury. The tests described above can be performed repetitively, or the patient can be required to hold the test position for a longer period of time to make it more challenging. Other advanced exercises are described in Chapter 12, Exercise, and the exercise positions can also be used as tests.

Neurological Exam

Thoracic Spine

Spinal nerve root impingement and peripheral nerve entrapment are rare in the thoracic spine.

Resisted Muscle Tests

Neurological involvement in the thoracic spine may cause weakness of the abdominal and/or intercostal muscles.

Sensation Testing

Sensation testing involves the dermatome patterns of the thoracic spinal nerves as they pass laterally and slightly inferiorly around the torso of the body (Fig 4-36).

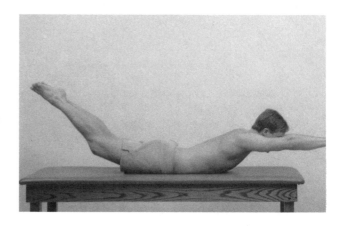

Figure 4-76. Testing lumbar paraspinal strength.

Lumbar Spine

Resisted Muscle Tests

Muscle strength of the lower extremities is tested bilaterally simultaneously whenever possible. This gives the clinician greater appreciation of very slight differences in strength and makes it more difficult for the patient to exaggerate weakness. Resisted muscle tests for the neurological exam of the lumbar spine involve the following muscle groups:

Hip flexion (L1-2) is done with the patient lying supine or sitting with the hip and knee flexed to 90° (Fig 4-79). The patient is asked to hold the position as resistance is applied. As noted earlier, increased pain with resisted muscle tests suggests muscular pathology. There is often an exception in the case of resisted hip flexion. Increased pain with this test can also mean joint pathology in the lumbar spine and/or hip. The attachment of the iliopsoas muscle on the anterior portion of the lumbar vertebral bodies causes an anterior pull on the lumbar spine as the iliopsoas contracts, often causing increased pain if there is pathology in the spinal segments. Tumors or metastatic lesions should always be suspected if a true neurological deficit is found in the upper lumbar spine since spinal nerve root impingement or peripheral nerve root entrapment or injury at this level is very rare.

Knee extension (L3-4) is tested with the patient sitting with the knees slightly flexed (Fig 4-80). This test is done bilaterally simultaneously whenever possible.

(Ankle dorsiflexion [heel walking] (anterior tibialis muscle, L4) is tested bilaterally with the patient sitting. The patient is asked to hold the position as resistance is applied (Fig 4-81). Heel walking is an another way of testing ankle dorsiflexion.

Great toe extension (L5) is tested bilaterally with the patient sitting. The patient is asked to hold the position as resistance is applied (Fig 4-82).

(Ankle plantarflexion (S1) [toe walking] is tested with the patient standing or walking on his toes. Since the gastrocnemius and soleus muscle group is quite strong, it is often necessary to test plantar flexion by having the patient repeat 10-20 repetitions of rising on his toe, first with the uninvolved side then with the involved side, before a true comparison can be made (Fig 4-83).

Knee flexion (S1-2) is tested bilaterally with the patient lying prone or sitting (Fig 4-84).

Sensation Testing

If specific sensation testing is indicated, it is carried out with the patient standing, sitting or lying in a position that is convenient to check the specific areas involved. The pin prick tests are done to map out the areas of numbness. The exact area is measured and

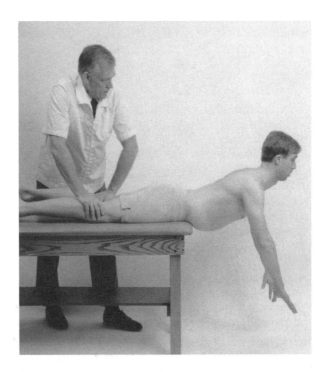

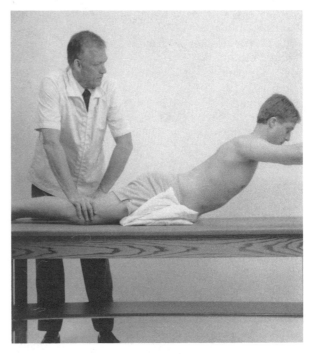

Figure 4-77. Alternate positions for testing lumbar paraspinal strength.

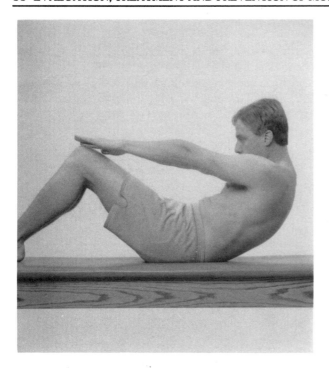

Figure 4-78. Testing abdominal strength.

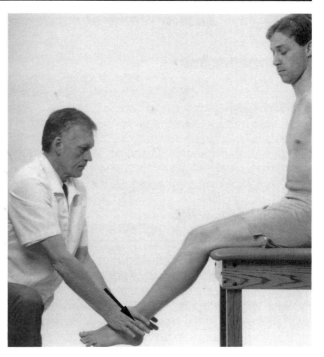

Figure 4-80. Testing knee extension.

indicated on the body diagram (Fig 4-2) and described in detail in the evaluation report. Neurological levels L1 through L3 provide sensation in oblique bands over the general area of the anterior thigh between the inguinal ligament to the knee. The L4 dermatome covers the medial side of the leg and foot. Neurological level L5 covers the lateral leg and dorsum of the foot with the crest of the tibia being the dividing line between L4 and L5 (all that is lateral to the crest including the dorsum of the foot is L5). The S1 dermatome covers the lateral side and a portion of the plantar surface of the foot. The S2 dermatome is on the posterior lateral heel. The dermatomes around the anus are arranged in three concentric rings (S2 outermost, S3 middle and S4-S5 innermost[16])(Fig 4-36).

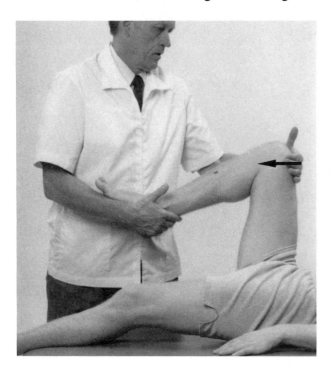

Figure 4-79. Testing hip flexion.

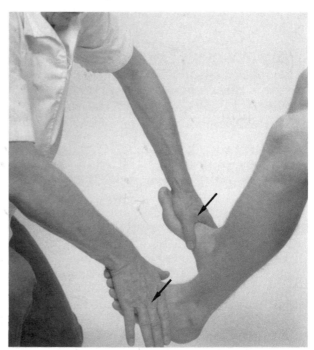

Figure 4-81. Testing ankle dorsiflexion.

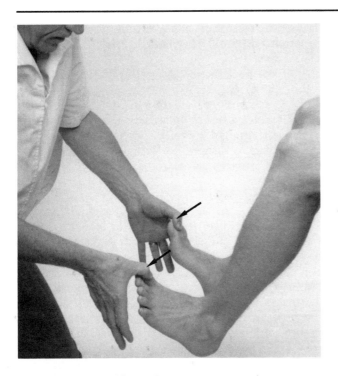

Figure 4-82. Testing great toe extension.

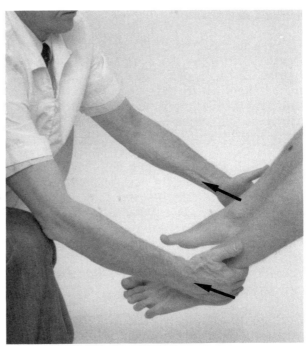

Figure 4-84. Testing knee flexion.

Muscle Stretch Reflexes

The quadriceps (L3-4) and gastrocnemius-soleus (S1-2) muscle stretch reflexes are tested in sitting (Fig 4-85). The ankle reflex is sometimes elicited better when the patient is prone with the knees flexed. The examiner may passively dorsiflex the ankles with one hand and quickly alternate a tap on each heelcord to pick up subtle changes in muscle stretch reflexes. The patient often tries to "help" by actively dorsiflexing the foot. This can be discouraged by asking the patient to plantarflex the ankle then relax, while the examiner quickly taps the heelcord during relaxation. There is no convenient muscle stretch reflex for the L5 nerve root, and the L4-5 intervertebral disc is sometimes known as the "silent disc."

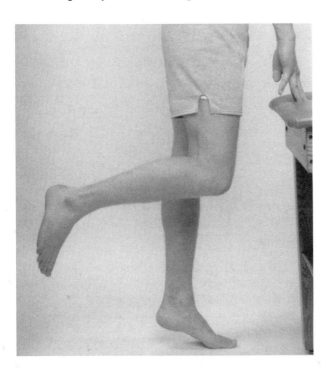

Figure 4-83. Testing ankle plantar flexion.

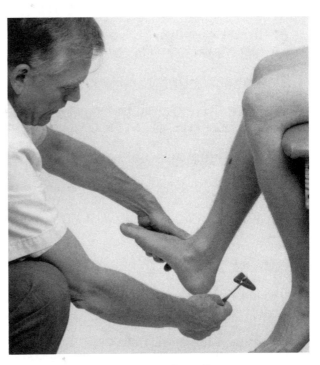

Figure 4-85. Testing reflexes.

Neural Tension Tests

As mentioned previously in this chapter, there is a need to consider the neural tissue tract as a contributing source of symptomatic complaints and limited mobility in the objective examination. Applying functional stresses to the neural tissues and their supporting connective tissue interfaces is critical to assessing their effect on the patient's symptoms.

There are four neural tension tests that are used in the physical examination of the lower limbs and trunk. They are passive neck flexion, prone knee bend, straight leg raise, and the Slump test.

The neural tension tests discussed in this section are generally recommended for all patients presenting with non-irritable conditions of the lumbar spine and lower extremities.

Contraindications to neural tension testing and treatment include the following:

1. Irritable conditions

2. Inflammatory conditions

3. Spinal cord signs

4. Malignancy

5. Nerve root compression signs

6. Severe, unremitting, constant night pain

7. Neurological signs (includes true numbness, weakness or reflex changes)

8. Recent paresthesia/anesthesia

9. Active spinal motions easily provoke distal symptoms, paresthesia or anesthesia

10. Reflex sympathetic dystrophy

It should be noted that any pathological process that causes less space for neural tissue to slide freely will produce an earlier onset of symptoms with the tension tests.[13]

Passive Neck Flexion

The passive neck flexion test is indicated for all spinal disorders and any headaches or extremity complaints of spinal origin. To perform the test, the patient can be either supine, sitting or standing. Neck flexion is induced passively by the examiner. Symptom response, range of motion and any resistance encountered should be noted (Fig 4-86).

Passive neck flexion should normally be painless, although a "pulling" sensation is occasionally encountered in the cervicothoracic junction. Passive neck flexion can be combined with other tension tests such as the straight leg raise to reproduce functional postures and to assess the effect of combined neural tension in provoking symptoms.

Prone Knee Bend

The prone knee bend is akin to the straight leg raise, with the prone knee bend putting selective tension on the upper lumbar segments. If the patient is complaining of pain or other symptoms in the upper lumbar spine and/or in the L1-4 dermatomal region, a femoral nerve stretch test (prone knee bend) should be done (Fig 4-87). As the femoral nerve is stretched by flexing the knee and hyperextending the hip, the nerve roots L 1, 2 and 3 are stretched across their respective intervertebral foramen. If there is reduced mobility or impingement of one of these spinal nerve roots, the symptoms will be increased as this test is done. One must be careful to distinguish between a painful quadriceps muscle and a true nerve root sign. If nerve root impingement is present, the symptoms may extend into the lateral aspect of the hip and into the upper lumbar spine as well as into the anterior thigh.

The prone knee bend is simply passive knee flexion with the patient lying prone. Symptom response, range of motion and resistance encountered should be noted and compared to the contralateral side.

The normal response for the prone knee bend is not well documented. However, common clinical findings include a "stretching" sensation in the rectus femoris and an anterior pelvic tilt with an increase in lumbar lordosis.

Straight Leg Raise

This is the most common tension test used by physical therapists. It is indicated for patients presenting with any spinal and/or lower limb complaints.

The straight leg raise test is traditionally performed to determine if there is compromise of the nerve roots or irritation of the sciatic nerve (radiculitis). One must be aware that any acute, painful condition in the lumbar spine or sacroiliac may be irritated by the straight leg raising test. Tight hamstring muscles, hip joint pathology or sacroiliac joint pathology also can

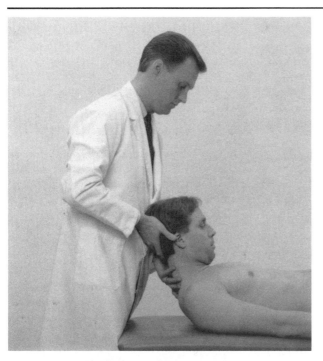

Figure 4-86. The passive neck flexion test.

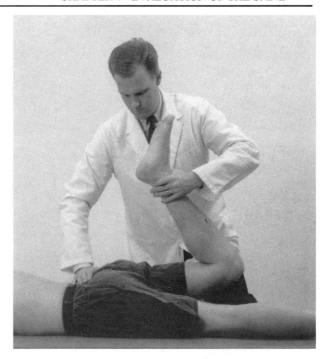

Figure 4-87. The prone knee bend test.

cause a painful response to the straight leg raise. An adherent nerve root will cause a positive straight leg raise test. Piriformis syndrome also can be irritated by the straight leg raise test. Therefore, considering all the variables associated with this test, one must use careful interpretation when determining if there is nerve root involvement if the only evidence is a positive straight leg raise test. Differentiation tests can help the clinician distinguish true radiculitis from other musculoskeletal conditions.

The patient is positioned supine for the straight leg raise. The examiner raises the leg while making sure the knee remains straight. As the straight leg is raised, progressive tension is applied to the sciatic nerve, which in turn places tension on the nerve roots. If compromise or irritation of the nerve roots exists, symptoms will be exacerbated by this maneuver. If the test increases pain in the posterior thigh, it may not truly be a positive neurological sign, but may still be a significant clinical finding.

The examiner should palpate the ASIS for the first sign of movement into posterior rotation. It is at this point that the hamstrings have engaged the pelvis, causing such movement to occur (Fig 4-88). By comparing both sides, the examiner can ascertain the degree of hamstring tightness of that patient. It is helpful to do hold-relax muscle stretching of the hamstring to distinguish between true nerve root signs and tight hamstrings. If the hold-relax stretching seems to increase the range of motion, the pain and restriction

are probably in the hamstring. If, on the other hand, the hold-relax technique does not seem to change the pain or restriction, spinal nerve root impingement or irritation may be involved. The hold-relax technique is not advised on patients presenting with a positive straight leg raise at less than 30° hip flexion, as it may provoke an irritable condition.

The bowstring test is a useful variation of the straight leg raise test. The clinician flexes the patient's hip and knee, each to 90°. With one hand, he palpates the sciatic nerve in the popliteal fossa. When the nerve is located, the clinician extends the knee to the point of hamstring tightness and then presses the sciatic nerve with the other hand (Fig 4-89), which causes increased neural tissue tension. If pain is produced proximally, this may be a sign of nerve root irritation.

Lasegue's sign helps to further differentiate true nerve root signs. After the clinician raises the leg to the point of symptomatic response, the leg is lowered 1/2 to 1 inch. The stress to all structures, including the nerve roots, should be relieved. With the leg stationary, the foot is then dorsiflexed. This applies tension to the nerve roots without affecting the other structures (hamstring, sacroiliac joint and hip joint). Exacerbation of pain on dorsiflexion of the foot is the true Lasegue's sign of radiculitis.[30]

Other differentiation tests are quite useful. Adding neck flexion, ankle dorsiflexion, hip rotation or adduction can alter the tension applied, and thus the

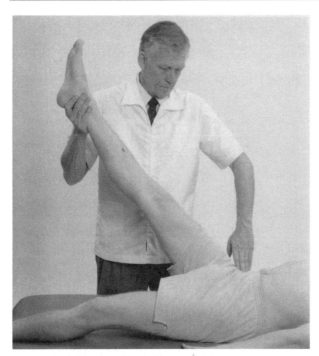

Figure 4-88. The straight leg raise test.

response observed. When the head is flexed, the dura is pulled superiorly, putting an added tension on the spinal nerve root, which may increase a positive sign of the straight leg raise. This is not always the case, however.

Normally, the positive straight leg raise test suggests more severe pathology when positive at 20°

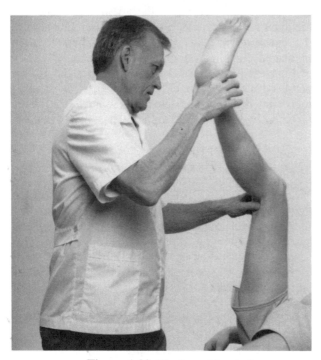

Figure 4-89. The bowstring test.

to 40° of hip flexion and less severe pathology if positive at 50° to 70°. It is difficult to interpret a straight leg raise as positive for radiculitis at ranges over 70°. The degree of hip flexion present when the symptoms occur should be recorded so the clinician can decide whether progress is made during a later reassessment.

Occasionally, symptoms are provoked as the opposite leg is raised. This may suggest a disc herniation with protrusion medial to the nerve root. If symptoms are relieved as the opposite leg is raised, a bulge lateral to the nerve root may be present.

Slump Test

The Slump test is a relatively new neural tension test. It combines the sitting straight leg raise, passive neck flexion and a "slump" or slouch of the lumbar spine in sitting. This test was first developed and researched by Maitland in 1979.[27] The test is indicated for any patient with low back pain and/or lower limb complaints.

The Slump test is performed in the following manner (Fig 4-90):

1. The patient sits comfortably at the end of an exam table.

2. The clinician asks the patient to slump or slouch. This is sustained by the clinician.

3. The patient performs neck flexion.

4. While sustaining passive neck flexion, the clinician asks the patient to straighten either of his or her legs.

5. The clinician then asks the patient to dorsiflex the ankle.

6. The neck flexion is released to neutral, and again any change in symptoms is noted.

7. The test is repeated with the opposite leg.

8. The test is repeated with both legs at once.

Normal responses to the Slump test are summarized below:

- When the patient initially slumps, no complaints are usually offered.

- When the neck is passively flexed, 50% of subjects report a stretch in the T8-T9 area.

- When the leg is straightened, a symmetrical limitation of range when compared bilaterally and a stretch feeling in the posterior hamstring and knee is normal.

- Likewise, a symmetrical restriction of dorsiflexion is normal.

- A release of the neck flexion may increase the available range of dorsiflexion at the ankle.

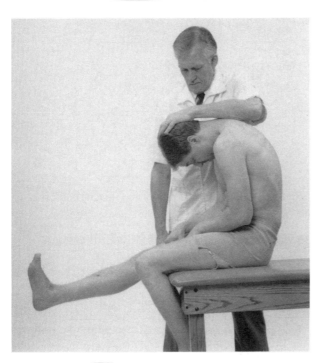

Figure 4-90. The Slump test.

It is important in any tension testing to consider the following:

- Before beginning, carefully identify all the patient's symptoms complaints.

- Note which symptoms are present in the starting position.

- Carefully note any <u>onset or change</u> in symptoms at each step of the test.

- Move the patient's limb in each step to the point of <u>onset or change</u> in symptom complaints.

- Compare the findings of the test to the contralateral limb and what is considered normal.

As with any musculoskeletal test, reassessment of the test at later intervals will help the clinician decide whether treatment is effective. To compare later findings, the clinician must document the following thoroughly:

- *The range of motion at which the symptoms first appear*

- *The nature and location of the symptoms*

- *Any abnormal resistance felt by the clinician during the test*

Babinski's Test

The Babinski test, as described under the neurological exam of the cervical spine, completes the neurological exam of the lumbar spine.

Palpation Exam

Due to the depth of many structures of the lumbar, mid and lower thoracic spine, palpation of the skin may not reveal temperature or color changes even though inflammation may be present.

A useful test to assess muscle guarding or spasm in the lumbar spine is the weight shift test. With the patient standing, the examiner places his or her thumbs on the patient's lumbar paraspinals. The patient is then asked to shift his or her weight from one foot to the other (Fig 4-91). Normally, the paraspinals on the side of the stance foot will relax, but if muscle guarding and/or spasm is present the muscle will not relax.

Chronic thoracic and lumbar problems are often accompanied by changes in the soft tissue. Asymmetrical toughened or ropy areas in the paraspinal or interscapular musculature may be clues to long-standing problems.

The piriformis, iliopsoas and quadratus lumborum muscles receive specific attention in the palpation examination.

The piriformis muscle (Fig 4-92) is palpated at the greater sciatic notch (halfway between the ischial tuberosity and the greater trochanter) with the patient lying prone.

With the patient lying supine, the iliopsoas (Fig 4-93) is palpated in three different areas: 1) Deep on the lateral border of the femoral triangle over the lesser trochanter; 2) On the inner border of the ilium behind the ASIS; and 3) Underneath the rectus abdominus (found by palpating approximately 2" lateral to the umbilicus and pressing downward and then medially).

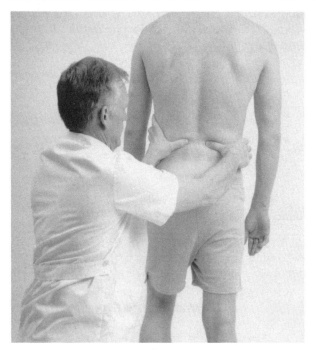

Figure 4-91. The standing weight shift test.

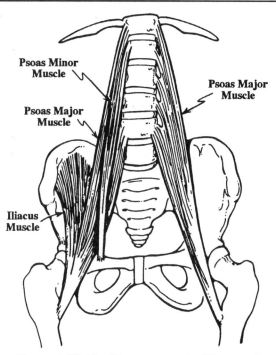

Figure 4-93. The iliopsoas muscle (iliacus and psoas).

The quadratus lumborum (Fig 4-94) is found by positioning the patient to separate the 12th rib from the iliac crest (mild sidebending and flexion to the opposite side) and palpating deep and just lateral to the paraspinals.

When palpating the lumbar, mid and lower thoracic spinal joints (ligament and bone), the spinous processes and the supraspinous ligament are all the examiner can feel. The information gained through palpating these structures is surprisingly valuable. The supraspinous ligament is normally springy and supple. If it is thick and hardened, the segment may be hypomobile. When palpation between the spinous processes elicits pain, it may indicate the spinal segment

(facet joints or intervertebral disc) is involved.

The position of the spinous processes is felt to determine alignment of the spine. If one spinous process is lateral to the one below it, the segment may be locked in rotation or sidebending. When the spinous processes are close together the segment may be locked in backward bending. If they are far apart the

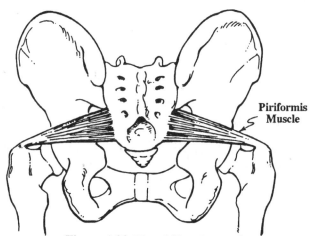

Figure 4-92. The piriformis muscle.

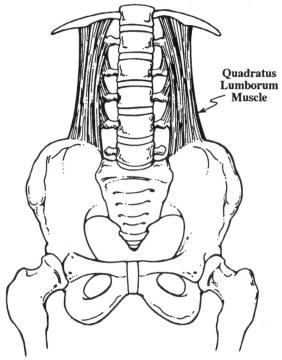

Figure 4-94. The quadratus lumborum muscle.

segment may be locked in forward bending or a compression fracture may be present. These changes in position of the bone are called "positional changes" and suggest the presence of facet joint impingement or facet joint hypomobility. Positional changes are usually felt with one finger placed between two spinous processes. The "pinch test" also is useful in finding rotational positional changes. The pinch test is done by pinching the spinous processes of two adjacent vertebræ between the thumb and index finger of each hand and looking to see if they are properly aligned (Fig 4-10).

Positional changes may be congenital in nature and when seen by themselves they do not necessarily mean a joint is locked or hypomobile. Mobility testing must confirm that a segment is locked or hypomobile before the final assessment is made.

The inexperienced examiner can make the best use of the segmental mobility and palpation examinations by successively palpating deeply at each interspinous space and/or spring testing at each level. When the patient complains of increased symptoms at a particular level, the clinician then examines that level more closely for signs of hypo or hypermobility, positional changes or subtle variations in soft tissue texture. This method is much more effective and less confusing and frustrating than trying to find the subtle problems "blindly."

Special Tests

Distraction Test

The distraction test is a neurological test and a mobility test. As traction is applied to the spine, certain symptoms may be altered suggesting a possible spinal nerve root impingement. For example, if traction relieves the patient's symptoms it may suggest that a spinal nerve root is impinged. Actually, facet joint or disc pain can be relieved with this test also and it is, therefore, not a completely reliable indication of spinal nerve root impingement. The test is valuable in that it gives the clinician an indication when traction might be an effective treatment or when it might aggravate the patient's condition (Fig 4-95). Furthermore, if distraction relieves or centralizes the patient's symptoms, it is an indication that a back support may be helpful.

Waddell's Tests

Gordon Waddell, et. al.,[40] have described a series of tests that are designed for use as a simple and rapid screening exam to help identify the patients who present with nonorganic, psychological and social elements to their pain syndromes (Fig 4-96). The screening test is not intended to be a psychological diagnostic test, only a screen for those who may need further evaluation. The physical therapist who treats low back pain patients should incorporate the tests described below into the normal lumbar examination.

If a patient tests positive for any individual sign, it counts as a positive sign for that type. A positive finding for three or more of the five types is clinically significant. Isolated positive signs are ignored. Positive findings are detailed below. For further details, see Waddell's article.[40]

Type I - Tenderness

Superficial
The skin is tender to light pinch over a wide area of lumbar skin. The exception would be a localized band of tenderness in a posterior primary ramus distribution, because it may be caused by nerve irritation.

Non-anatomic
Deep tenderness is felt over a wide area, and is not localized to one structure. It often extends to the thoracic spine, sacrum or pelvis.

Type II - Simulation

These tests give the patient the impression that a particular examination is being performed when in fact it is not.

Axial Loading
Low back pain is reported when the examiner uses his or her hands to vertically load the patient's skull while the patient is standing.

Rotation
Low back pain is reported when the patient's shoulders and hips are passively rotated in the same plane (the lumbar spine is not actually moved).

Type III - Distraction

Straight Leg Raising
A positive straight leg raise is found when tested in supine, but when the patient is in a sitting position and is distracted from the purpose of the test (with clinician apparently examining the foot or ankle), the finding is negative.

Type IV - Regional Disturbances

These involve complaints in a widespread region of neighboring parts such as the whole leg below the

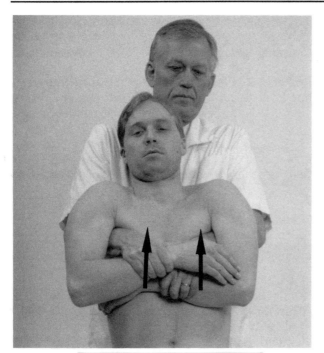

Figure 4-95. Lumbar distraction.

Type I - *Tenderness*
• Superficial
• Non-anatomic

Type II - *Simulation*
• Axial Loading
• Rotation

Type III - *Distraction*
• Straight leg raising

Type IV - *Regional*
• Weakness
• Sensory

Type V - *Overreaction*

Figure 4-96. Waddell's five types of physical signs indicating non-organic source of symptoms.

knee, the entire leg or the whole left side of the body, where the complaints diverge from normally accepted neuroanatomy. Care must be taken not to mistake multiple root involvement for a regional disturbance. Multiple level spinal stenosis or repeated spinal surgeries may cause multiple root involvement.

Weakness

The patient demonstrates weakness on formal testing by a partial cogwheel "giving way" of many muscle groups that do not fit a particular myotome.

Sensory

Patient has sensory disturbances that do not fit a normal dermatomal pattern.

Type V - Overreaction

This may take the form of disproportionate verbalization, facial expression, muscle tension and tremor, collapsing or sweating. Judgments should be made with caution, as there are considerable cultural variations or examiners can inadvertently provoke overreactive responses.

Waddell's tests should be performed with *every* patient complaining of lumbar pain. The tests do not take much time to perform and can lend valuable information about the patient's true status. They should not be performed as a separate group but should be spread throughout the objective evaluation, following the natural sequence discussed in Chapter 3.

REFERENCES

1. AMA: <u>Guides to the Evaluation of Permanent Impairment,</u> 3rd Edition, Revised. AMA, Chicago IL 1990.
2. Aspinall W: Clinical Testing for Cervical Mechanical Disorders which produce Ischemic Vertigo. JOSPT 11:5, November 1989.
3. Biering-Sorenson F: Physical Measurements as Risk Indicators for Low Back Trouble Over a One-Year Period. Spine 9:106-119, 1984.
4. Burdett R, et al: Reliability and Validity of Four Instruments for Measuring Lumbar Spine and Pelvic Positions. Physical Therapy 66:677-684, 1986.
5. Butler D: <u>Mobilization of the Nervous System.</u> Churchill Livingstone, Edinburgh 1991.
6. Butler D: The Effects of Age and Gender on the Slump Test (unpublished thesis). South Australian Institute of Technology, Adelaide 1985.
7. Cailliet R: <u>Neck and Arm Pain.</u> FA Davis, Philadelphia

PA 1964.

8. Cloward R: Cervical Discography: A Contribution to the Etiology and Mechanism of Neck, Shoulder and Arm Pain. Annals of Surgery 150(6) 1052-1064, 1959.

9. Cyriax J: Diagnosis of Soft Tissue Lesions. Textbook of Orthopædic Medicine, Vol 1, 8th edition. Bailliere-Tindall, London 1982.

10. Finneson B: Low Back Pain. JB Lippincott, Philadelphia PA 1973.

11. Grant A: The Slump Test. South Australian Institute of Technology, Adelaide 1983. Unpublished thesis.

12. Griffin A and Troup J: Tests of Lifting and Handling Capacity. Ergonomics 27:305-320, 1984.

13. Groom D: Cervical Spine and Shoulders. The Saunders Group, Minneapolis MN 1992. Course Manual.

14. Halbach J and Tank R: The Shoulder. In Orthopedic and Sports Physical Therapy, Vol 2. J Gould and G Davies, eds. CV Mosby, St Louis MO 1985.

15. Hirsch C, Ingelmark B and Miller M: The Anatomical Basis for Low Back Pain. Acta Ortho Scanda 33:1-17, 1963.

16. Hoppenfeld S: Physical Examination of the Spine and Extremities. Appleton-Century- Crofts, Norwalk CT 1976.

17. Jackson D and Brown M: Is There a Role for Exercise in the Treatment of Low Back Pain Patients? Clin Orthop and Rel Res 179:39-45, 1983.

18. Jackson N, Winkelman R and Bickel W: Nerve Endings in the Lumbar Spinal Column. JBJS 48A:1272-1281, 1966.

19. Jensen G: Musculoskeletal Analysis: The Thoracic Spine. In Physical Therapy. R Scully and M Barnes, eds. Lippincott, Philadelphia PA 1989.

20. Kahanovitz N, et al: Normal Trunk Muscle Strength and Endurance in Women and the Effect of Electrical Stimulation and Exercises to Increase Trunk Muscle Strength and Endurance. Spine 12:112-118, 1987.

21. Kapandji I: Spine. Vol 3 of The Physiology of the Joints, 2nd edition. Churchill-Livingstone, London-New York 1974.

22. Keeley J, et al: Quantification of Lumbar Function Part 5: Reliability of Range of Motion Measures in the Sagittal Plane and in Vivo Torso Rotation Measurement Techniques. Spine 11:31-35, 1986.

23. Kendall F and McCreary E: Muscles: Testing and Function. Williams and Wilkins, Baltimore MD 1983.

24. Kenneally M, et al: "The Upper Limb Tension Test: The Straight Leg Raise Test of the Arm." In Physical Therapy of the Cervical and Thoracic Spine, Vol 17 of Clinics in Physical Therapy. R Grant, ed. Churchill Livingstone, Edinburgh 1989.

25. Koontz C: "Thoracic Outlet Syndrome, Diagnosis and Management." In Orthopedic Physical Therapy Forum series. AREN, Pittsburgh, PA 1987. Videotape .

26. Maitland G: Vertebral Manipulation, 5th edition. Butterworth, London 1986.

27. Maitland GD: Negative Disc Exploration: Positive Canal Signs. Australian Journal of Physiotherapy 25:129-134, 1979.

28. Mayer T and Gatchel R: Functional Restoration for Spinal Disorders: The Sports Medicine Approach. Lea and Febiger, Philadelphia PA 1988.

29. McKenzie R: The Lumbar Spine. Spinal Publications, Waikanæ New Zealand 1981.

30. Mennell J: Back Pain. Little-Brown, Boston MA 1964.

31. Mooney V and Robertson J: The Facet Syndrome. Clin Orthop and Rel Res 115:149-156, Mar/Apr 1976.

32. Nachemson A: Exercise, Fitness and Back Pain. In Exercise, Fitness and Health: A Consensus of Current Knowledge. C Bouchard, et al, eds. Human Kinetics Books, Champaign IL 1990.

33. Rocabado R and Inglarsh A: Musculoskeletal Approach to Maxillofacial Pain. Lippincott, Philadelphia PA 1991.

34. Roofe P: Innervation of the Annulus Fibrosis and Posterior Longitudinal Ligament: Fourth and Fifth Lumbar Level. Arch Neurol Psych 44:100-103, 1940.

35. Saal J, et al: High Levels of Inflammatory Phospholipase A_2 Activity in Lumbar Disc Herniations. Spine 15(7):674-678, 1990.

36. Spangford E: Personal Communication. Orthopædic Surgeon. Huddinge, Sweden 1982.

37. Stokes H: The Seriously Uninjured Hand - Weakness of Grip. Joul of Occ Med 25(9):683- 684, Sept 1983.

38. Toby EB and Koman LA: Thoracic Outlet Compression Syndrome. In Nerve Compression Syndromes. RM Szabo, ed. Slack, Thorofare, London 1989.

39. Troup J, et al: The Perception of Back Pain and the Role of Psychophysical Tests of Lifting Capacity. Spine 12:645-657, 1987.

40. Waddell G: Non-Organic Physical Signs in Low Back Pain. Spine 5:117-125, Mar/ Apr 1980.

41. Waitz E: The Lateral Bending Sign. Spine 6:388-397, 1981.

42. White A and Panjabi M: Clinical Biomechanics of the Spine, 2nd edition. Lippincott, Philadelphia PA 1990.

43. Zohn D and Mennell J: Musculoskeletal Pain: Diagnosis and Physical Treatment. Little, Brown and Company, Boston MA 1976.

CHAPTER 5

TREATMENT OF THE SPINE BY DIAGNOSIS

INTRODUCTION

The physical therapist is becoming increasingly interested in and involved with evaluating and assessing the patient with musculoskeletal disorders. Understanding the causes of these disorders is essential before an accurate assessment can be made. Assessment and treatment planning are cognitive processes. The assessment must be based on correlation of the patient's comparable signs and symptoms in a "rule out" process. This chapter is not intended to provide "cookbook" answers to difficult problems. Rather, it is intended to be a guide to intelligent decision making for appropriate treatment. Remember that it is not always possible to fully evaluate a patient on the first visit or to determine a specific pathological entity, in which case the therapist must assess the various problems the patient has that may be contributing to his or her symptoms. These problems can then be treated, often with excellent results. Chapter 6 discusses the philosophy of treating by "problem" rather than by diagnosis.

A difficulty with preparing a text of this sort is the wide difference of opinion and placement of emphasis found in the literature. All theories postulated about musculoskeletal disorders cannot possibly be discussed, but the object is to present the major "schools of thought" and some of the more recent trends in this area.

Many questions remain unanswered about spinal pathology. Consider the following two cases. In one instance, a disc protrusion is identified by myelography and is determined to be the cause of the patient's complaint. The disc protrusion is surgically removed but the patient's signs and symptoms remain unchanged. In the other instance, a disc protrusion is identified by CT/MRI scan, appropriate physical therapy measures or another form of treatment is applied, and the patient's signs and symptoms disappear. Yet on a follow-up CT/MRI scan, the disc protrusion remains unchanged.

The point is that there is often no clear-cut cause and effect relationship between what we see, or think we see, and what may actually be causing the patient's problem. Certainly many of the things we observe, especially radiological findings, are difficult to assess and are probably unrelated to the actual problem.[3, 22, 42, 47, 48, 49, 67, 90, 93] What exactly is taking place when one patient with a documented nerve root syndrome secondary to foraminal encroachment improves with spinal traction and another patient, with presumably the same disorder, does not improve? What is really happening to the disc when a lateral shift correction maneuver is done and is followed by extension exercises? We think that the disc is reducing. Furthermore, there is some scientific evidence to support such a hypothesis. However, much of what we practice has its basis in the hypothetical realm. We must use caution when basing our treatment on our hypotheses. The same caution applies when assuming anything that shows up on the patient's radiological examination is causing the patient's complaint.

This is not to suggest or imply that just because we do not have all the answers, we should not discuss what we think may be happening. We certainly should not stop using effective treatment methods just because at this point we do not understand everything about spinal pathology. However, because specific etiologies may not be fully understood or recognized, and because much of our treatment is based in theory, we must be cautious in our approach to a patient's problem. We must work our way through the problem with each patient, individualizing treatment appropriately.

Musculoskeletal disorders are of primary importance because they are the largest group of complaints seen by health care practitioners, and by the physical therapist in particular. However, the therapist should be capable of recognizing systemic and visceral problems that can mimic musculoskeletal disorders and also appreciate that musculoskeletal disorders can produce visceral responses as well.

GENERAL TREATMENT CONSIDERATIONS

Generally, treatment in the acute and subacute stages of musculoskeletal dysfunction should be directed to: 1) Relieve pain; 2) Restore normal anatomy and biomechanics; 3) Promote healing; 4) Prevent joint stiffness; 5) Prevent muscle weakness; and 6) Prevent postural changes. Often, too much attention is focused on relief of pain (medication, rest and passive modalities and treatments) with little or no attention directed toward prevention of joint stiffness, muscle weakness and adaptive postural changes and the resulting disabilities that these disorders will ultimately produce. One should realize that pain is only a symptom of underlying pathology and that healing, in most instances, will eventually take place in spite of any treatment. Therefore, the emphasis of treatment of musculoskeletal disorders should be the restoration of full joint mobility, muscular strength and flexibility and normal posture rather than the overuse of modalities and other passive treatments that is sometimes seen.

Unless otherwise indicated, the evaluation findings and treatment described for the various conditions below apply to all areas of the spine – cervical, thoracic or lumbar.

MUSCLE DISORDERS

Spinal disorders primarily of muscular origin are uncommon. While it is true that muscle guarding and/ or intrinsic muscle spasm usually accompanies spinal pain regardless of the underlying cause, there is no neurophysiological reason for a normal muscle to spontaneously begin to spasm.

To convince oneself of this principle, one should compare how injury or pathology occurs in other muscles of the body, such as the biceps brachialis, and use common sense to decide if the muscles of the spine are really any different. For example, any therapist who has treated low back injuries knows that a lower back injury commonly occurs when a patient bends over or rises up from a bent position with no weight ("I just bent over to tie my shoe!") Upon physical examination, the muscles may be tender to palpation, and the patient's range of motion and strength may be limited due to pain. In the absence of other objective findings, a diagnosis of muscle strain is tempting. This would be equivalent to diagnosing biceps strain in a patient who simply bent his elbow to take a drink! We know that biceps strains do not occur in this way. Why, then, do we accept the assumption that a paraspinal muscle strain can occur in such a fashion? In other words, it does not make sense that an individual who is in average physical condition would strain a back muscle during a simple bending motion. Taking this concept a step further, it does not make sense that a heavy construction worker, who is used to lifting hundreds of pounds a day, would strain a back muscle while shoveling his or her driveway. Therefore, without a thorough evaluation and assessment, it is often an easy "cop-out" to incriminate the muscles as the source of the patient's complaint.

There are, of course, primary muscular disorders that are legitimate diagnoses. These can be classified as strains, contusions and inflammations. In addition, "trigger points" will develop in muscles as a result of dysfunctional biomechanics; stressful, prolonged or repetitive positions; or in response to irritation or injury of a muscle.

This section will describe the identifying features of general muscle guarding, muscle strains and muscle inflammation. The clinician can apply the principles discussed to all muscles of the trunk.

In addition, specific findings for pathology of the piriformis, the iliopsoas and the quadratus lumborum will be discussed separately in some depth, as it is common for the clinician to overlook pathology in these muscles because of their relative inaccessibility.

Finally, treatment for all muscle disorders will be discussed. The treatment principles can be applied to all general muscle disorders, including muscle guarding and spasm; muscle strains and contusions; and muscle inflammation. The same principles apply to specific muscle pathology, such as occurs in the piriformis, iliopsoas and quadratus lumborum muscles.

Findings

General Muscle Disorders

Muscle Guarding and Intrinsic Muscle Spasm

Muscle guarding nearly always accompanies pain, regardless of the underlying cause. Muscle guarding may develop wherever pain is felt, even if it is referred from elsewhere in the body. Acute muscle spasm is probably the most painful part of many back disorders. One must remember, however, that the amount of pain present is no indication of the seriousness of a problem. We have all experienced excruciating muscle cramps that were painful yet harmless. Prolonged muscle guarding or spasm, on the other hand, leads to circulatory stasis and the retention of metabolites. The muscle then may become inflamed (myositis) and a localized tenderness develops in the muscle. This intrinsic muscle spasm adds additional pain and discomfort (Fig 5-1).

Muscle guarding and intrinsic muscle spasm may be noted during the palpation exam by the tension and tenderness of the muscles. A positive weight shift test indicates muscle spasm (Fig 5-2). Prolonged intrinsic

muscle spasm tends to cause generalized pain along the spine and may aggravate areas of degenerative joint and disc disease.

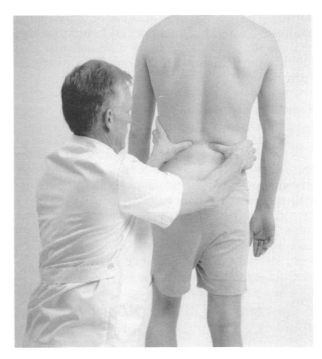

Figure 5-2. The weight shift test for muscle spasm.

Without a thorough evaluation, it is easy to incriminate muscle guarding and the resulting in intrinsic muscle spasm as the primary cause of the patient's problem. It is unwise to make this assumption as there is always an underlying cause of the muscle guarding. It is, however, often necessary to treat muscle guarding and intrinsic muscle spasm before treating the underlying problem.

Muscle Strains and Contusions

Musculotendinous strains and contusions have a definite history of trauma such as a blow to the back, a tearing sensation while lifting or another traumatic event, or a more subtle history of aggravation such as constant repetition of a new activity. With rest, the patient will claim relief of pain but will complain of "stiffening." He will usually report movement initially hurts but activity will often "loosen up" the stiffness. The patient complains of pain and a general, vague loss of active and passive movements. The patient does not describe any particular positions or activities, such as standing or sitting, that stand out as being especially painful. Movement is usually more painful than rest, so walking may be worse than standing or sitting.

Pain is usually referred over several spinal levels and the patient has difficulty "pinpointing" the pain.

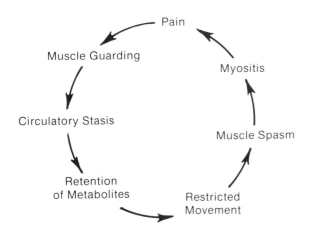

Figure 5-1. The vicious cycle that often develops with musculoskeletal disorders.

One of the most significant objective findings will be pain upon palpation of the muscle but no pain upon palpation of the joint or upon spring testing the spinal segment passively. The neurological exam will reveal no true positive findings. Mennell describes these patients as having a torturous recovery from the forward bent position.[54] The patient may have radicular pain following the sensory distribution of the associated nerve root.[37, 56]

Muscle Inflammation (Myositis)

Muscle inflammation, or myositis, occurs by itself only on rare occasions. The patient may describe the onset after sleeping in a draft or sitting too close to an air conditioner. Muscle inflammation more commonly follows muscle strain or contusion or develops secondary to prolonged muscle guarding or chronic stress. It essentially has the same characteristics as a muscle strain except that myositis will be of insidious onset and may show temperature and color changes over the involved musculature.

Specific Muscle Disorders

Piriformis Muscle

Referred pain of myofascial origin from the piriformis may radiate to the sacroiliac region laterally across the buttock and hip to the proximal two-thirds of the posterior thigh. Symptoms of piriformis involvement may be caused by referral from trigger points within the muscle, entrapment of the neurovascular bundle within the substance of the muscle, or against the rim of the greater sciatic foramen and by sacroiliac dysfunction. Since the muscle functions to restrain vigorous internal and external hip rotation, activation of these myofascial trigger points in the piriformis results from acute overload as when catching oneself from a fall or running.

The patient with piriformis muscle involvement will tend to squirm and shift weight frequently when seated. Pain can be referred into the posterior thigh. In the supine position, the foot of the involved side is externally rotated. Internal rotation of the hip will be restricted and painful, and resisted external rotation will be painful. In the prone position, pelvic asymmetry may be noted. Standing examination may reveal an uneven sacral base. The piriformis muscle will be painful to palpation, and painful nodules (trigger points) may be evident.

Iliopsoas Muscle

Myofascial pain in the iliopsoas can result from acute overload, stress or prolonged sitting with the hips acutely flexed. Referred pain from the iliopsoas may extend along the spine from the thoracolumbar junction to the sacroiliac joint and upper gluteal region. The iliacus portion may refer symptoms into the groin and anterior thigh.[85]

The patient with iliopsoas involvement will have pain and restriction with hip extension. Resisted hip flexion will be painful. Pain with palpation and/or painful trigger points will be seen.

Quadratus Lumborum Muscle

Myofascial pain from the quadratus lumborum is easily mistaken for radicular pain of lumbar origin. Activation of myofascial trigger points in the quadratus lumborum often occurs as a result of simultaneously bending forward and reaching to one side to pull or lift something or as a consequence of a trauma such as a fall or motor vehicle accident.

Pain from the quadratus lumborum is usually deep and aching, although it may be sharp during movement. Referred pain will be felt along the crest of the ilium and sometimes in the lower quadrant of the abdomen and into the groin. The greater trochanter, buttock and sacroiliac joint can also be areas of referred pain. The areas of referred pain can also be tender, thus mimicking local pathology.[85]

The patient with quadratus lumborum pathology may have a functional lumbar scoliosis that is convex away from the involved side. The normal lumbar lordosis may appear flattened due to the vertebral rotation that accompanies the scoliosis, even though the quadratus lumborum is a spinal extensor.[85] Lumbar flexion and extension are limited and painful, and sidebending is restricted toward the painfree side, and sometimes bilaterally. Rotation is usually limited and painful toward the side of involvement. In supine or prone, shortness of the muscle may distort pelvic alignment. The patient may have marked tenderness, but it is easily missed unless the examiner takes care to position the patient so that the ribs are separated from the iliac crest during palpation, and palpates deep through the lumbodorsal fascia to reach the quadratus lumborum.

Treatment of Muscle Disorders

Treatment of primary muscular disorders should initially include rest with gentle activity within the pain free range. Posture support with a lumbar pillow or corset is often helpful. One may progress to mild activities and mobilization when tolerated. Gentle or vigorous stretching is indicated, depending on the irritability and chronicity of the condition. Even when in pain, the patient should be encouraged to perform mild activities that do not aggravate the condition.

Ice massage, cold packs and electrical stimulation are usually preferred in the acute stage, changing to moist heat and electrical stimulation in the subacute stage. Massage is also a useful modality for treatment of muscular disorders, especially those of the chronic strain variety. Ultrasound combined with electrical stimulation also gives the sensation of a warm massage and is very helpful with many patients in the subacute or chronic stages. If definite trigger points are found (i.e., in the piriformis, iliopsoas or quadratus lumborum), they will respond to intermittent cold with stretch (spray and stretch) techniques or injection.

As the patient progresses, the activity and mobilization treatment should also progress. Restoration of full function (strength and mobility) and normal posture should be the most important aspects of treatment. Primary muscle disorders will probably heal in spite of the care given to them, but stiffness, weakness and postural changes may take place while healing is occurring. These losses of function and adaptive postural changes can lead to more serious chronic problems and, therefore, should be of primary concern to the therapist treating these disorders. It is not necessary to wait until the patient is pain free to begin active exercise. If pain with exercise is present, it is not necessarily a harmful sign. If the pain is not severe, does not last and is not progressive, the exercise should be encouraged.

Experience shows that more long-term harm is caused by too little activity than by too much.

JOINT DISORDERS

For classification purposes, the following structures are considered to be a part of the three-joint vertebral complex (two facet joints and the intervertebral disc): 1) Disc; 2) Cartilaginous endplate; 3) Hyaline cartilage; 4) Subchondral bone; 5) Meniscoid bodies; 6) Synovial lining; 7) Joint capsule; and 8) Ligament. Joint disorders considered in this section are impingement, sprain, inflammation, hypomobility, hypermobility and degenerative disease. Disc disorders are discussed in a separate section.

Facet Impingement

Facet blockage, subluxation, fixation, locking and acute cervical torticollis are all terms sometimes used to describe facet joint impingement. Impingement is one of the disorders that has made chiropractors popular because manipulation is usually an effective treatment. The mechanism of injury is usually a sudden, unguarded movement involving backward bending, sidebending and/or rotation with little or no trauma. Kos and Wolf describe it as a nipping of the intervertebral menisci.[41] Kraft and Levinthal describe a mechanism in which the synovial and capsular tissue that line the facet joint capsule become impinged between the joint surfaces[42] (Fig 5-3). Maitland[50] and Sprague[80] have accurately described cervical joint locking, its signs and symptoms and its treatment.

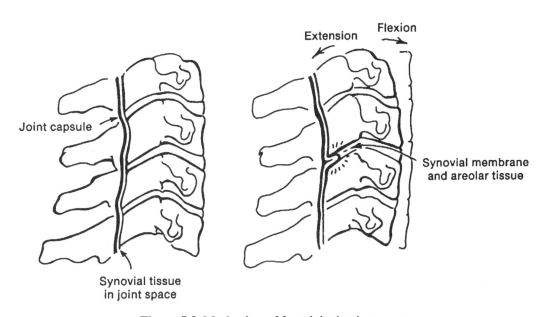

Figure 5-3. Mechanism of facet joint impingement.

Findings

The patient with a facet impingement will report that rest relieves, movement hurts and certain passive and active movements will be restricted and/or painful. The patient will often be "locked" into a protective posture. The protective posture will involve sidebending and rotation to the same side in the cervical spine and often sidebending and rotation in opposite directions in the thoracic and lumbar spine. The rotary component may not be readily observable but occurs according to Fryette's Laws of Spinal Motion (see Chapter 2, Spinal Biomechanics, for review).

In the lumbar or thoracic spine, rotation and sidebending can be limited in either the same or opposite directions, depending upon whether hyperflexion or hyperextension is present along with the rotatory and sidebending components. For example, if the spine is "stuck" in either extension or flexion at the same time it is rotated and sidebent, the rotation and sidebending will be in the same direction.

Pain and/or restriction of movement will be present when the patient attempts movement in the direction opposite the position in which he or she is locked. For example, with acute cervical facet impingement, if the patient is locked in left sidebending and left rotation, he will have pain and/or restriction of movement with sidebending and rotation to the right. Further movement to the left is usually free and painless. An example of facet impingement in the thoracic or lumbar spine, however, might involve a patient locked in a position of sidebending to the left and rotation to the right and the pain and/or restriction will be noticed when the patient sidebends to the right and rotates to the left. Pain may follow the corresponding dermatomal distribution.[56] Cailliet states that pain arising from the facet joint may be felt as pain in the entire sensory distribution of the corresponding spinal nerve root.[9]

Facet joint impingement and other facet disorders should not present true positive neurological signs. However, considering the findings of Mooney and Robertson, the definition of "true" neurological signs must be discussed. They found that injection of hypertonic saline solution into a lower lumbar facet joint not only produced local pain, but also pain that radiated distally in a pattern corresponding to the dermatomal distribution of the adjacent spinal nerve roots (posterior buttock and thigh[56]). Similar pain patterns have been demonstrated by injecting irritants into spinal muscles, interspinous ligaments and the intervertebral disc.[28, 29, 30, 34, 35, 69, 85] However, perhaps of even greater significance, Mooney and Robertson also found increased myoelectrical activity in the hamstring muscles, painful straight leg raising and depressed quadriceps muscle stretch reflexes to be associated with the referred pain stimuli. These so-called "positive" neurological findings were found in a group of patients diagnosed as having herniated nucleus pulposus (HNP). However, upon injection of a local anesthetic into the appropriate soft tissue or facet joints, these "positive" findings returned to normal. Based on this preliminary experience, these researchers no longer consider painful straight leg raising or reflex changes of the quadriceps group to necessarily implicate nerve root compromise. The only true neurological signs they will now accept are specific motor weakness or specific dermatomal sensory loss.[56]

As with muscle problems, one of the keys to finding joint involvement is the palpation exam. When the examiner palpates between the spinous processes or along the articular pillars (cervical), the single involved segment will be tender. Good judgment is necessary with palpation because of muscle guarding and spasm. If the patient has had pain for more than one or two days, the muscles may also be tender from guarding and spasm alone. As previously pointed out, this reflexive guarding and spasm may sometimes be incorrectly interpreted as being the primary disorder.

The positional changes previously discussed can occasionally be felt by palpating the spinous processes (Fig 5-4). For example, if the segment is locked in rotation and sidebending, the superior spinous process will not be in alignment with the adjacent inferior spinous process. If the segment is locked in forward bending, the space between the spinous processes will be wider at that level. If the segment is locked in

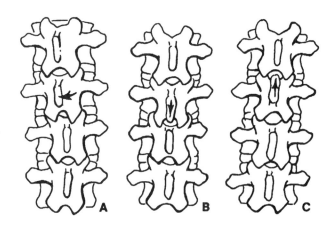

Figure 5-4. Positional changes related to facet joint impingement. A) Rotation; B) Backward bending; C) Forward Bending.

backward bending, the space will be narrower. However, if the segment is locked in mid-range, a positional fault may not be evident upon palpation.

Lab findings and routine x-rays will be negative. Mobility x-rays, which are special techniques that show spinal motion and position, may be helpful in demonstrating a locked or immobile segment. However, such procedures seem unnecessary since the clinical exam will also demonstrate this loss of mobility and/or positional change. Clinical confirmation of the other signs and symptoms must also be made before the diagnosis is clear.

Treatment

Facet joint impingements respond well to mobilization therapy and manual or mechanical traction (see Chapters 9 and 10). It is often wise to precede the mobilization or traction with ice or heat and soft tissue techniques to relieve the muscle guarding and spasm that may accompany the facet disorder. Treatment for cervical facet impingement involves manual traction and gentle rotation and sidebending, first in the pain free direction, then gradually working toward the painful directions while the traction is being maintained. A similar effect can be achieved in the lumbar spine if a three-dimensional mobilization table is used in combination with traction. While the traction force is being applied, the table can be moved slowly to provide a gentle mobilization force in the desired plane and direction of motion.

Facet Joint Sprain

It is necessary to distinguish between facet joint impingement and facet joint sprain because the treatment for these two disorders differs. The two disorders are, of course, quite different, but their objective signs and symptoms are often hard to distinguish during the musculoskeletal examination.

Findings

The key to differential diagnosis is found in the patient's history. With facet joint sprain, the patient has a history of moderate to severe trauma, enough so that the examiner must consider the possibility of joint sprain with effusion in and around the joint. Facet joint impingement can be treated with mobilization as soon as the disorder is confirmed. Facet joint sprain, on the other hand, must be treated with a more conservative approach using physical therapy modalities, pain free movements, support and rest. The joint sprain needs time to heal.

It is possible for facet joint impingement to occur with trauma. In this case, the examiner must assume that the soft tissue around the joint has also been injured and must take a more conservative approach to treatment. Mobility tests, palpation and other signs and symptoms of joint sprain will be similar to those found with facet joint impingement, except that movement may be generally more restricted and may involve more than one specific segment. Positional faults are not as common.

Treatment

If the patient gradually increases activity as the joint sprain heals or if the injury is treated with mild to moderate mobilization and range of motion during the subacute stage, the joint is likely to have normal mobility by the time complete healing occurs. If the patient has been immobile during the subacute stage and/or there has been a great deal of muscle guarding, the joints are likely to become hypomobile (stiff) as they heal. If, on the other hand, the joint capsule and/or supportive ligaments are torn or over-stretched during injury, the joint may be hypermobile (unstable) when healed.

One must especially guard against the development of postural changes such as forward head in a cervical sprain or slumped sitting (flat back) in a lumbar sprain. During the acute and subacute stages, it may be painful to sit or stand erect, or hold the head and neck in normal postures. Thus, the patient may tend to stand and sit slumped or develop a stooped, forward head posture. As healing occurs and as the muscles and ligaments adapt to their new positions and the faulty posture is maintained, the muscles weaken and a chronic postural strain develops. Supports such as a soft cervical collar, a lumbosacral corset or a lumbar pillow often help prevent these postural changes. Modalities and medications may help relieve the pain, making normal posture possible. Above all, patient awareness that long term postural problems, stiffness and weakness can develop is imperative.

Joint Inflammation

Findings

Joint inflammation will have a history of insidious onset, frequently following acute joint sprain or chronic postural sprain. It will also occur secondary to aggravation or overuse in the presence of degenerative joint/disc disease. As in all joint disorders, movement will hurt. If joint inflammation is present, however, the patient may also complain of pain and stiffness at rest. The involved segments will be tender to palpation. Active and passive movement will generally be restricted. Joint inflammation often presents bilateral symptoms. The color and temperature changes characteristic of inflammation may not be noticeable because of the depth of the joints in the spine. Rheumatoid arthritis is not a consideration here since it is classified as a systemic disease and requires specialized management.

Treatment

Treatment consists of modality therapy (ice, electrical stimulation), gentle movement, support, rest and anti-inflammatory medications to promote healing. Movement exercises can be somewhat painful, as long as they do not cause pain that lasts or that progressively gets worse. Support can consist of a lumbar pillow, cervical collar or corset. As with the other musculoskeletal disorders, passive treatments are followed by gradual reconditioning to restore strength, mobility and normal posture.

Degenerative Joint/Disc Disease (Osteoarthritis, Spondylosis)

Degenerative joint/disc disease is a chronic and commonly progressive degeneration of the facet joints and/or the intervertebral disc (Fig 5-5). There is frequently an associated osteophytosis of the adjacent vertebræ. Neurological complications can also be seen with degenerative joint/disc disease due to the foraminal encroachment that sometimes occurs. The term spondylosis is also used to describe various degenerative disorders of the spine. The term osteoarthritis is commonly applied to a degenerative disorder of synovial joints only. Degenerative joint/disc disease is more common in the cervical spine than in the lumbar spine (Fig 5-6).

There are four characteristics of degenerative joint disease in synovial joints: 1) Proliferation of calcific deposits in, and especially around, the periphery of the joint; 2) Wearing away of the hyaline cartilage; 3) Thickening of the synovial lining and joint capsule; and 4) Thickening of the subchondral bone. Degenerative disc disease is characterized by: 1) Dehydration of the nucleus pulposus; 2) Narrowing of the intervertebral space; 3) Weakening and degeneration of the annular rings; and 4) Approximation of the facet joints.

Although degenerative joint/disc disease is a natural process of aging and is often asymptomatic, it sometimes develops as the result of hypomobility because of the loss of joint/disc nutrition. The intervertebral discs and the hyaline cartilage surfaces of synovial joints do not have a blood supply. The movement of body fluids is necessary for these structures to receive their normal nutritional supply.[5, 6, 31, 32, 38, 40] Therefore, loss of mobility contributes to early development of joint/disc degeneration. Joint hypermobility or instability also leads to early joint/disc degeneration because of the increased wear and tear to which the disc and joints are subjected when hypermobility exists.[38] Thus, both joint hypomobility and joint hypermobility can contribute to the development of degenerative joint/disc disease. When degenerative disease develops, the joint/disc is vulnerable to increased aggravation and strain, thus a progressive cycle develops as the disorder worsens.

Findings

The patient with degenerative joint/disc disease usually presents a history of joint injury with episodes of joint pain and/or stiffness. X-ray will reveal the degenerative process and/or a narrowing of the disc space. The patient will have tenderness at the segmental levels involved. A thickened supraspinous ligament can often be palpated. Active and passive movements are usually restricted, but because hypermobility or instability of the joint sometimes develops, active and passive movements are occasionally excessive. In advanced stages, pain is present with any movement. However, it should be emphasized that this disorder is asymptomatic in many cases. The joint is more vulnerable to facet impingement, sprain and inflammation when degenerative joint disease is present. The disc can also be injured more easily. Many factors are thought to contribute to joint/disc degeneration; thus, the etiology is sometimes obscured. As previously stated, joints that are hypomobile or hypermobile, as well as joints continually subjected to repeated trauma, are susceptible to early development of degenerative joint disease.

We have seen conflicting radiological evidence in patients who seem to have degenerative joint/disc disease. Some individuals remain asymptomatic (except for hypomobility) despite radiological evidence of advanced degenerative joint/disc disease. On the other hand, physical therapists often see those patients who have no radiological evidence of disease but who have both mobility problems and pain. In such cases, it is the soft tissue stiffness that must be the source of pain, since the hyaline cartilage of the joint surfaces is aneural.

Discogenic pain related to degenerative joint/disc disease is difficult to assess clinically, but also seems

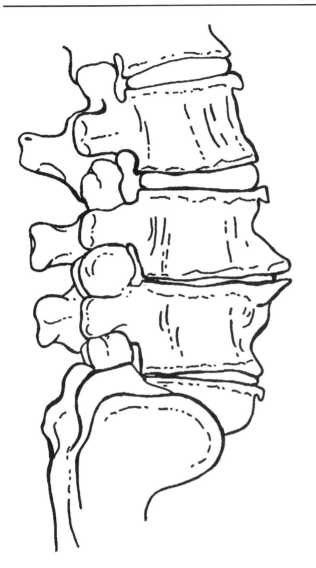

Figure 5-5. Degenerative joint/disc disease of the lumbar spine.

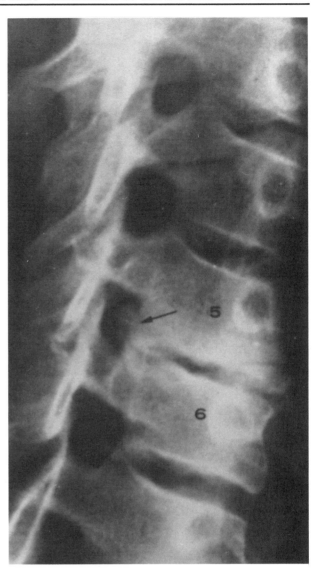

Figure 5-6. Degenerative joint/disc disease of the cervical spine (reprinted with permission from Peterson and Kieffer[66]).

to be intermittent in nature and is related to certain stressful activities. When evaluating a patient, it is often difficult, if not impossible, to determine if the pain the patient is experiencing is coming from the disc or from the facet joints. If the pain is discogenic, it may be because of mechanical irritation or inflammation of the outer wall of the annulus. Discogenic pain may also arise because of a chemical irritation.[70] The mechanism of aggravation and/or analysis of the most painful positions (flexion versus extension) may give the most reliable clues. If flexion (sitting and forward bending) is more painful and/or is the mechanism of aggravation, the disc is probably the irritated structure. If the reverse is true and extension (standing and walking) is most aggravating, the facets are probably involved.

It must be emphasized that one cannot assume that a patient with degenerative joint/disc disease will be either hyper- or hypomobile. One could theorize that a segment with degenerative joint/disc disease would be hypermobile because of ligamentous laxity due to the narrowing of the joint and disc space. Another could argue that adaptive shortening will occur as the gradual narrowing takes place and the segment will be hypomobile. Dr. William Kirkaldy-Willis believes that the segment first goes through a hypermobile stage, then later becomes hypomobile.[38] At any rate, the good clinician will determine the actual mobility of the segment through segmental mobility testing and/or mobility x-rays rather than blindly accepting one of the above theories. Patients should not be told that they have instability or hypomobility just because they have radiological evidence of degenerative joint/disc disease.

Treatment

Mild to Moderate Stages

If the patient has joint hypomobility, treatment may involve ultrasound; mobilization; manual or mechanical traction; and flexibility exercises. In the case of hypermobility, back supports are often necessary. Muscle strengthening and postural training may be indicated in either case, and modality therapy and medication may be necessary for relief of pain and inflammation. Usually, at least initially, the patient should exercise in the direction opposite that of the aggravation. In other words, if flexion aggravates, extension exercises are indicated. Conversely, if extension aggravates, flexion exercises are indicated. The amount of lordosis will also help determine which exercises are appropriate with each patient. If the patient is hyperlordotic, flexion exercises are indicated; if hypolordotic, extension exercises are indicated.

Severe Stage

If the patient has joint hypomobility, it is usually beneficial to mobilize the involved segments. If this can be done without aggravating the patient's pain, it is probably the treatment of choice. If, on the other hand, any attempt to increase mobility or activity results in increased pain and/or increased inflammatory responses, another approach should be considered. This approach involves bracing or support to reduce movement and vertical loading, which reduces irritation.

Bracing or support is sometimes used when the patient with degenerative joint/disc disease suffers from frequent episodes of aggravation due to an activity, or has a job involving heavy physical labor, or participates in sports. Bracing may be used in all three stages (mild, moderate or severe).

DISC DISORDERS

Disc disorders that are treatable by the physical therapist usually involve some variation of herniated nucleus pulposus (HNP). Other disc disorders such as infections or congenital abnormalities will not be discussed.

Herniated nucleus pulposus (HNP) is classified as the disorder in which there is displacement of the nuclear material and other disc components beyond the normal confines of the annulus. Four degrees of displacement are recognized: 1) Intra-spongy nuclear herniation; 2) Protrusion; 3) Extrusion; and 4) Sequestration.[23]

HNP-protrusion occurs gradually over time. In the early stages, it is asymptomatic. As the protrusion progresses, the patient first experiences back pain, then back and leg pain, and finally, back and leg pain with signs of neurological involvement indicating impingement or irritation of the nerve root. We choose to classify HNP-protrusion as occurring in two stages. In the first stage (mild to moderate), the signs and symptoms are purely discogenic in nature. In the second stage (moderate to severe), the signs and symptoms also indicate involvement of the nerve root. These classifications are based on treatment concepts that often change as the condition changes.

It is recommended that all other terms dealing with disc displacement such as hard disc, soft disc, disc derangement, disc prolapse, ruptured disc and slipped disc be discarded due to their imprecise meaning or because these terms do not describe a verifiable condition.[23]

Intra-Spongy Nuclear Herniation

Intra-spongy nuclear herniation refers to displacement of the nucleus into the vertebral body through the cartilaginous endplate. It is similar to a Schmorl's node except that it is a traumatic defect rather than a developmental one.[23] Schmorl's nodes represent small invasions of the vertebral body by the nucleus protruding superiorly. According to Cyriax, they never cause any symptoms, either at their time of occurrence or later in life. In fact, Schmorl's nodes are thought to stabilize the nucleus and diminish the intra-articular centrifugal force, thus rendering posterior displacement less probable. Unfortunately, they are rarely seen where they are most needed, i.e., at the fourth and fifth lumbar levels. They occur most commonly in the lower thoracic and upper lumbar spine and are purely an adolescent phenomenon as no increased frequency is observed as age advances.[12]

Traumatic intra-spongy nuclear herniation is also thought to be of little clinical importance. There are few references in orthopædic literature to indicate that it is of clinical significance.

Farfan describes a disc injury that deals with the fractured endplate of the vertebral body due to a compression injury. He maintains that these injuries can be a source of pain and that they occur in four grades:

Grade 1 = Subchondral fractures in the vertebral body.

Grade 2 = Small cracks in the endplates.

Grade 3 = A crack in which a piece of bone has shifted.

Grade 4 = A crack in which a piece of bone has shifted and disc material is forced through the crack (intra-spongy nuclear herniation).[18]

Findings

Traumatic intra-spongy nuclear herniation usually occurs as the result of moderate to severe flexion trauma. The patient with intra-spongy nuclear herniation has pain with flexion activities, including forward bending and sitting. Actual diagnosis is by radiological examination.

Treatment

Treatment consists of rest and avoiding compressing forces on the disc. Controlling protective muscle guarding with physical therapy modalities is important because muscle guarding contributes a compressive force. Hyperextension and mild traction may help to restore the anatomy of a Grade 3 or 4 injury. Support with a corset or brace may also be indicated.

Herniated Nucleus Pulposus - Protrusion (Without Spinal Nerve Root Involvement)

Herniated nucleus pulposus (HNP) protrusion describes the condition in which there is displacement of the nuclear material beyond the normal confines of the inner annulus, producing a discrete bulge in the outer annulus. No nuclear material escapes, however.[23] There are divergent opinions about the role of the disc in spinal pain where there is no evidence of nerve root impingement. Until recently, most literature stated that, except for the outermost rings of the annulus, the intervertebral disc itself is not a source of pain because of its lack of a sensory nerve supply.[28, 29, 30, 34, 35, 69] In more recent articles, Jeffrey Saal, et. al., describe the disc as a source of pain resulting from chemical inflammation[70] or mechanical deformation of the outer annulus.

Lumbar Spine

In the lumbar spine, HNP-protrusion is most common in the L4-L5 and L5-S1 discs and is rarely seen above those levels (less than 5%). This disorder is rarely associated with a single injury or incident. Rather, it is caused by the cumulative effects of months or even years of forward bending and lifting and/or sitting in a slumped, forward bent posture. One usually sees a generalized loss of mobility, especially spinal extension,[53, 89] and an overall decline in general physical fitness.[8, 44] Since mobility is necessary to maintain adequate nutrition to the disc, this loss of mobility leads to further weakening of the annular rings.

Findings

The typical patient will be 25-45 years old. HNP-protrusion is uncommon in younger people—probably because the causative factors of stiffening, weakening and degeneration have not progressed enough. It is uncommon in older individuals because there is a tendency for the fluid nucleus to become more fibrous with age. Because the disc is less fluid and more fibrous it will be less likely to rupture through the small cracks in the annular rings.

In the early stages, the patient will complain of pain, usually in the lower back, but sometimes in the posterior buttock and thigh. The presence of leg pain usually indicates a larger protrusion than that of back pain alone.[53] Usually, the patient will not hesitate when asked, "Which hurts more – sitting, standing, walking or lying down?" The answer will be "sitting." The patient will also often report that prolonged sitting will cause the pain to move from the lower back into the leg. He will also report difficulty when assuming an erect posture after sitting or lying down. However, after standing up and walking around, he usually obtains some relief of pain. When asked to locate the pain, the patient usually says that it is greater on one side of the lower back than the other, but it may be bilateral. Referred pain into the leg is usually unilateral and will correspond to the dermatomal pattern of the involved segment. The reason that spinal pain tends to be bilateral in these cases is that a connecting branch of the sinuvertebral nerve joins the right and left portions of that nerve.[19] It is the sinuvertebral nerve that innervates the outer annulus.

Although the patient may report a sudden onset of symptoms, usually relating to forward bending or prolonged sitting, this sudden onset is believed to be "the straw that broke the camel's back." It is much more logical to assume that the onset was insidious and related to the repetition of forward bending or sitting activities over time (Fig 5-7). The patient may not feel a gradual onset because the disc interior is not innervated.

The patient will report an occupation or activity that relates to a long history of a flexed lumbar posture.[15, 53, 62, 79] For example, truck drivers have a higher incidence of this disorder than persons in most other occupations.[62] Typically, the patient will describe having had multiple episodes over several months or years, with episodes occurring more frequently and more painfully. The patient may describe a gradual worsening of symptoms with each episode, with pain spreading from the back to the buttock and then to the posterior thigh and calf.

Patients may need to be questioned closely about previous episodes of pain. They may not relate previous episodes of what may have been diagnosed as "muscle strain" to their current complaints. We believe, however, that many of these minor episodes are related, particularly when the mechanism of injury is similar. Previous diagnoses of muscle strain or mechanical low back pain may actually have been "pre-disc syndromes." It is imperative that these patients realize this, as the importance of preventing future episodes of HNP will be more evident to them.

Figure 5-8 shows the development of the HNP-protrusion. The first drawing is that of a normal disc; the second depicts the development of a slight posterolateral protrusion (this condition would be painless); the third drawing shows a protrusion into the posterior rings of the annulus. It is at this stage that the patient begins to experience discogenic pain and symptoms. Note also that the nerve root is not involved at this stage. Therefore, it seems reasonable to assume that the patient's pain comes from the sensory innervation of the outer annulus or the surrounding soft tissues.

The clinical examination will reveal a patient who sits in a slumped posture with the lumbar spine in flexion. He or she will often reach down to the chair

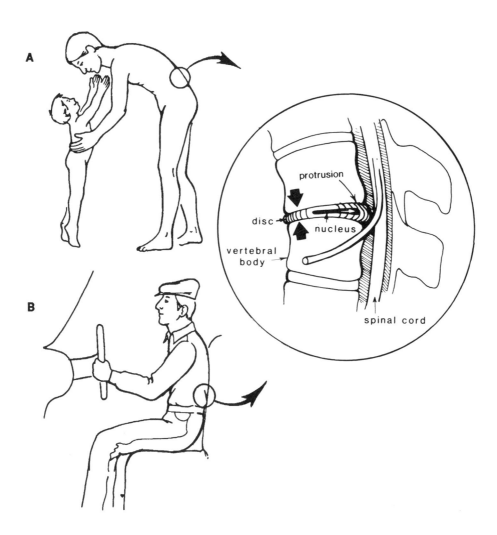

Figure 5-7. Disc mechanics with A) Forward bending; B) Slumped sitting (the bulge is not yet touching the nerve root).

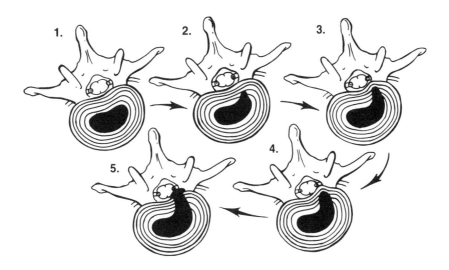

Figure 5-8. Stages of disc herniation.

seat with the hands to take the weight of the trunk off the lower back. The patient may have a lateral shift (lumbar scoliosis). Technically, there is a difference between a lateral shift as described by McKenzie[53] and a lumbar scoliosis. In a true scoliosis, there will be a more pronounced secondary curve and the patient's head and shoulders will probably be positioned directly over the pelvis. With a lateral shift, the center of the patient's shoulders will be lateral to the center of the patient's pelvis.

McKenzie states that 50% of the patients with HNP-protrusion have a lateral shift because of the tendency for the nuclear gel to move posterolaterally. As the gel moves posteriorly, the patient tends to shift his weight in an anterior direction, flattening the lumbar lordosis (Fig 5-9). The patient also shifts the shoulders away from the side of nuclear movement, thus producing a lateral shift (Fig 5-10). Therefore, the most important clinical features of this disorder are the flattening of the lordosis and the shift of the torso away from the painful side. Flattening of the thoracic kyphosis is also characteristic of the disorder.[12, 53, 89] There will be no positive neurological signs at this stage. The involved spinal segment will be tender to palpation and routine x-rays will usually be negative.

Some investigators imply that HNP-protrusion represents the early stages of disc degeneration. The exact source of pain is not well established, but there is evidence that upon intradiscal injection of hypertonic saline, it is often possible to reproduce pain similar to that which occurs naturally.[30, 69] Since the recurrent sinuvertebral nerve supplies the outermost rings of the annulus, the posterior longitudinal ligament and the dura mater, it must be involved in this syndrome. The involvement of this nerve would also explain the referred pain into the extremities.

According to McKenzie, HNP-protrusion involves a disturbance of the normal resting position of the articular surfaces of two adjacent vertebræ as a result of a change in the position of the fluid nucleus between these surfaces. The alteration in the position of the nucleus (derangement) may also disturb the annulus.

This will cause disturbance of the normal mechanics of movement. The particular pattern will depend upon the exact area where the disturbance lies. The nucleus is always under positive pressure that

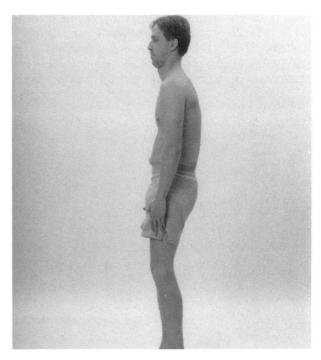

Figure 5-9. Flattened lumbar lordosis commonly found in patients with lumbar-HNP with a posterior or posterolateral protrusion.

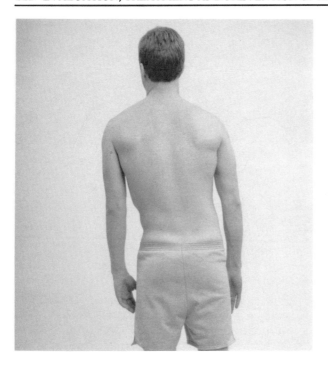

Figure 5-10. Lateral shift commonly found in patients with lumbar-HNP with a posterolateral protrusion.

slightly deforms the elastic annulus. The position of the spine in flexion or extension will add to or subtract from the pressure exerted at the posterior and posterolateral borders of the annulus. The center of the nucleus is all gel and the periphery of the annulus is all collagen fiber; one merges into the other, with the fibers becoming less dense near the interior of the nucleus[53] (Fig 5-11). On extension of the spine, the intervertebral disc spaces tend to open anteriorly and close down posteriorly, thus exerting pressure on the nucleus to move it anteriorly. The converse is true with flexion.[36, 53, 73]

McKenzie[53] theorizes that prolonged flexed lumbar posture and/or lifting and walking with the lumbar spine flexed will make the nucleus migrate posteriorly or posterolaterally. As this condition progresses, pain sensitive structures are encountered and the patient begins to have pain in the lumbar spine (stage three of Figure 5-8). If the condition is not corrected, it may continue to progress until the patient begins to have pain in the buttock and thigh. This may eventually progress to involve nerve root impingement.

Mechanical correction of the lateral shift will usually cause increased pain. It is important to note, however, whether the increase in pain is central in the lower back or if the increase in pain is toward the periphery. If the bulge is mild or moderate, correction of the lateral shift will cause increased pain in the <u>central</u> low back. Increased central pain is acceptable. If attempts to correct cause increased pain toward the periphery, however, they should be discontinued, at least for the present. Theoretically, if the bulge is small and the nuclear material is not displaced beyond the posterolateral edge of the vertebral body, the correction should not increase leg symptoms (Fig 5-12).

Standing forward bending is sometimes limited due to the severity of the pain and muscle guarding that may be present, but it is not uncommon for the patient to have full lumbar flexion mobility. The lumbar spine is actually often fully flattened or flexed when initially examined.

When tested in the standing position, flexion will cause the pain to move peripherally. This is especially true if forward flexion is repeated several times. The pain that is produced will tend to linger for a while after the repeated forward bending movements have been stopped. In other words, repeated forward bending

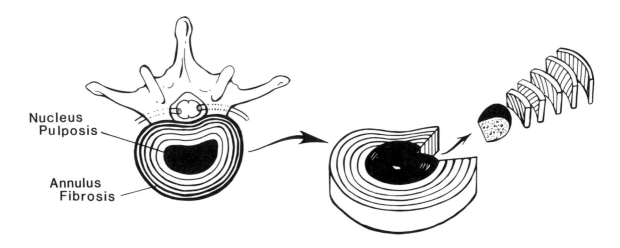

Nucleus Pulposis

Annulus Fibrosis

Figure 5-11. The intervertebral disc.

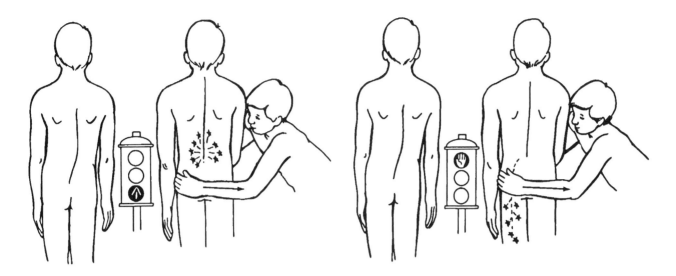

Figure 5-12. One of these two reactions is usually seen when one attempts to correct lateral shift caused by HNP-protrusion. Increased central pain is acceptable, but increased peripheral pain is not.

causes the protrusion to enlarge, producing increased pressure on the annular wall. This enlargement does not subside immediately, thus the tendency for the pain to linger even after the movement has stopped (Fig 5-13).

If a lateral shift is present, it should be corrected before testing extension. Extension or backward bending after the lateral shift has been corrected will almost always be restricted and will cause increased pain. It is important to note whether the increase in pain centralizes or peripheralizes. If the bulge is mild

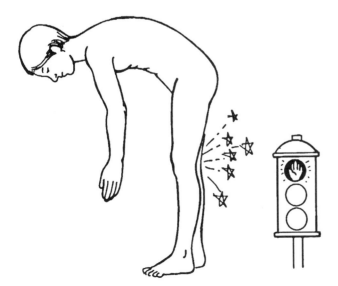

Figure 5-13. Flexion will cause pain to move peripherally in patients who have HNP-protrusion.

to moderate (not displaced beyond the posterolateral edge of the vertebral body), extension may cause increased pain, but it will be <u>central</u> in the lower back. Let us assume for the present that extension causes increased central pain with no increase in leg symptoms (Fig 5-14). Occasionally, extension will dramatically relieve peripheral pain.

In summary, patients with mild to moderate HNP-protrusion usually have more pain with sitting than with walking, standing or lying down. They will also have a reduced lumbar lordosis and limitation of lumbar extension, and about 50% will have a lateral shift. If the patient is asked to perform repeated flexion movements, the symptoms will worsen and <u>peripheralize</u> from the center of the spine into the leg. Once aggravated, the peripheralized pain will tend to linger for a while. On the other hand, correction of the lateral shift and extension will <u>centralize</u> the pain.

Treatment

McKenzie[53] advocates correction of the lateral shift and passive extension exercises to move the nucleus of the disc centrally. He also advocates constant maintenance of the correction to allow healing of the annular fibers to occur. The cardinal rule to always follow with correction of a lateral shift and the passive extension exercises that follow is: Correction may cause increased pain in the back but must not increase the leg pain. If the peripheral pain is increased by this corrective maneuver, it indicates that either the bulge is not being reduced by the maneuver or that the nerve

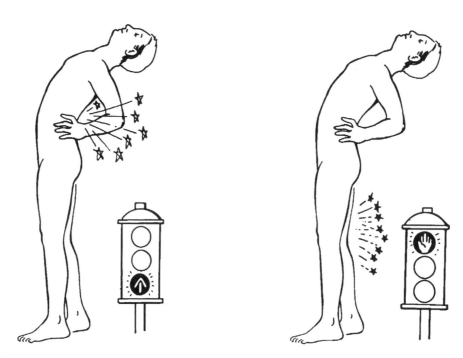

Figure 5-14. One of these two reactions is usually seen when lumbar extension is attempted in the presence of HNP-protrusion. Increased central pain is acceptable, but increased peripheral pain is not.

root is being pulled or pushed onto the bulge by the maneuver. In either case, it is wrong to proceed. Any activity that peripheralizes the pain is probably making the condition worse, whereas something that causes pain to centralize in the lower back may not be harmful and may, in fact, be the correct thing to do. If the patient has a mild to moderate bulge, an attempt to correct should be successful.

If attempts to correct the lateral shift in the standing position are unsuccessful, correction is attempted lying down. Sometimes elimination of the compressive force of gravity is enough to allow successful correction of the lateral shift.

Assume, then, that attempts to correct the lateral shift are successful, in either the standing or prone position. Figure 5-15 shows what is believed to be happening when one can correct the lateral shift without increasing the peripheral signs and symptoms. One must understand that the correction is not made with one simple maneuver. Shift correction may need to be performed several times before the patient can hold the correction on his own. It then becomes the patient's responsibility over the next few days to constantly keep correcting the shift until he or she has successfully reduced the bulge (Fig 5-16). All the methods show overcorrection, which is acceptable. A three-dimensional mobilization table is very helpful in passive correction of a lateral shift. It can subsequently be used for passive extension (Fig 5-17). When the

lateral shift has been successfully corrected, or if the patient does not have a lateral shift, the next step in treatment of the mild to moderate disc protrusion is passive extension exercises.

Passive extension exercises are usually started in the prone position and are progressed to the standing position as tolerated. These exercises are described in detail in Chapter 12, Exercise. The first passive extension exercise simply consists of lying prone on a hard surface for a few minutes. This may not be necessary except for the very acute patient with a severely forward bent posture. The second passive extension exercise is the "elbow prop." Here, the patient simply props himself on his elbows to allow the lower back to passively extend. As described above, a three dimensional mobilization table is excellent for passively extending a patient in this rest position.

As the patient progresses with the passive extension exercises, he begins to do the passive press-ups. The stomach and back muscles must be completely relaxed as the patient pushes himself into an arched position. The patient is encouraged to do this exercise five to ten times, several times a day.

Often, this program will cause the patient to have dramatic relief of the leg pain and it is natural for the patient to become enthusiastic about doing the program because he or she experiences success. However, one

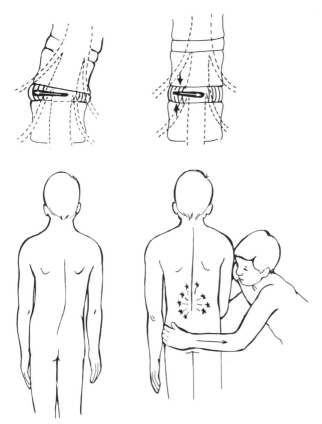

Figure 5-15. Disc mechanics with lateral shift correction (small to moderate bulge).

should caution the patient not to do the exercises excessively at first because the back may become very sore. This, in turn, may cause increased muscle guarding and work against the patient's overall progress. It is better to do the exercises gently but very frequently throughout the day than to do the exercises vigorously only once or twice a day.

As soon as the patient has had success with the passive extension exercises in the prone position, he or she can begin to do them in the standing position. Again, the patient is encouraged to do this exercise several times a day. It is very important to remember that if there is a lateral shift, it must be corrected before extension is done.

Figure 5-18 shows what is believed to happen when the patient can do passive extension exercises without increasing the peripheral signs. The patient must be given clear instructions about the exercises and must have an understanding of what is being accomplished with these exercises.

Figure 5-19 shows the work of Shah,[74] which demonstrates the posterior movement of the nucleus with flexion and anterior movement with extension on a cadaver specimen.

To move the nucleus anteriorly, the patient must be taught to maintain the lordosis at all times and hold it there until healed. This means that a lumbosacral corset or a lumbar roll must be used behind the back at all times while sitting. The purpose of these external supports is to maintain and support the lordosis and to remind the patient that he or she must not forward bend. Figure 5-20 shows a lumbar roll that can be given to the patient. It is a foam roll approximately five inches in diameter. Small straps are attached which allow the roll to be tied to a chair or automobile seat.

Patient instructions for acute stages of HNP-protrusion consist of the following points:

- Maintain lordosis at all times.

- Avoid forward bending as it will stretch the supporting structures of the back and lead to further weakening.

- When in acute pain, sit as little as possible, and then only for short periods of time.

- While sitting, sit with a lordosis. This can be accomplished by placing a supportive roll in the small of the back.

- Try to sit on a firm, high chair if possible.

- Avoid sitting on low, soft chairs or couches.

- When rising from a sitting position, maintain lumbar lordosis.

- When in acute pain, drive as little as possible.

- When driving a car, keep the seat close enough to the steering wheel to allow maintenance of the lordosis.

- When in acute pain, avoid all bending and lifting.

- If lifting cannot be avoided, use correct lifting techniques:

  - Keep the head and chest upright

  - Stand close to the load

  - Have firm footing and a wide stance

  - Bend the knees and keep the back straight

  - Have a secure grip on the load

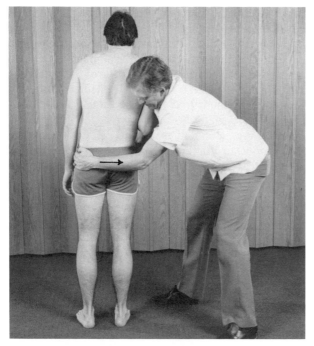
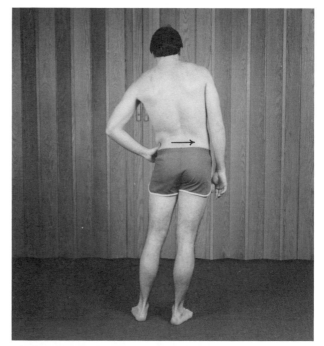
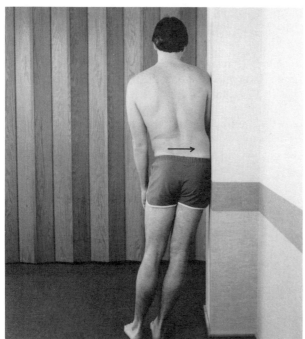
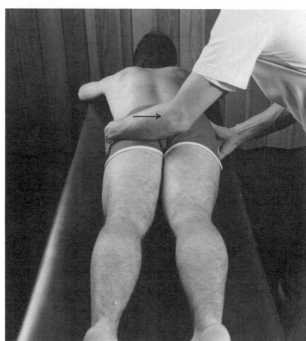
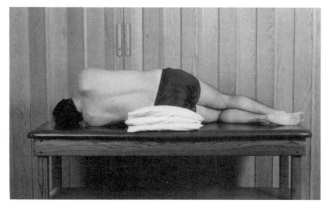

Figure 5-16. Various methods of correcting a lateral shift. Over correction is acceptable.

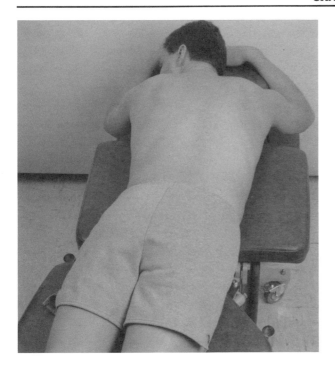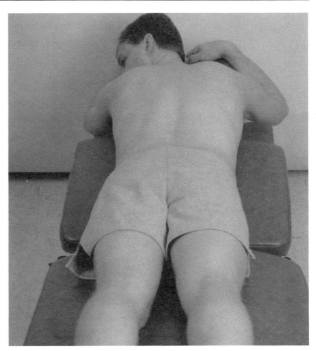

Figure 5-17. Using a 3-D mobilization table to correct a lateral shift.

- Lift by straightening the knees, keeping the chest upright

- Lift steadily - do not jerk

- Pivot with the feet - do not twist

• Use a firm support for resting and sleeping.

• When coughing or sneezing, stand up, bend slightly backwards and increase the lordosis to lessen the strain.[53]

The patient must absolutely avoid positions and activities that increase the intradiscal pressure or that cause a posterior force on the nucleus (flexion exercises, forward bending and slumped sitting). Exercises, mobilization or activities involving rotation must be avoided initially for two reasons. First, rotation causes a narrowing of the intervertebral space and produces increased intradiscal pressure.[61] Also, as rotation of the spine occurs, there is a relaxation of one-half of the oblique annular fibers while the other one-half are drawn taut. This puts the disc in a vulnerable position for injury.

There must be strict compliance with this program for two to ten weeks. The severity of the disorder and the initial success the patient has with the treatment program will determine the speed of recovery. There is evidence that healing of the disc can occur.[29] The key is to reduce the bulge and then to maintain the posterior aspect of the disc in close approximation so

the scar that is formed will protect from further protrusion.[53] It is important to emphasize to the patient that one can recover from a disc injury and that healing can and will take place. Teaching the patient that the nucleus will become more fibrous with age and will therefore naturally tend to stabilize is important for the patient's confidence.

Additional treatment should also be directed at pain relief and restoration of function and mobility. Modality therapy may relieve pain which, in turn, will reduce muscle guarding. Since spinal muscle guarding is a compressive force on the disc, it is important to control such guarding. Traction may also effectively reduce the bulge.[14, 52, 63] A support or corset may be used to allow the patient more pain free activities, to aid postural correction and to reduce compressive forces on the disc.[57, 59]

Patients with HNP-protrusion lose range of motion because of the bulge itself but may also become restricted because of scarring and thickening of collagen tissue in and around the disc and the facet joints (joint hypomobility). Restoration of full mobility is a necessary component of treatment as soon as the protrusion is stable. Passive extension and flexion exercises, joint mobilization and traction are indicated if mobility is restricted. A particularly helpful technique is to passively extend the patient to the level of restriction using a three dimensional mobilization table and apply P/A mobilizations to the restricted segment(s). Later, active back extension exercises should be used to increase spinal strength and further

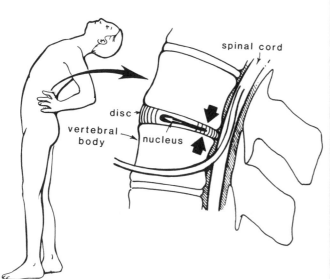

Figure 5-18. Disc mechanics with extension (small to moderate bulge).

promote correct posture. Finally, since many of these patients have been in poor physical condition for a long time, a full physical fitness program should be implemented.

Cervical Spine

In the cervical spine, HNP-protrusion without nerve root involvement is seen less commonly or, at least, the clinical picture is less well defined.

Findings

The patient with a mild to moderate HNP-protrusion in the cervical spine will usually report increased pain with sitting and with neck flexion. Standing up and walking around will tend to lessen the symptoms. As the condition worsens, a progression of pain from central to peripheral (neck to shoulder to arm) is seen. Interscapular symptoms corresponding to Cloward's areas (see Chapter 4) can help identify a particular disc level (see Fig 4-1). The patient will often lack extension and extension will cause increased central pain, while lessening peripheral pain. The forward head posture previously discussed will almost always be present. Often, postural correction will increase central cervical pain but decrease peripheral pain (Fig 5-21).

Treatment

Treatment is directed toward: 1) Returning the patient to normal posture and flexibility; and 2) Maintaining correct posture to allow the disc to heal.

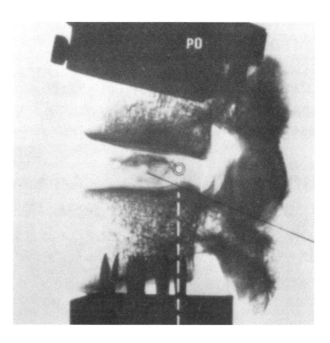

Figure 5-19. Posterior movement of the nucleus with flexion (top) and anterior movement with extension (bottom) as demonstrated by Shah (reprinted with permission[74]).

This is accomplished by starting with the head back, chin in exercises shown in Chapter 12 and progressing to passive cervical extension exercises. Normal cervical lordosis must be maintained. This requires a fiber or feather pillow that can be shaped to maintain the desired amount of support while sleeping. Solid foam pillows are not recommended because some muscular tension is required to maintain the head position and the solid foam does not conform adequately to the natural cervical lordosis.

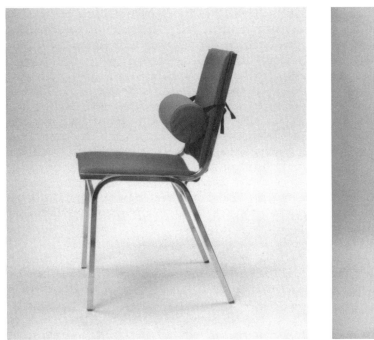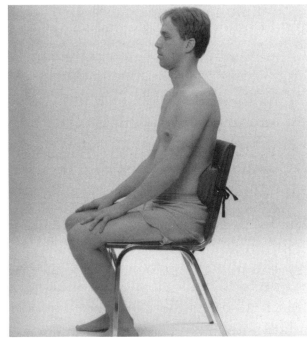

Figure 5-20. Lumbar roll to encourage normal sitting posture.

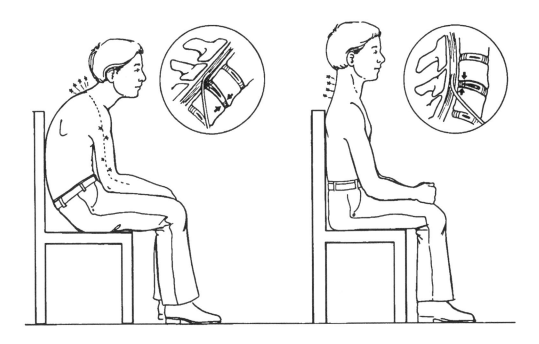

Figure 5-21. For a patient with cervical HNP-protrusion, treatment is directed toward normalizing posture.

As the patient improves, full flexibility and strength must be restored. Since slumped sitting is often associated with forward head posture, use of a lumbar roll and a full back and neck strengthening and flexibility exercise program is necessary (see Chapter 12, Exercise).

Herniated Nucleus Pulposus - Protrusion (With Spinal Nerve Root Involvement)

HNP-protrusion with nerve root involvement is described as a condition in which the nucleus is bulging but is still contained within the annulus and/or posterior longitudinal ligament. The bulge is large enough to encroach into the spinal canal and/or the intervertebral foramen and is capable of impinging upon or irritating the nerve root.[23]

The patient with a lumbar HNP-protrusion who was a candidate for mechanical correction with extension exercises and principles was presented earlier. This patient was a candidate for lateral shift correction and extension exercises because when these were attempted, there was no increase in peripheral signs. Now, however, the bulge or protrusion worsens and attempts to correct the lateral shift or to do extension exercises increase the peripheral signs and symptoms. If the patient otherwise has all the signs and symptoms of a disc protrusion, it is possible that the protrusion is now bulging beyond the posterior edge of the vertebral bodies and that extension or correction of the lateral shift cannot reduce the bulge. When this is the case, traction and other management techniques may be necessary before extension principles are applied. In other words, the patient has exactly the same disorder that was presented earlier, but the protrusion is simply larger (Fig 5-22), and is probably pinching or irritating the nerve root.

Figure 5-23 shows the bulge in relation to the nerve roots. In nearly all cases, the bulge will encroach upon the nerve root that is descending in the spinal canal to make its exit at the segmental level below the bulge. An L5-S1 bulge impinging upon the S1 nerve root is the most common example. An L4-L5 protrusion would probably impinge directly upon or laterally upon the L5 nerve root. While it is possible that the bulge can encroach upon the nerve root that is making its exit at the same level as the bulge, this is unusual. If such is the case, the bulge is usually medial and inferior to the nerve root. It is important to understand the relationship of the bulge to the nerve roots because this provides another explanation of why a patient may develop a lateral scoliosis. Finneson theorizes that if the bulge lies laterally to the nerve root, the patient may shift to the opposite side to take the nerve root away from the bulge. If the bulge is encroaching upon the nerve root as shown in Figure 5-23A, the patient would shift to the right. When the bulge is medial to the nerve root, the patient may shift toward the side of the symptoms. The example in Figure 5-23B shows a bulge medial to the nerve root with the patient shifting to the left. Finneson calls this phenomenon "protective scoliosis."[19] One can see that any attempt to correct the protective scoliosis will cause the nerve root to be forced back onto the bulge which would probably increase peripheral signs and symptoms. One should also be aware that if traction is attempted with a patient in a protective scoliosis, the spine will be straightened which, again, would cause increased peripheral signs and symptoms.

Figures 5-24 and 5-25 show what may happen when correction of a lateral shift or extension is attempted with a large protrusion. As these maneuvers are attempted, some of the disc material may be trapped instead of reduced. This is likely to cause the bulge to protrude further and peripheral signs and symptoms will increase. In any case, if lateral shift correction or extension causes increased peripheralization of signs and symptoms, further attempts to do these maneuvers should be stopped.

Lumbar Spine

Findings

The patient will have all the signs and symptoms of an HNP-protrusion previously discussed, with the addition of positive neurological signs and symptoms such as strength loss, decreased muscle stretch reflexes, loss of sensation and a positive straight leg raise test. An x-ray may now show a narrowed disc space. As discussed, attempts to correct a lateral shift or to implement extension exercises may increase peripheralization of symptoms. Also, spinal flexion in the recumbent position may afford relief of some symptoms.

Occasionally, the onset is sudden with no previous history of spinal pain, but it is more common to see disc herniation with signs of nerve root involvement as a gradually worsening condition that first appears without nerve root involvement.

Treatment

Traditionally, at least in America, conservative treatment of HNP-protrusion has consisted of flexion positions, flexion exercises, bed traction and rest. Our rate of success has been poor when we recognize that there is an average of 300,000 to 400,000 back

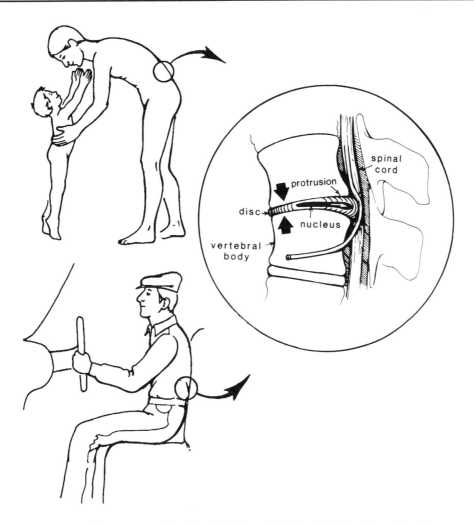

Figure 5-22. Disc mechanics with A) Forward bending; B) Slumped sitting (the bulge is touching the nerve root). The patient will probably have central and peripheral symptoms.

operations done in this country every year. [62] These figures are eight times higher per capita than in European or Scandinavian countries. [91]

It is now evident that flexion positions and exercises are potentially harmful for the patient with HNP-protrusion. [12, 36, 53, 61, 74] However, there are some reasons why the recumbent flexed posture may give the very acute disc patient some relief. If the spine is flexed, the posterior wall of the annulus is drawn taut, which could very well take the bulge off the nerve root (Fig 5-26). This posture may afford the patient some initial relief, but while there is separation posteriorly, there is also compression anteriorly and this could stop the disc from returning to its normal position. Nachemson[61] has shown that flexed positions increase intradiscal pressure and, from his studies, one must assume that the overall intradiscal space is also decreased (Fig 5-27). However, if the patient is in an acute state of pain with muscle guarding and spasm, this flexed, recumbent posture may be necessary to

allow initial relief. The recumbent position also eliminates the compressing force of gravity when compared to sitting or standing postures, and slight flexion provides a mild stretch to the lumbar musculature. Since the patient is often medicated with muscle relaxants, anti-inflammatory and pain medications while undergoing this type of treatment, all of these combined factors may give the patient considerable relief.

However, the flexed position is not productive in the long run and should only be used for the very acute patient. Once some pain relief is accomplished, attempts should be made to bring the patient out of the flexed posture and to restore the normal lordosis (extension principles).

During the past 30 years, the Americans were treating the HNP-protrusion patient with rest, bed traction and flexion principles, while Dr. James Cyriax and other English, European and Scandinavian

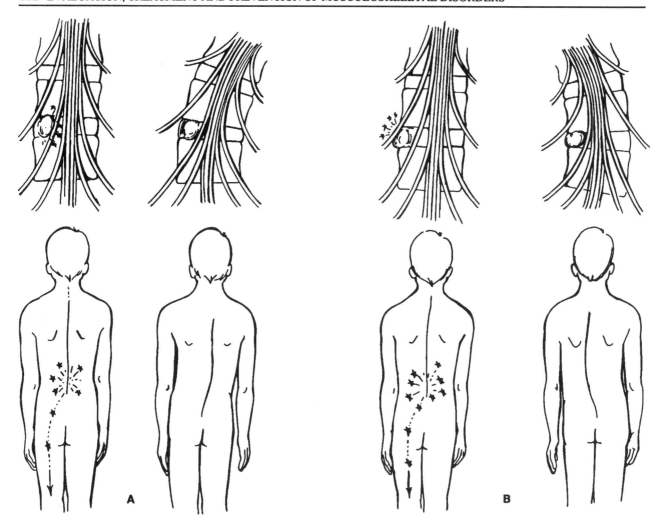

Figure 5-23. Protective scoliosis. A) The bulge is lateral to the nerve root it is encroaching upon, so the patient achieves relief by leaning <u>away</u> from the symptoms; B) The bulge is medial to the nerve root it is encroaching upon, so the patient achieves relief by leaning <u>toward</u> the symptoms.

physicians and physical therapists were using a different approach. In 1950, Cyriax reported that at St. Thomas Hospital in London the laminectomy rate for patients diagnosed as having a herniated disc had fallen from 1 in 40 to 1 in 300. In an article published in the British Medical Journal, he advocated sustained, prone pelvic traction of up to 200 pounds for 10-20 minutes as the treatment of choice for the herniated disc. After the traction reduced the bulge, he stated that the patient should be locked into an exaggerated hyperlordosis until the disc was healed.[14] Similar references can be found in Canadian and European literature. [27, 65]

Dr. James Mathews, another English physician, did studies using epidurography to show that traction forces reduce the extent of a lumbar disc protrusion. Of even more importance, Mathews showed that there was a movement of the contrast medium beyond the line of the posterior longitudinal ligament into the disc space. This suggests that the traction causes a suction force on the bulging nucleus. Fig 10-1, from Mathews's work, shows convincing evidence that the traction force creates a suction force on the nuclear material. This work was done with a prone static traction force of 120 pounds for 20 minutes. [51, 52]

In 1978, Gupta and Ramarao[27] reported clinical improvement in 11 of 14 patients with HNP who were treated with traction. Using epidurography, these researchers showed evidence of reduced protrusion in the patients who demonstrated clinical improvement, while they were unable to show a change in the protrusion in the patients who did not improve clinically. They also included extension exercises in the treatment protocol.

A recent study by Onel[63] shows more convincing evidence that mechanical traction can reduce HNP-protrusion. He studied the effects of a traction load of

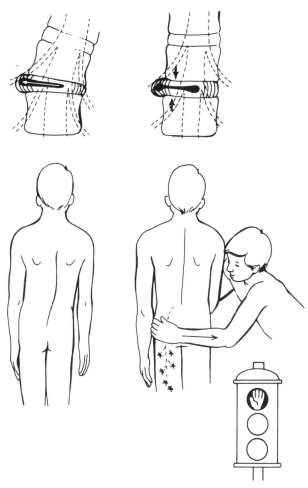

Figure 5-24. Disc mechanics with lateral shift correction (large bulge).

45 kg (100 lb) in 30 patients with lumbar disc herniation. In 21 of 30 patients, the traction treatment caused a retraction of the herniated disc material. He found that both the retraction rate and the incidence of clinical improvement were far greater in medial and posterolateral herniations than in lateral herniations. He theorized that the disc space widening that occurs during traction causes a temporary decrease in intradiscal pressure that "sucks" the herniated nuclear material back into place. Indeed, Nachemson's work shows that a traction load of 30 kg causes a reduction in intradiscal pressure from 30 to 10 kg in the L3 intervertebral disc.[58]

Because medial and posterolateral protrusions respond better to traction than lateral protrusions, Onel further theorized that the effect of traction is partially due to the pushing effect that the posterior longitudinal ligament would have on the posterior aspect of the disc as the ligament is drawn taut. [63]

When a protective scoliosis is present, traditional traction techniques may cause the spine to straighten, forcing the nerve root onto the disc bulge. In such as case, traction may still beneficially reduce the bulging disc but it must be done so it preserves the protective scoliosis. In other words, unilateral or three dimensional traction is necessary in these cases to apply the traction force without straightening the spine[72] (see Chapter 10).

If a protrusion is reduced with traction, it is still unstable and the patient must not aggravate the

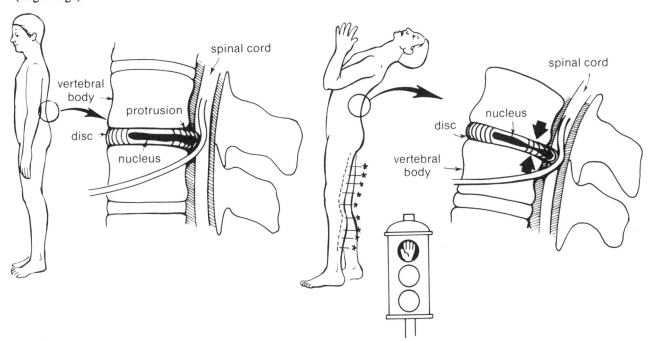

Figure 5-25. Disc mechanics with extension (large bulge).

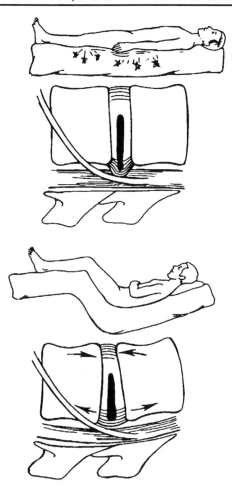

Figure 5-26. The effect of supine flexion on a disc protrusion that is touching the nerve root. Flexion draws the bulge away from the nerve root. In the long-term, however, it further stretches the posterior annulus and encourages further protrusion.

condition for a time. It must be emphasized that traction alone is usually ineffective and that a total treatment regimen must be followed or the patient will not achieve a lasting benefit. As with all the previously discussed treatments and techniques, if traction increases peripheral signs and symptoms, it must be modified or discontinued.

Total management usually involves passive extension exercises as soon as they can be done without increasing peripheral signs and symptoms. In other words, if the traction successfully reduces the extent of the bulge, the patient may then become a candidate for extension exercises and extension principles. At the very least, attempts should be made to restore the normal lordosis as the patient is able. Sometimes, passive extension principles can begin immediately after the first traction treatment. Often, however, patients are slow to return to the passive extension exercises, but they do respond well to sitting

with the lumbar roll and attempting to increase their lordosis gradually when sitting or standing. Obviously, they should avoid slumped sitting and forward bending completely at this stage.

In separate studies, Nachemson and Morris[59] and Morris, Lucas and Bresler[57] have shown that with a garment such as a lumbosacral corset, which compresses the abdomen, intradiscal pressure is diminished by approximately 25%. This significant unloading of the disc occurs in both the standing and the sitting positions. It is accomplished because the corset increases the intra-abdominal pressure and causes the abdominal cavity to become a weight bearing structure. The steel stays within the corset should be bent into a normal or hyperlordotic position and the patient should be instructed to maintain that posture at all times. The corset is especially helpful because it reminds the patient to avoid forward bending, to avoid slumped sitting and to maintain good posture (Fig 11-9).

Attention again must be directed toward positions and activities that cause increased intradiscal pressure. Fig 5-27 shows that forward bending and sitting are the most hazardous positions. Rotation is avoided initially because of the compressive forces it causes. Also, active exercises such as straight leg raising, active back extension and, especially, sit-ups are contraindicated in the early stages.[61]

Figure 5-28 summarizes the treatment considerations for HNP-protrusion. When combined with a comprehensive educational program, these principles can be effective in treating moderate to severe protrusions. Usually, one will know within a few treatments if this program is going to be effective. There is no set time that is necessary to effect a complete cure, but it will usually take 6-10 weeks before the patient can return to strenuous activities, especially those involving forward bending and/or prolonged sitting. The number of traction treatments necessary are few as excessive treatments of traction may cause increased soreness in the back.

For the first two or three weeks, the lumbosacral corset is used at all times when the patient is up. The patient is gradually weaned from it and may then begin using a more active back support or none at all. An active back support such as the S'port All (Fig 11-14) can allow more comfortable exercise and function sooner, which ultimately benefits the patient. Back strengthening exercises should begin as soon as the patient can perform them without increasing peripheralization of symptoms. The patient should start these exercises carefully and gradually build into a vigorous back strengthening program. Tight hamstring muscles can prevent the pelvis from flexing

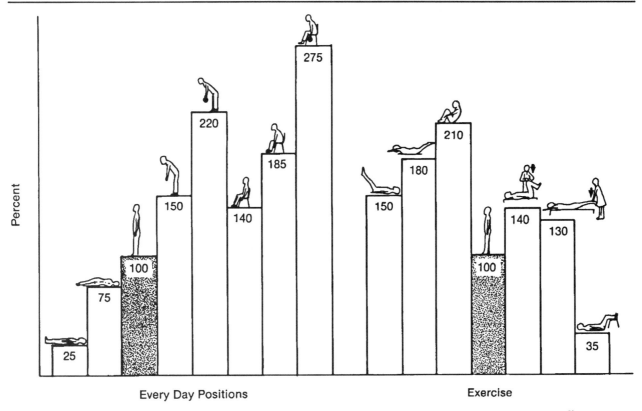

Every Day Positions   Exercise

Figure 5-27. Intradiscal pressure with various positions and activities (adopted from Nachemson[59]).

over the hip joint during forward bending, causing increased stress on the disc. If the patient has tight hamstrings, stretching becomes a vital part of the rehabilitation program. Eventually, overall physical fitness for the improvement of flexibility, strength and endurance should become the goal of this total program. Surgical intervention (discectomy or chemonucleolysis) may be indicated if this management program fails and if there are signs of progressive neurological deficits, or loss of bowel and/or bladder function. In certain cases, however, a "wait and see" attitude is justified because spontaneous regression of HNP has been documented.[83]

Cervical Spine

In the cervical spine, HNP-protrusion with nerve root involvement is less common than in the lumbar spine and the clinical picture is less well defined. Cervical nerve root syndromes are most common at

1.	Relieve compressive forces
2.	Reduce herniation
3.	Maintain correction
4.	Rehabilitate

Figure 5-28. Successful management of HNP-protrusion involves a comprehensive approach.

the C5-C6 segment and involve the C6 nerve root. In most cases, cervical nerve root syndrome is caused by degenerative joint/disc disease rather than by disc protrusion. Often, an x-ray, CT/MRI scan or myelogram may be necessary to determine the diagnosis.

Findings

The clinical picture of cervical HNP-protrusion with nerve root involvement is usually one of gradual worsening with the symptoms starting centrally at the base of the neck, then spreading to the shoulder and the arm as the condition worsens. Pain is also referred to the upper thoracic spine. Interscapular pain corresponding to Cloward's areas may be found. Later, positive neurological signs appear. The slumped, forward head posture is usually seen with HNP-protrusion and attempts to correct the posture or to perform extension of the cervical spine increase the peripheral signs and symptoms because the protrusion is too large to be reduced with this maneuver (Fig 5-29). The x-ray may be normal or may show very slight narrowing of the disc space. This is a clue that one is dealing with HNP-protrusion rather than degenerative joint/disc disease. Degenerative joint/disc disease significant enough to cause neurological signs will usually cause more significant changes in the radiological exam.

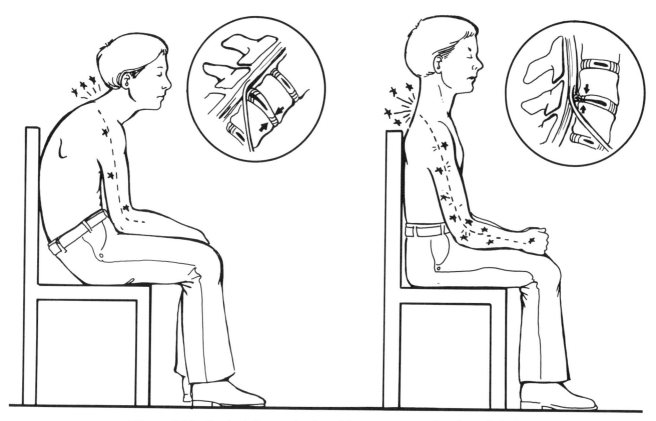

Figure 5-29. Cervical disc mechanics with posture correction (large bulge).

The following differentiation test helps distinguish nerve root irritation due to HNP-protrusion from nerve root irritation due to encroachment within the neural foramen. Cervical compression with the neck in slight flexion will reproduce symptoms if HNP-protrusion is causing the patient's symptoms. Cervical compression with the neck in slight extension will reproduce symptoms if the nerve root is being impinged in the neural foramen.

Treatment

Treatment goals are to reduce the protrusion with traction and maintain the correction by restoring normal posture until the disc heals. Initial attempts to restore normal posture may be unsuccessful, but when combined with traction, may be possible. Manual traction combined with passive axial extension and/or passive backward bending exercises is often effective (see techniques in Chapters 10 and 12). If initial attempts at traction do not relieve the patient's peripheral pain, the therapist should try to modify the angle of pull. Sometimes, a little more flexion or a slight lateral angle may achieve the desired results. As improvement is noted, the angle of pull should be reduced to regain normal posture. Other treatment, as outlined earlier under the section on cervical HNP-protrusion without nerve root involvement, is indicated as the patient progresses.

Herniated Nucleus Pulposus - Extrusion/Sequestration

HNP extrusion is defined as the disorder in which the displaced nuclear material extrudes into the spinal canal through disrupted fibers of the annulus (Fig 5-30). HNP sequestration is defined as the condition in which the nuclear material escapes into the spinal canal as free fragments that may migrate to other locations.[23]

Findings

Patients with an extrusion or sequestration will have similar histories, signs and symptoms as patients with HNP-protrusion except that the peripheral signs and symptoms will probably predominate the spinal signs and symptoms.[54] However, this is not always the case, as the symptoms are often unpredictable. They may change suddenly, become intermittent or follow an inexact or incomplete dermatomal pattern. The patient will often have a gradually worsening history, beginning with HNP-protrusion without nerve root signs and symptoms, progressing to HNP-protrusion with nerve root signs and symptoms, and finally to HNP extrusion or sequestration. At this stage, there is no longer pressure on the annular wall and the pain arising from the disc bulge itself will be diminished while the signs and symptoms of nerve root irritation and/or impingement may be increased. For example, at the extrusion/sequestration stage, the patient's back pain may be gone and sitting may be comfortable.

Treatment

No particular form of physical therapy treatment is effective at this stage except, perhaps, electrotherapy and other modalities for pain relief. Flexion exercises and the flexed recumbent position may afford relief but will not be of lasting benefit and could theoretically cause further extrusion of nuclear material. If extension causes increased <u>peripheral</u> signs and symptoms, it is contraindicated, but if extension principles can be applied without increasing the peripheral signs and symptoms, they should be cautiously implemented. Restoring and maintaining normal lordosis may close the defect in the annulus, giving the disc a better chance to heal. A lumbosacral corset should be used to help reduce intradiscal loading and to remind the patient to avoid forward bending and slumped sitting. Again, surgery is not always necessary because these disorders have been shown to regress spontaneously.[83] Rehabilitative exercise should be implemented as the patient's symptoms stabilize (stop worsening). After 7-10 weeks, the exercise can often get very aggressive.

Even if some of the activities cause increased pain, the patient should begin to gradually work through the pain. However, if there are signs of progressive neurological involvement, a less aggressive approach or surgical intervention may be indicated.

Clinically, one occasionally sees what appears to be an extruded or sequestered disc (predominance of peripheral signs and symptoms) respond well to a combination of traction and extension principles. This causes one to conclude that the condition may have only been a protrusion and points out the importance of a trial of physical therapy in all such cases. In other words, one cannot be certain clinically whether a condition is a disc protrusion, extrusion or sequestration and the trial of physical therapy treatments helps establish the final diagnosis.

Summary of the Stages of Disc Herniation

Figure 5-8 summarizes the stages of disc herniation. Stage one is normal. Stage two shows slight movement of the nuclear gel. The patient would be pain free at this stage. Stage three shows a mild to moderate protrusion. At this stage the patient may

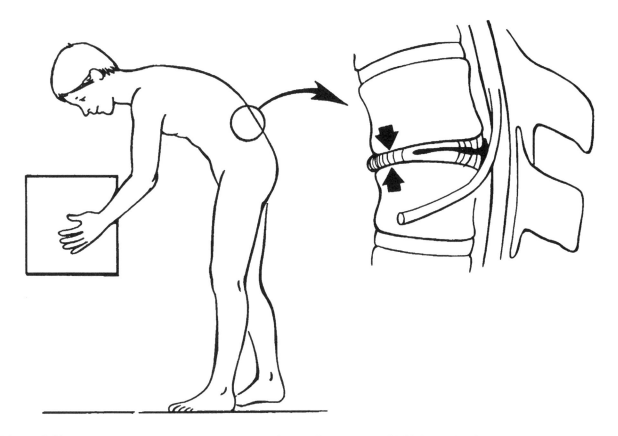

Figure 5-30. HNP-extrusion. Clinically, peripheral signs and symptoms will likely predominate over central symptoms.

have back and leg pain but no positive neurological signs. Postural correction and extension exercises and principles are usually effective treatments at this stage. Stage four shows a protrusion that is bulging and impinging against the nerve root. The patient has back pain, leg pain and positive neurological signs. Treatment includes traction; back support; extension exercises and principles; and the other measures presented in this chapter. Stage five shows disc extrusion and sequestration. In this stage, back and leg pain diminishes as neurological signs usually increase and traction becomes ineffective.

Post-Laminectomy/Discectomy/ Chemonucleolysis

Long term results from laminectomy/discectomy and chemonucleolysis are very often disappointing. Several follow-up studies of patients who underwent laminectomies show that five years later, 50% of them were no better or worse than they were before the operation.[24, 67, 68, 87, 88] This may be because little or no attention was directed toward restoring normal posture, flexibility, strength and physical fitness. Often, nothing is done to educate or motivate the post-surgical patient about proper body mechanics or other lifestyle changes that will be necessary if he or she is to have a reasonably healthy back following surgery. The surgical procedure may remove or dissolve the disc herniation, but it does nothing to correct the poor posture; faulty body mechanics; stressful living and working habits; loss of strength and flexibility; and poor physical fitness – the real causes of the problem.

Therefore, a full rehabilitation program should be implemented for all patients who have had surgery. Straight leg raise stretching to prevent nerve root adhesions and dural tightness should be implemented quite soon in the rehabilitation process. Gentle stretching can even begin while the patient is still in the hospital. The patient should also be instructed in restoration and maintenance of normal posture (extension principles) and should eventually be instructed in a full flexibility, strengthening and fitness program, as well as a complete back care educational program.

Sometimes patients who have previously had back surgery begin to have signs and symptoms indicating that another disc disorder is developing. In such cases, treatment protocol need not be altered because the patient has had surgery. In other words, if extension principles and/or traction are indicated because of the signs and symptoms, they should be given. The only exception is the patient who has had a recent (within one year) spinal fusion or a complete laminectomy. In

these cases, the surgeon should be consulted about specific treatment before proceeding.

NEURAL DISORDERS

Nerve Root Syndromes

Nerve root syndromes are classified as disorders caused by impingement or irritation of the spinal nerve root. They are characterized by production of true neurological signs and symptoms.

As previously discussed, referred pain may arise from any pain-sensitive structure in the spine. It can be felt along the general distribution of the nerve roots involved. Referred pain alone is certainly not a true neurological finding. Nerve root pain tends to be felt as a deep, burning pain that is specific to one spinal nerve root sensory distribution, whereas referred pain is felt as a superficial aching pain that is somewhat more diffuse, tending to cover two or three dermatomes. For example, if one is experiencing referred pain because of a disc protrusion of the L5-S1 disc, the pain may be felt in the sensory distribution of both the L5 and S1 spinal nerves. This is because branches of the recurrent sinuvertebral nerve from both the L5 and S1 levels supply the L5-S1 disc. If a disc protrusion at the L5-S1 level is impinging or irritating the S1 nerve root, the nerve root pain produced is specific to the S1 sensory distribution. Of course, in the latter example, referred pain would also be present along with the spinal nerve root pain.

Nerve Root Compression

Findings

Nerve root compression is often caused by HNP-protrusion. The management of HNP-protrusion was discussed previously. Other less common causes of nerve root compression include congenital anomalies, tumors and fractures. Advanced degenerative joint/disc disease is the most common cause of nerve root compression. This condition is often called lateral spinal stenosis. The patient with nerve root compression will have true neurological signs (true numbness, weakness and reflex changes).

Treatment

Since nerve root compression is usually accompanied by degenerative joint/disc disease, its treatment is nearly identical to the treatment described in that section. This consisted of mobilization, manual or mechanical traction, flexibility and strengthening exercises and modalities. In the case of nerve root compression, however, caution should be used with joint mobilization because it may increase nerve root irritation. Traction is probably safer than mobilization at this stage.

Since many of these patients are restricted in both spinal flexion and extension (forward and backward bending), exercises to increase mobility in both directions are indicated, provided they do not aggravate the nerve root irritation. Many practitioners have avoided extension exercises with these patients because they believed that extension would close the foramen, further irritating the nerve. While it is true that extension does close the foramen in a normal, healthy spine, it is questionable whether the foramen closes at a spinal segment where there is already narrowing of the disc space and the facet joints are already in their maximum close packed position (full extension). If the facet joints are indeed in maximum extension, then further extension will take place about an axis at the facet joints themselves and only widening can occur at the intervertebral foramen and disc spaces (Fig 5-31). Therefore, both flexion and extension exercises should be attempted with this disorder and those relieving the signs and symptoms should be used. Clinical experience shows the response to these exercises can

only be determined by assessing the patient's reaction to them individually.

Nerve Root Swelling and Inflammation (Neuritis)

Findings

Nerve root swelling and inflammation may be severe enough to cause impingement or irritation within the intervertebral foramen; this will produce true positive neurological signs. Nerve root swelling and inflammation can have an insidious onset or can accompany joint and muscle inflammation. This condition is usually seen within a few days following severe injury as an inflammatory response to the injury. Symptoms are the same as with any nerve root syndrome and consist of positive neurological signs as well as referred pain.

Treatment

Treatment should be similar to that used for other inflammatory disorders. Measures to maintain normal posture and promote healing and a gradual return to

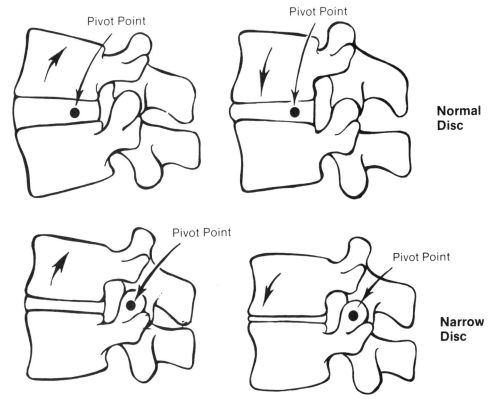

Figure 5-31. In a segment with a normal disc, flexion and extension occur about an axis slightly posterior to the nucleus. Therefore, flexion widens and extension narrows the intervertebral foramen. When a narrowed disc is present, flexion and extension may occur about an axis within the facet joint. Therefore, flexion may narrow and extension may widen the intervertebral foramen in this situation.

full strength and mobility as healing occurs are the important aspects of treatment. Although traction is sometimes prescribed for this disorder when it accompanies an acute cervical strain (whiplash), it should be avoided because the extent of any ligamentous damage cannot be determined at this stage and traction may over-stretch already damaged ligaments.

Adverse Mechanical Neural Tension (AMNT)

Nerve Root Adhesions

One type of abnormal mechanical neural tension results from a spinal nerve root becoming entrapped by scar tissue. Probably this disorder is most commonly seen following spinal surgery. As a preventive measure following surgery, many surgeons now advocate mobilizing the spinal nerve root by a program of passive straight leg raising starting the day after surgery and continuing until there is appreciable healing. Nerve root adhesions may also form following an episode of disc herniation. As the body attempts to heal the bulge or defect in the annulus, collagen tissue is laid down. If the nerve root is lying close by, it may become entrapped by the scar tissue.

Findings

Historically, the patient with nerve root adhesion is likely to have had spinal surgery or, at least, a history of disc herniation. The patient probably still has some of the signs and symptoms of the previous disability, but he or she may have had a period of complete recovery with subsequent insidious onset of spinal pain and/or referred pain with or without positive neurological signs.

The outstanding diagnostic characteristic of this syndrome is the marked absence of lumbar flexion in standing versus little or no restriction of lumbar flexion when tested in sitting or supine. The straight leg raising test will also show the restriction. In other words, when the lumbar spine alone is flexed, no restriction is present, but when the spinal nerve is pulled through the intervertebral foramen, such as in forward bending while standing or straight leg raising, the restriction will be shown. Other classical disc protrusion signs and symptoms, such as increased pain with sitting, will not be present.

Treatment

Treatment for this disorder consists of mobilizing the nerve root adhesion by passive straight leg raise stretching and/or Slump stretching. The following

section on general AMNT disorders should also be reviewed, as many of the techniques discussed there are applicable as well. Unilateral lumbar traction is also beneficial for this disorder. Prevention of this disorder, by passive straight leg raising exercises soon after surgery and other rehabilitation measures described earlier for the post-laminectomy/discectomy patient, is of the greatest importance.

It should be noted that mobilization of the nerve root either by passive stretching or traction will cause a temporary increase in peripheral symptoms. This is an unfortunate but necessary result of the treatment itself. The symptoms should, however, subside quickly after the stretch is discontinued. If the stretch causes increased symptoms that last for more than a few seconds to minutes, indicating an irritable condition, it should be performed less strenuously. The patient should perform frequent, mild, prolonged stretching at home to complement the treatment performed in the clinic. Persistence is needed, as improvement is often slow. After the patient is familiar with the stretches, the majority of the treatment should be continued at home.

Adverse Mechanical Neural Tension

Findings

The therapist should test for AMNT when a patient presents with the following clinical picture:

1. Symptoms present in the spine, head or extremities

2. No neurological signs (true numbness, weakness or reflex changes)

3. No significant irritability present (the tests themselves may cause further irritation and should be approached cautiously when the patient describes a highly irritable condition)

Long-standing pins and needles in the upper or lower extremities is often a clue that AMNT may be present. The therapist should also test for AMNT in all neuromusculoskeletal patients before discharge to ensure proper neural tissue mobility.

Adverse Mechanical Neural Tension (AMNT) is present when a positive response is seen to the Upper Limb Tension Test (ULTT) in the upper limbs or to the Slump tests in the lower limbs. These tests were discussed in detail in Chapter 4.

Painful or dysfunctional neuromusculoskeletal conditions can be either irritable (with various degrees of irritability seen) or non-irritable. This is true of all neuromusculoskeletal conditions, but is of particular clinical importance in the case of conditions involving abnormal mechanical neural tension (AMNT). As discussed in Chapter 4, an irritable condition is one in which symptoms linger after a provocative position or activity is ceased. Neural tissue is by nature highly irritable. Therefore, treatment of AMNT that causes irritability should be approached cautiously, and the treatment guidelines discussed in this section are classified according to whether the condition is irritable or non-irritable. Both the irritable and non-irritable problems discussed here are at opposite ends of a continuum. In reality, the therapist sees varying degrees of irritability. Therefore, the treatment guidelines discussed are not definitive techniques ("cookbook") which always work for either problem, and the therapist is encouraged to continually reassess the patient to determine the degree of aggressiveness with which the techniques can be applied. The therapist is cautioned to monitor and advise the patient to be aware of the possibility of latent symptom responses.

There are several other considerations that will help determine the amount and type of actual treatment. The therapist should consider and develop a clinical picture of the following:

- What are the site(s) of altered neural tissue mechanics?

- What are the specific neural tissues involved?

- What structures are juxtaposed with neural tissues along the neural tissue tract that could interfere with their normal mechanics?

Treatment

Contraindications to neural tension testing and treatment include the following:

1. Irritable conditions

2. Inflammatory conditions

3. Spinal cord signs

4. Malignancy

5. Nerve root compression signs

6. Severe, unremitting night pain

7. Neurological signs

8. Recent paresthesia/anesthesia

9. Active spinal motions easily provoke distal symptoms/paresthesia/anesthesia

10. Reflex sympathetic dystrophy

The treatment goals of AMNT disorders are decreased symptom response and improved functional mobility of the neural structures.

Butler[7] suggests three related ways of treating neural tension problems through movement:

1. *Direct Mobilization*

This approach consists of treating a neural tension problem through direct mobilization of the neural tissues. This can be accomplished by reproducing the neural tension tests (including the Upper Limb Tension Test (ULTT), the Slump test, the straight leg raise, passive neck flexion and prone knee bend), their components, and through joint mobilization techniques.

2. *Related Tissue Treatment*

This type of treatment involves mobilization of the mechanical interfacing components of neural tension problems. These "related" tissues may include joints, muscles, fascia, and skin interfaces. Techniques can involve soft tissue mobilization, joint mobilization, and modalities and exercise used in conjunction with other techniques.

3. *Indirect Treatment*

This approach uses indirect methods to decrease the adverse effects of the patient's occupation and daily activities on the tissue components. Postural advice and ergonomic assessment are the significant features here. These are discussed in detail in Chapter 6.

Successful treatment using mobilization consists of many features. The therapist must develop the ability to feel or appreciate tissue resistance met during treatment, to assess the patient's symptom response and its relationship to movement, and to decide whether treatment should be strong or gentle. The therapist must continually reassess the patient and compare progress with the goals of decreased symptom response and improved functional mobility of the neural structures.

Butler[7] states, "We can do much better than crudely stretching the nervous system." Thus, it would seem appropriate that "mobilization" techniques traditionally used for the joints can apply to the neural tissues as well.

Maitland[50] describes five grades of mobilization:

Grade 1 = Gentle movements of small amplitude done at the beginning of available range.

Grade 2 = Gentle movements of larger amplitude done into available mid-range of a joint.

Grade 3 = Moderate movements of large amplitude done through the available range of the joint and into the resistance.

Grade 4 = Oscillating movements of small amplitude done at the end of range and into the resistance.

Grade 5 = Thrusting movements done to the anatomical limit of the joint.

We can use these grades when describing the direct mobilization techniques described in this section. For example, a Grade 3 mobilization technique used in reference to a straight leg raise might involve the therapist flexing the patient's hip with the knee extended into the point where resistance is felt. A Grade 2 mobilization would stop short of the point where resistance is felt, and a Grade 4 mobilization would involve oscillation at the point where resistance is felt.

As discussed above, treatment techniques will differ depending upon whether or not the disorder is irritable, and to what degree it is irritable.

1. *Irritable Problem* - Usually consists of an inflammatory reaction where pathophysiological responses dominate the clinical picture (i.e., constant pain which is easily provoked and takes a long time to settle).

   a. The therapist may start by using a Direct Technique, but one which is well removed from the symptom area.
   For example, the therapist can use a straight leg raise or opposite limb ULTT initially to treat an acute cervical problem with upper extremity symptoms with a neural tension

component on the right. This can establish a starting point or base technique on which others can be added as tolerated.

   b. Initially, the techniques should be non-provoking. Clinically, this means treatment should stop short of symptom response or increase. Most physical therapists would agree that it is best to "undertreat" or be conservative with any potentially irritable problem. Caution should be taken to monitor and advise the patient regarding latent symptom responses.

   c. Suggested grades of treatment are the large amplitude, non-resistance Grade 2 mobilizations performed through range with minimal symptom provocation. It may be possible to eventually "sneak up" to resistance at a very conservative Grade 4 that gently nudges the resistance, as long as symptom responses are monitored.

   d. Monitoring of symptom responses is essential. Avoid gnawing, deep, constant pain.

   e. Proper postural positioning allows the patient to be in a position of "ease" or pain relief. The patient can be taught to replicate the positioning used in the clinic for self-treatment at home.

   f. When the problem becomes less irritable, the therapist can begin applying direct techniques to the symptom area using gentle techniques, starting with Grade 2 amplitude mobilizations. If we apply this to the previous example, the acute cervical problem with right upper extremity symptoms could be mobilized with Grade 2 right shoulder depression/elevation with the patient positioned comfortably supine. The cervical spine and distal limbs would be positioned to take the body off tension (i.e., right cervical sidebending, right elbow flexion, pillows under knees, etc.). As the patient improves, tension onto the distal components of the ULTT can be progressively added (i.e., left cervical sidebending, elbow extension, shoulder abduction, etc.).

2. *Non-Irritable Problem* - Usually consists of biomechanical compromise by nature, where pathomechanical problems dominate the clinical picture (i.e., stiffness and tissue resistance with abnormal mechanical features).

   a. Initially, techniques applied should be into the resistance, but should still stop short of symptom provocation. Grade 3 or 4 mobilizations can be used here. If symptoms are provoked, they should resolve when the treatment is discontinued. Care needs to be taken to monitor any latent symptom provocation.

b. Functional movements that vary from the test positions can be added. Tension onto distal components can be added, which better mimics function and provokes symptoms. The limiting factor is the clinician's clinical creativity. Reassessment should still be performed in the standard test positions.

c. Relative irritability should be considered. Eventual treatment progression to the symptom source is the goal, but initial treatment may still need to start away from the cause of the problem(s).

d. Reassessment is critical after neural mobilization techniques have been applied. Take care to note any changes in functional mobility, resistance encountered, and symptoms provoked.

Treatment Progression

As clinicians, we understand that no two patients' signs and symptoms will be the same. Since each patient will require treatment specific to his or her individual problem, no recipes are available when treating neural tension problems. However, some suggestions may be helpful for the clinician just learning to address AMNT treatment.

1.   Gradually increase the number of repetitions. Oscillatory mobilizations lasting 20-30 seconds may be a good starting point.

2.   Gradually increase the amplitude of the technique. This may include adding more resistance until symptoms are reproduced.

3.   Symptom response should continually be monitored. Asking the patient if the symptoms are changing or building during treatment is as important as similar questioning on follow-up visits. Latency should be monitored.

4.   Treatment should progress to adding more tension to the system, while taking into account the irritability of the condition.

5.   Muscle energy techniques offer a careful way to add tension to interfacing components in a controlled manner.

6.   Soft tissue massage techniques can be applied to nerves, where accessible, and their surrounding myofascial tissues. The techniques should be applied with all applicable tissues under tension.

7.   The importance of reassessment during and after treatment application and at follow-up visits should not be underestimated.

Self-Treatment

It is usually helpful and necessary to teach patients to perform self-mobilization at home, at work, and during recreation. Symptoms should be monitored carefully to avoid an unnecessary flare-up or latent symptom response. Preventive self-stretches should then be considered for maintaining neural tissue mobility.

Neural tissue mobilization and neural tension testing are exciting new areas in physical therapy. Current clinical research is evolving in these areas. The definitive text on this subject is Mobilization of the Nervous System by David Butler.[7] We highly recommend it as essential to understanding this topic better.

Thoracic Outlet Syndrome

When thoracic outlet compression syndrome (TOS) causes neurological symptoms, it can actually be thought of as a type of adverse mechanical neural tension (AMNT) disorder. Thus, many of the treatment principles for neurological manifestations of TOS are similar to those presented in the AMNT section of this chapter. However, because TOS can cause arterial or venous symptoms as well as neurological symptoms, its treatment is discussed separately.

Thoracic outlet syndrome can involve compression or stretching of the subclavian artery, subclavian vein and/or the brachial plexus as they pass through the thoracic outlet. Neurological symptoms account for at least 90% of thoracic outlet compression problems,[39, 84] which is why the evaluation and treatment of TOS must involve neural tension testing. Mechanical tissue interfaces where compression can occur include the area between the scalenus anticus and medius, between the clavicle and the 1st rib (or a cervical rib) or between the pectoralis minor and the ribs. Diagnostic tests can help the clinician differentiate where the compression is occurring, and how best to treat it.

Findings

Subjective findings may vary depending upon whether artery, vein or brachial plexus is being compressed. With arterial compression, the patient will report pain and fatigue during activity that goes away with rest. Often, symptoms will start distally and proceed proximally. In later stages, cold sensitivity may be present. Any signs of possible emboli, such as cyanosis in one or more fingers, are considered serious and require immediate medical attention.[39]

Venous compression may lead to edema, skin tightness, cyanosis, pain and fatigue. After activity, venous distention may be seen in the extremity. The edema should decrease after a change in the precipitous activity. If the edema does not diminish, it is a sign of a possible venous thrombosis, and requires the attention of a physician for further evaluation.

Nerve compression causes various symptoms including pain, tingling or numbness that usually follows the nerve trunk. Ulnar nerve symptoms are more common than median nerve symptoms.[39] Night pain is common.[39, 54]

When arterial compression is present, positive objective findings may include any of the following: A positive Adson's test, costoclavicular test, hyperabduction test or Roo's test (described in Chapter 4). If a patient complains of symptoms with a particular position or activity, the therapist should monitor the patient's radial pulse while attempting to reproduce the position or activity. Bilateral brachial blood pressure comparisons showing a difference of more than 20-30 mm Hg is suspicious for arterial stenosis. Arteriography and other objective tests not readily available to most physical therapists can also point toward arterial stenosis.

Venous compression is diagnosed objectively through plethysmography and other medical diagnostic tests not available to the physical therapist. The presence of edema; skin tightness; and cyanosis or venous distention after activity are clues to venous compression. When possible, the therapist should try to reproduce the position or activity that causes the symptoms. Other possible causes of peripheral vascular symptoms should be ruled out before a definitive diagnosis is made.

Diagnosis for brachial plexus compression in the thoracic outlet is primarily done through ruling out other pathology in the cervical spine and upper extremities that could cause similar symptoms.[39] Objectively, if Adson's test, the costoclavicular test, the hyperabduction test or Roo's test reproduces neurological symptoms, and if other pathology is ruled out, thoracic outlet syndrome is a likely cause of the patient's neurological symptoms. The neural tension tests for the upper limb discussed in Chapter 4 are important as well.

Treatment

If signs of possible venous or arterial emboli are present, the patient's condition should be considered serious and immediate medical attention is required.

When the patient's symptoms are not serious, but the condition is very irritable, careful stretching into the direction of the restriction is indicated. For example, the patient with a positive hyperabduction test should stretch into hyperabduction. The patient with a positive costoclavicular test should stretch the shoulders and anterior chest area. The stretches should be performed often (every one to two hours) but gently throughout the day. Symptom reproduction as a result of the stretching is acceptable, but not if it lasts for more than a few minutes after the stretch is discontinued. Patience and perseverance are necessary to find just the right amount of stretching tolerable to the patient whose condition is very irritable.

For patients who present with positive neural tension tests, the treatment principles presented in that section apply.

It is also necessary to stretch other tight structures. For example, the patient with TOS often has a generally tight upper and mid thoracic spine. Therefore, stretching the thoracic spine into extension and rotation can be very beneficial.

Simultaneously, the patient should begin strengthening the postural muscles. Forward head, rounded shoulder posture almost always accompanies thoracic outlet compression and is often its cause. For this reason, exercises encouraging proper posture are extremely important, particularly those encouraging interscapular and lumbar strengthening.

Mobilization techniques for tight thoracic segments or for the 1st rib are often highly beneficial. Soft tissue stretching is also beneficial but does not substitute for the patient's diligence with a home stretching program. Cervical traction is usually not beneficial and may be contraindicated.[39]

The patient must be taught early on that TOS usually takes several weeks or months to resolve. Careful, consistent attention to the patient's home exercise program is necessary for long term resolution.

In some cases, surgical resection of a cervical rib or other surgical release techniques can be successful. However, successful surgical management must include patient education and exercise to prevent factors such as poor posture, repetitive activities and poor ergonomic conditions from causing the patient's symptoms to recur.

MISCELLANEOUS DISORDERS

Congenital Abnormalities

One often sees patients with various disorders such as lumbarized sacral vertebræ, sacralized lumbar vertebræ, asymmetry of the facet joints or other congenital anomalies. The clinical signs and symptoms these patients have are quite varied and do not seem to present a clear clinical picture that can be consistently related to a definable pathological disorder. In other words, except for the radiological evidence, it is difficult to determine the real significance of many of these congenital anomalies. We believe that, except as these anomalies contribute to joint hypermobility or hypomobility or perhaps to degenerative joint/disc disease, they are insignificant and are often unrelated to the patient's real problem. In fact, there is a certain danger in diagnosing the patient's condition by the radiological findings when there is no direct cause and effect relationship established during a complete evaluation and assessment. When a patient is told about a congenital anomaly or "birth defect," will the patient be as likely to carry out the self-help program that he or she has been given? Perhaps everyone would be better off not knowing that these probably insignificant abnormalities exist in the first place. One should always be on guard against the temptation to use one or two isolated findings as the basis for a diagnosis.

Traumatic Fractures

X-rays need not be taken of every patient who complains of spinal pain. However, when trauma is involved, a radiological exam is absolutely necessary to determine if a fracture is present.

Findings

The patient will report a traumatic incident, such as a fall or an accident. The fracture is diagnosed by x-ray.

Treatment

Spinal fracture management is outside the scope of practice for a physical therapist. When a spinal fracture has healed, however, it is important to evaluate strength, mobility and posture, and to rehabilitate the patient as needed.

Compression Fractures/Osteoporosis

Although osteoporosis is associated with dorsal and lumbar spinal pain, it is not likely to cause symptoms by itself. The pain associated with osteoporosis is probably caused by fractured bones (compression fractures) and the resulting pressure on nerve roots or sensory fibers in the periosteum. Osteoporosis has many known causes; the majority are classified as post-menopausal and senile. Genetic abnormalities, nutritional dysfunctions, endocrine disorders, corticosteroids, pregnancy, prolonged immobilization, inactivity and weightlessness are all known causes of osteoporosis.[1, 19]

Findings

Diagnosis of compression fracture is by x-ray. The patient will often have sharp pain with or without signs of nerve root compression. In the acute state the pain will be especially sharp with movement. Flexion of the spine is usually painful, is harmful and should be avoided. A single thoracic compression fracture will be characterized by the presence of a prominent spinous process and a wide interspinous space below the prominent spinous process. Multiple thoracic compression fractures are characterized by progressive increase of kyphosis, which can eventually lead to severe disability.

Treatment

In most cases, only the anterior portion of the vertebral body fractures, creating a wedge. If the posterior aspect of the body has fractured, management must be directed by an orthopædic surgeon on an individual basis. Therefore, the treatment principles discussed here apply to an anterior compression fracture only, with the posterior edge of the vertebral body structurally intact.

Educating the patient about positions and activities that are beneficial or potentially harmful is absolutely necessary.[1] The rule is to encourage positions or activities that promote spinal extension and avoid positions or activities that encourage flexion. In particular, the patient should avoid using large pillows under the head or sleeping in a flexed position. The patient should be taught how to roll to the side to get up from a recumbent position. Good lumbar support when sitting will help the patient avoid flexed sitting postures. Walking and other weight bearing activities will help prevent further demineralization of the bone. Active and passive extension exercises are indicated as soon as the patient's pain has decreased to the point that he or she can tolerate them. All positions and activities involving spinal flexion must be avoided. Modalities such as moist heat and electrical stimulation may relieve some of the pain.

A spinal brace or support is often helpful in the management of acute compression fractures. The function of the brace or support is to help the patient maintain extension and to prevent flexion. The type of brace or support selected will vary from a rigid three-point hyperextension brace such as the Cash or Jewett brace to a semi-rigid Taylor-type brace or a dorsolumbar corset (see Chapter 11).

An older or senile patient with an osteoporotic compression fracture will probably not tolerate a rigid hyperextension or even a Taylor brace and may only be comfortable in a dorsolumbar corset. The dorsolumbar corset, of course, does not provide as much support but in this case is the only reasonable solution. In contrast, a younger patient with a traumatic compression fracture probably would need more rigid support and would tolerate a hyperextension brace well.

The hyperextension brace serves only one purpose — that of preventing flexion. A corset or brace that provides circumferential support, however, will reduce vertical loading on the lumbar spine because of the effect of abdominal compression. Therefore, a lumbar compression fracture may be best managed with a support or brace that provides both abdominal compression and protection from flexion. A chair back or Taylor-type brace best serves this dual purpose.

Certain patients who are strong, alert and able to carefully maintain proper extension positions and postures and avoid flexion may only need to use a brace for a very short time, or in some cases will not need a brace or support at all.

Spondylolysis/Spondylolisthesis

Spondylolysis is a defect involving the pars interarticularis of the neural arch of the vertebra. When the defect in the neural arch is bilateral, separation of the anterior and posterior elements at the site of these defects may occur. This displacement is called spondylolisthesis. The most common site for occurrence is L5 on S1. There is almost certainly a congenital weakness associated with this disorder, and it is thought that the defect actually occurs as a stress fracture. Many people have spondylolysis or spondylolisthesis and are symptom free.

It is important to remember that once a diagnosis of this nature is made, the diagnosis may follow the patient and be implicated as the source of all symptoms. There may, however, be another cause for the patient's complaints.

Findings

Diagnosis is by x-ray, but clinically, a "step-off" of the spinous processes can sometimes be felt. The patient will often have hyperlordosis and complain that prolonged standing increases pain, sitting relieves it and various types of vigorous physical activities aggravate the condition. The original onset of symptoms can often be traced back to athletic or other vigorous physical activities during adolescence.

If a spondylolisthesis is the true cause of a patient's symptoms, it will probably be because the segment is unstable and aggravation is due to the excessive movement and stress at the segment when physical activities are attempted. If, on the other hand, a spondylolisthesis is stable, it will probably not be the source of the patient's complaint. Frequently, in the presence of an unstable spondylolisthesis, the patient will describe a slipping sensation or movement occurring in the back when assuming a certain position or doing certain activities. Some patients learn to self mobilize to correct this. As previously mentioned, a step-off can often be felt when palpating the spinous processes. If the spondylolisthesis is unstable the step-off can usually be felt when the patient is standing and side lying, but it will disappear when the patient lies prone with pillows under the lumbar spine.

Treatment

The presence of an unstable spondylolisthesis makes the patient more vulnerable to joint sprains and muscular strains, and such a patient may need to avoid heavy labor and vigorous physical activities. General postural improvement is necessary, especially abdominal muscle strengthening and other flexion exercises. It is often necessary to fit the patient with a lumbosacral support or brace to be used when performing any activities that may aggravate the condition. In such cases, a lumbosacral support or brace may not immobilize the involved segments effectively but at least may remind the patient to limit vigorous activity. A support or brace that provides abdominal compression will also help reduce vertical loading of the spine which may further reduce stress and aggravation due to physical activity.

In a hyperlordotic state, or in the case of obesity and weak abdominals, the vertical shear forces are greatly magnified. Reduction of the hyperlordosis can reduce the shear forces. These patients can often be effectively managed in a brace designed to reduce the lumbar lordosis and/or with flexion exercises with an emphasis on abdominal strengthening.[76] Any type of support that helps reduce a protruding abdomen has the effect of moving the center of gravity posteriorly, thus reducing the lumbar lordosis.

Teen-agers indulging in contact sports and preteen children participating in sports requiring excessive lumbar lordosis (i.e., gymnastics) and are more frequently found to have spondylolysis. Traumatic spondylolysis/spondylolisthesis should be suspected and ruled out in any physically active preteen or teenage patient who has persistent back pain for more than two or three weeks. An acute spondylolysis (stress fracture) may not be evident on x-ray and a bone scan may be necessary to make the diagnosis. When a break in the pars interarticularis is found on x-ray, a bone scan can be performed to determine whether the break represents a stress fracture. If a bone scan demonstrates increased metabolic activity over the pars interarticularis, a stress fracture is the cause. Such patients can be treated with the use of a brace that reduces the lumbar lordosis in an attempt to heal the stress fracture. There is evidence that healing can take place, and the pain can readily be eliminated.[55] In patients whose scans are not "hot," the assumption is made that nonunion has resulted. If pain is a problem in these cases, a lumbar brace or support often provides relief.[19, 20] During acute episodes, rest and modality treatments are also indicated. If the displacement is great enough there may be signs of neurological impingement of the cauda equina. In such cases, Cyriax advocates traction.[13] Surgical fusion may be necessary in severe cases.

Spinal Stenosis

In the past two decades, encroachment upon the cervical spinal cord resulting from a stenotic cervical spinal canal has been generally accepted as a recognizable clinical entity. This disorder is characterized by neurological symptoms that may initially lead to diagnosis of multiple sclerosis or other neurological diseases.[77]

There are a number of ways encroachment can occur. Annular protrusions of the cervical disc; osteophytes; folding or bulging of the ligamentum flavum; subperiosteal thickening over the vertebral body and the laminal arch; and congenital smallness of the spinal canal are all factors. Smith states that a combination of these factors is frequently involved.[77]

Lumbar spinal stenosis is also known as neurogenic intermittent claudication of the cauda equina. Spinal stenosis occurs much the same way in the lumbar spine as it does in the cervical spine in that it is usually associated with degenerative joint disease and a combination of factors that act together to diminish the size of the spinal canal (Fig 5-32). Blau and Logue state that the ultimate mechanism producing the symptoms is vascular insufficiency of the cauda equina nerve roots.[4]

Findings

Cervical

Mixed hyper- and hypoactive reflexes are sometimes observed in the upper extremities, depending upon the level of encroachment. Hyperactive reflexes may be observed in the lower extremities. There may be paresthesia, pain and motor weakness in the extremities. Symptoms are aggravated by extension of the neck.

Lumbar

The chief symptoms are pain in the lower back and one or both legs, numbness and tingling in the feet and legs, decreased muscle stretch reflexes and motor weakness in the legs. Often these symptoms are present only after walking and are relieved by rest and/or flexing the lumbar spine. Spinal extension decreases the volume of the lumbar spinal canal and increases nerve root bulk. Bulging of the ligamentum flavum is also most pronounced in spinal extension. With this information, it is easy to see why the symptoms are most pronounced when the patient is standing or lying flat with the lumbar spine extended.

The therapist should be aware of a condition known as vascular intermittent claudication, caused by decreased circulation to the musculature of the lower extremities. Vascular intermittent claudication produces some of the same symptoms as lumbar spinal stenosis. However, it does not cause back pain and is not necessarily relieved by spinal flexion. It is diagnosed by assessing peripheral circulation to the lower extremities.

Treatment

Treatment centers around educating the patient to avoid aggravating or irritating the disorder. A soft collar or lumbar support is often helpful. Physical therapy modalities may provide temporary pain relief. Measures to increase mobility and flexibility (exercises

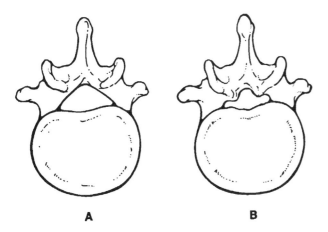

A   **B**

Figure 5-32. A) Normal spinal canal. B) Narrowed spinal canal.

and traction) sometimes help. A decompression laminectomy is indicated in severe cases.

Ankylosing Spondylitis

Ankylosing spondylitis is characterized by progressive joint sclerosis and ligamentous ossification which first appears in the sacroiliac joints and later spreads into the lumbar and thoracic spine and rib cage. In severe cases the cervical spine, hip and shoulder joints may also become involved. Complete ankylosis of the involved joints may eventually occur. This eases pain, but may lead to disability depending upon the position the joints are in when they become fixed. The younger the patient is at onset, the worse the prognosis; men usually do worse than women.[12]

Findings

Onset typically occurs between 20 and 35 years of age and first appears as a vague lower back pain and stiffness that is usually worse upon waking and eased by exercise. The symptoms are intermittent with episodes lasting for weeks or months at a time. The onset of each acute episode seems to be insidious, unrelated to exertion or activities.

Clinically, one sees a flattening of the lumbar lordosis and increased rounding of the thoracic and cervical spine. Since the two upper cervical joints are affected later, hyperextension may be seen here in contrast to the tendency otherwise for a spinal flexion deformity to develop. In severe cases, if the hip joints also become fixed in flexion, the patient may become seriously disabled. Certain laboratory tests (elevated sedimentation rates) may be helpful in diagnosis. X-ray diagnosis may be possible only after several years, with the earliest abnormalities being seen in the sacroiliac joint. [12, 19]

Treatment

Patient education is of great importance. If the patient is young at onset, it is important to direct him or her toward a career that does not involve heavy work. It is best to tell the patient that the spine will eventually stiffen in a way that does not interfere with sedentary work, and that the pain is controllable.

Certainly, positioning and exercises to resist the gradual development of the flexed spine (and hip joints, in severe cases) play an extremely important part. The patient must sleep on a firm mattress and should avoid lying curled up on his side or using more than one pillow when lying supine. Some prone lying is necessary and both passive and active extension exercises should be emphasized. Use of the lumbar roll (Fig 5-20) when sitting and avoidance of prolonged sitting and flexion postures is recommended. Manual mobilization to maintain spinal extension is also indicated and can often be taught to family members. Use of a lumbar support, medication and physical therapy modalities may be helpful during acute episodes.[12]

Coccyx Injuries

Injury to the sacrococcygeal joint may occur as a sprain, subluxation or fracture. As healing occurs, the joint gradually becomes sclerosed and passive movement becomes restricted.[86] The classic patient will be one who has been to many doctors and has had very little help.

Findings

The patient will have a history of a fall directly on the coccyx or a childbirth injury. The x-ray may show a healed fracture. The patient will be unable to sit on both buttocks at the same time. External and internal examination will reveal tenderness to palpation of the coccyx and mobility of the coccyx may be very limited or absent.

The normal coccyx flexes while sitting and extends when standing. When the coccyx is injured or subluxed, it may heal in the more extended position. If this happens, the soft tissue directly over the end of the coccyx develops a painful pressure point when the patient sits.

The coccyx can also be dislocated or fractured and heal in a flexed position or become fragmented or unstable in a flexed position. This disorder can be diagnosed by palpating the position of the coccyx and testing the passive mobility of the sacrococcygeal joint, or it may be diagnosed by radiological exam.

Treatment

Surgical removal of the coccyx may be indicated if it is hypermobile (unstable) or dislocated in a flexed position. The physical therapist can expect good results with ultrasound and passive mobilization along with other conservative management, such as a coccyx pillow, if the joint is hypomobile/subluxed and positioned in extension (see Chapter 9).

Leg Length Inequality (LLI)

Leg length inequalities are classified as either being true (actual bony asymmetry due to fracture, growth abnormalities, coxa vara/valga, etc.) or functional (positional due to a pronated foot, genu valgus, tight adductor muscles, sacroiliac lesions, etc.). They are included in the discussion of treatment of spinal disorders because of the frequent interrelationship between a leg length discrepancy and a functional asymmetry in the spine. One must determine the cause of the leg length discrepancy before deciding if the disorder can be treated.

The contribution of leg length inequality to low back pain and hip arthrosis remains controversial. One reason for the controversy is that LLI often escapes observation during the clinical examination. Many practitioners do not routinely check for LLI or may use inadequate assessment techniques (see Chapter 4 for details on assessing leg length inequalities). We feel that LLI is indeed a contributing factor in back and hip pain.

A lumbar scoliosis (convexity toward the short leg) will develop secondary to an uneven leg length (Fig 5-33). This will cause unequal biomechanical stresses on the structures of the spine and can, over a long time, contribute to the development of adaptive muscle shortening, ligamentous and capsular hypomobility, degenerative joint disease and, at least theoretically, to disc protrusion. The adaptive muscle shortening and joint hypomobility will develop on the concave (long leg) side. Degenerative joint disease develops in the facets on the concave side and osteoarthritic (traction) spurring has been observed on the convex side. If a disc protrusion develops, it will probably be toward the convex (short leg) side.

Friberg[21] studied 798 subjects with low back or hip pain and 359 subjects who were symptom free. He found highly significant statistical correlation between the symptoms and leg length inequality. In 79% of the cases of low back pain with sciatica, and in 89% of the cases of hip pain, the symptoms were present on the side of the longer leg. When the LLI was corrected with a shoe lift on the short leg side, complete or nearly complete relief of symptoms occurred in the majority of cases that were followed up to six months.

Findings

If a true leg length difference exists, the iliac crests will be uneven in a standing position. However, tests implicating sacroiliac joint dysfunction will be negative (see Chapter 7). Leg length can also be measured using a cloth tape measure and comparing the distance from each ASIS to medial or lateral malleoli, but these methods are generally thought to be less accurate and precise when compared to the method comparing standing iliac crest heights. X-ray measurement as described by Friberg and others should not be necessary in most cases because the method described in Chapter 4 has been shown to be sufficiently accurate.[21]

Treatment

Treatment involves compensating for the leg length difference with the use of a shoe lift. If the problem has been long-standing and adaptive muscle shortening and joint hypomobility are present, one must be absolutely certain that balanced mobility, strength and normal posture are restored. Correcting uneven leg length in the presence of joint hypomobility will not correct the lumbar scoliosis and may, in fact, increase the compensatory or secondary thoracic curve. Therefore, treatment such as ultrasound, unilateral lumbar traction, positional traction, joint mobilization and home exercises are necessary to restore full mobility in these cases.

Although full correction of any consistently measurable leg length discrepancy is the final goal, it may be advisable to make corrections gradually as mobility, strength and normal posture are being regained. Sometimes small corrections are made with a heel lift only. While this does correct standing leg length, it does not correct the discrepancy at toe-off during gait. Therefore, correction with a heel lift only is often not adequate treatment. Correction of more than 1/2" discrepancy usually requires shoe modification.

Systemic Disease and Referred Pain from the Viscera

Venereal disease, gout, lupus erythematosus, rheumatoid arthritis and urological infections are among the systemic diseases that can cause spinal pain. Metastatic lesions can be a source of pain and pain can also be referred from visceral structures.

Findings

Increased pain with rest and during the night, pain that is not associated with movement or body position, pain of insidious onset, pain covering large, non-specific areas and pain migrating from one joint to another are all signs of systemic or visceral origins and should alert the physical therapist that he may not be dealing with a musculoskeletal disorder. Changes in the patient's general health such as weight gain or loss, fever or previous carcinoma is indications of systemic diseases. Perhaps of most importance, any patient who does not respond in a timely fashion to a reasonable trial of physical therapy treatment should be suspected of having a systemic disease or a visceral problem. Although the diagnosis of these disorders is the responsibility of the physician, the physical therapist should be aware of signs and symptoms unique to these disorders. In the absence of any

A   **B**

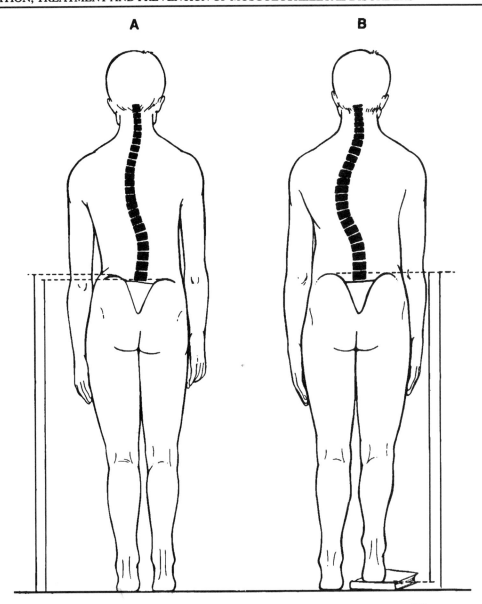

Figure 5-33. A) Long term leg length discrepancy with adaptive muscle shortening and joint stiffness occurring on the side of the long leg (left). B) Correction of the discrepancy with a lift on the right causes the lumbar scoliosis to stay the same or worsen unless full spinal mobility is restored concurrently.

musculoskeletal findings, the patient should be referred to the physician for further evaluation and assessment.

Treatment

Systemic disease and referred pain from the viscera are not musculoskeletal disorders and are therefore not treated by the physical therapist.

SUMMARY

This chapter has shown that many factors contribute significantly to spinal pathology, that each disorder has its own unique pathology and each should

also have its own unique treatment plan. We have tried to show many unique disorders are related, in that one disorder may eventually progress to another more serious disorder if left untreated (Fig 5-34). It also must be stressed that clinically, the patient often presents more than one of these disorders at the same time.

There is no substitute for a complete and thorough evaluation and assessment of the patient before planning an effective treatment program. Likewise, there is no substitute for complete and thorough knowledge of spinal pathology before making a meaningful evaluation and assessment.

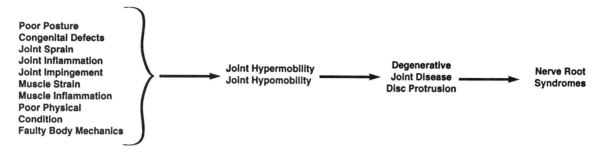

Figure 5-34. Spinal disorders often follow a natural progression, with seemingly minor disorders (left) leading to more serious disorders (right).

REFERENCES

1. Aisenbrey J: Exercise in the Prevention and Management of Osteoporosis. Physical Therapy 67:1100-1104, July 1987.

2. Asfour S, et al: Effects of an Endurance and Strength Training Program on Lifting Capabilities of Males. Ergonomics 27:435-442, 1984.

3. Bigos S, et al: Back Injuries in Industry: A Retrospective Study III: Employee Related Factors. Spine 11:252-256, 1986.

4. Blau J and Logue V: The Natural History of Intermittent Claudication of the Cauda Equina. Brain 101:211-222, 1978.

5. Brodin H: Paths of Nutrition in Articular Cartilage and Intervertebral Disc. Acta Orthop Scand 124:171-183.

6. Brown J: Studies on the Permeability of the Intervertebral Disc During Skeletal Maturation. Spine 1:240-244, 1976.

7. Butler D: <u>Mobilisation of the Nervous System</u>. Churchill Livingstone, Edinburgh 1991.

8. Cady L et al: Strength and Fitness and Subsqent Back Injuries in Firefighters. Joul of Occ Med 21:269-272, 1979.

9. Cailliet R: <u>Low Back Pain Syndrome</u>, 4th edition. FA Davis, Philadelphia PA 1988.

10. Chaffin D: Manual Materials Handling. Joul of Environmental Pathology and Toxicology 2:31-66, 1978.

11. Cummings G: <u>Proceedings of the Ninth Annual Dogwood Conference</u>. Dogwood Institute, Alpharetta GA 1984.

12. Cyriax J: Diagnosis of Soft Tissue Lesions. <u>Textbook of Orthopædic Medicine,</u> Vol 1, 8th edition. Bailliere-Tindall, London 1982.

13. Cyriax J: Treatment by Manipulation. Massage and Injection. <u>Textbook of Orthopædic Medicine</u>, Vol 2, 10th edition. Bailliere-Tindall, London 1980.

14. Cyriax J: Treatment of Lumbar Disk Lesions. Brit Med Joul 2:14-34, 1950.

15. Davis P: Reducing the Risk of Industrial Bad Backs. Occupational Health and Safety (May/June 1979) 45-47.

16. DePalma A and Rothman: <u>The Intervertebral Disc</u>. Saunders, Philadelphia PA 1970.

17. Farfan H: <u>Mechanical Disorders of the Low Back</u>. Lea and Febiger, Philadelphia PA 1973.

18. Farfan H: <u>Proceedings of the International Federation of Orthopædic Manipulative Therapists</u>. B Kend, ed. Vail CO 1977.

19. Finneson B: <u>Low Back Pain</u> 2nd edition. Lippincott, Philadelphia PA 1980.

20. Flemming J: Spondylolysis and Spondylolisthesis in the Athlete. In <u>The Spine in Sports</u>. S Hochschuler, ed. Hanley and Belfus, Philadelphia PA 1990.

21. Friberg O: Clinical Symptoms and Biomechanics of Lumbar Spine and Hip Joint in Leg Length Inequality. Spine 8(6):643-651, 1983.

22. Gall E: Lumbar Spine X-rays - What Can They Reveal? Occ Health and Safety 48:32-35, 1979.

23. <u>Glossary of Spinal Terminology</u>. American Academy of Orthopædic Surgeons, Chicago IL.

24. Gottlieb H, et al: Comprehensive Rehabilitation of Patients Having Chronic Low Back Pain. Arch Phys Med Rehab 58:101-108, 1977.

25. Griffin J: Physiological Effects of Ultrasonic Energy As It Is Used Clinically. Phys Ther 46:18-21, 1966.

26. Groom D: <u>Cervical Spine and Shoulders</u>. The Saunders Group, Minneapolis MN 1992. Course Manual.

27. Gupta R and Ramarao S: Epidurography in Reduction of Lumbar Disc Prolapse by Traction. Arch Phys Med Rehabil 59:322-327, 1978.

28. Harris R and McNab I: Structural Changes in the Lumbar Intervertebral Discs. JBJS 36B:302-322, 1954.

29. Hirsch C, Ingelmark B and Miller M: The Anatomical Basis for Low Back Pain. Acta Ortho Scanda 33:1-17, 1963.

30. Hirsch D and Schajowicz F: Studies of Structural

Changes in the Lumbar Intervertebral Discs. JBJS 36B: 304-322, 1954.

31. Holm S and Nachemson A: Variations in the Nutrition of the Canine Intervertebral Disc, Induced by Motion. Spine 8:866-873, 1983.

32. Holm S and Nachemson A:Nutritional Changes in the Canine Intervertebral Disc After Spinal Fusion. Clin Orthop and Rel Res 169:243-258, 1982.

33. Hood L and Chrisman D: Intermittent Pelvic Traction in the Treatment of the Ruptured Intervertebral Disc. J Am Phys Ther Assoc 48:21-30, 1968.

34. Jackson N, Winkelman R and Bickel W: Nerve Endings in the Lumbar Spinal Column. JBJS 48A:1272-1281, 1966.

35. Jayson M and Barks J: Structural Changes in the Intervertebral Disc. Annuls Rheum Dis 32:10-15, 1973.

36. Kapandji I: Spine. Vol 3 of The Physiology of the Joints, 2nd edition. Churchill-Livingstone, London-New York 1974.

37. Kellegren J: Observations on Referred Pain Arising From Muscle. Clinical Science 3:175, 1938.

38. Kirkaldy-Willis W: The Three Phases of the Spectrum of Degenerative Disease. In Managing Low Back Pain. WH Kirkaldy-Willis and C Burton, eds. Churchill Livingston, New York NY 1992.

39. Koontz C: "Thoracic Outlet Syndrome, Diagnosis and Management." In Orthopedic Physical Therapy Forum series. AREN, Pittsburgh, PA 1987. Videotape .

40. Kornberg C and Lew P: The Effect of Stretching Neural Structures on Grade I Hamstring Injuries. JOSPT 10(12):481-487, 1989.

41. Kos J and Wolf J: Intervertebral Menisci and Their Possible Role in Intervertebral Blockage. Bul of the Orth Sec Amer Phys Ther Assn, Winter 1976.

42. Kraft G and Levinthal D: Facet Synovial Impingement. Surg Gynecol and Obstet 93:439-443, 1951.

43. Kramer J: Pressure Dependent Fluid Shifts in the Intervertebral Disc. Ortho Clinics of N Amer 8:211-216, Jan 1977.

44. Kramos P: New Rules to Fight Back Injuries. Health and Safety 44:42-44, 1975.

45. Levernieux J: Traction Vertebrate. Expansion Scientifique, 1960.

46. Lipson S and Juir H: Proteoglycans in Experimental Intervertebral Disc Degeneration. Spine 6:194-210, 1981.

47. Magora A and Schwartz A: Relation Between Low Back Pain and X-ray Changes IV: Lysis and Olisthesis. Scand J Rehabil Med 12:47-52, 1980.

48. Magora A and Schwartz A: Relation Between the Low Back Pain Syndrome and X-ray Findings I: Degenerative Findings. Scand J Rehabil Med 8:115-126, 1976.

49. Magora A and Schwartz A: Relation Between the Low Back Pain and X-ray Findings II: Transitional Vertebra

(Mainly Sacralization). Scand J Rehabil Med 10:135-145, 1978.

50. Maitland, G: Palpation Examination of the Posterior Cervical Spine: The Ideal, Average and Abnormal. Aust J Physiother 28:3-12, 1982.

51. Mathews J: Dynamic Discography; A Study of Lumbar Traction. Ann Phy Med 9:275-279, 1968.

52. Mathews J: The Effects of Spinal Traction. Physiotherapy 58:64-66, 1972.

53. McKenzie R: The Lumbar Spine. Spinal Publications, Waikanae New Zealand 1981.

54. Mennell J: Differential Diagnosis of Visceral From Somatic Back Pain. Joul of Occ Med 8:477-80, Sept 1966.

55. Micheli L: Back Injuries in Gymnasts. Clin Sports Med 4(1):85-93, 1985.

56. Mooney V and Robertson J: The Facet Syndrome. Clin Orthop and Rel Res 115:149-156, Mar/Apr 1976.

57. Morris J, Lucas D and Bresler M: Role of the Trunk in Stability of the Spine. J Bone and Joint Surg 43A:327-351, 1961.

58. Nachemson A and Elfstrom G: Intradiscal Dynamic Pressure Measurements in Lumbar Discs. Scand J Rehabil Med (Suppl)1:1-40, 1970.

59. Nachemson A and Morris J: In Vivo Measurements of Intradiscal Pressure. J Bone Joint Surg 46A: 1077-1092, 1964.

60. Nachemson A: Low Back Pain, Its Etiology and Treatment. Clinical Medicine 18-24, 1971.

61. Nachemson A: The Lumbar Spine, An Orthopædic Challenge. Spine 1:50-71, 1976.

62. Nordby E: Epidemiology and Diagnosis in Low Back Injury. Occupational Health and Safety. 50:38-42, Jan 1981.

63. Onel D, et al: Computed Tomographic Investigation of the Effect of Traction on Lumbar Disc Herniations. Spine 14(1):82-90, 1989.

64. Park W: Radiological Investigation of the Intervertebral Disc. In The Lumbar Spine and Back Pain. Jayson, Grune and Stratton, eds. 1976.

65. Parson W and Cummings J: Mechanical Traction in the Lumbar Disc Syndrome. Can Med Assoc Joul 77:7-11, 1957.

66. Peterson H and Kieffer S: Introduction to Neuroradiology. Harper and Row, Philadelphia PA 1972.

67. Quebec Task Force Study: Scientific Approach to the Assessment and Management of Activity Related Spinal Disorders. Spine 12:7S, 1987.

68. Quinet R and Hadler H: Diagnosis and Treatment of Backache. Sem in Arth and Rheu 8:261-287, 1979.

69. Roofe P: Innervation of the Annulus Fibrosis and Posterior Longitudinal Ligament: Fourth and Fifth Lumbar Level. Arch Neurol Psych 44:100-103, 1940.

70. Saal J, et al: High Levels of Inflammatory

Phospholipase A2 Activity in Lumbar Disc Herniations. Spine 15(7):674-678, 1990.

71. Saunders H: The Use of Spinal Traction in the Treatment of Neck and Back Conditions. Clin Orthop and Rel Res 179: 31-38, Oct 1983.

72. Saunders H: Unilateral Lumbar Traction. Phys Ther 61:221-225, Feb 1981.

73. Schnebel B, et al: A Digitizing Technique for the Study of Movement of Intradiscal Dye in Response to Flexion and Extension of the Lumbar Spine. Spine 13(3):309-312, 1988.

74. Shah J: Shift of Nuclear Material With Flexion and Extension of the Spine. In The Lumbar Spine and Low Back Pain. M Jayson, ed. Pitman Medical, London 1980.

75. Sheon R, et al: The Hypermobility Syndrome. Postgrad Med 71:199-209, 1982.

76. Sinaki M, et al: Lumbar Spondylolisthesis. Archives of Phy Med 70:594-598, August 1989.

77. Smith B: Cervical Spondylosis and Its Neurological Complications. Thomas, Springfield IL 1968.

78. Snook S: The Design of Manual Handling Tasks. Ergonomics 21:963-985, 1978.

79. Spangford E: The Lumbar Disc Herniation. Acta Orthop Scand (Suppl 142):5-95, 1972.

80. Sprague R: The Acute Cervical Joint Lock. Phys Ther 63:1439-1444, Sept 1983.

81. Tabary J, et al: Experimental Rapid Sarcomere Loss in Concomittant Hypoextensibility. Muscle Nerve 4:198-203, 1981.

82. Tabary J, et al: Physiological and Structure Changes in the Cat's Soleus Muscle Due to Immobilization by Plaster Casts. Joul Physiol 224:231-244, 1972.

83. Teplick J and Haskin M: Spontaneous Regression of Herniated Nucleus Pulposis. AJNR 6:331-335, May/June 1985.

84. Toby EB and Koman LA: Thoracic Outlet Compression Syndrome. In Nerve Compression Syndromes. RM Szabo, ed. Slack, Thorofare, London 1989.

85. Travell J and Simons D: Myofascial Pain and Dysfunction - The Trigger Point Manual. Vol 2. Williams and Wilkins. Baltimore MD 1992.

86. Turck S: Orthopædics. 2nd edition. Lippincott, Philadelphia PA 1967.

87. Turk D and Flor H: Etiological Theories and Treatments for Chronic Back Pain II: Psychological Models and Interventions. Pain 19:209-233, 1984.

88. Waddell G, et al: Failed Lumbar Disc Surgery and Repeat Surgery Following Industrial Injury. JBJS 61A(2):201-207, March 1979.

89. Waitz E: The Lateral Bending Sign. Spine 6:388-397, 1981.

90. Weisel S et al: A Study of Computer-Assisted Tomography - The Incidence of Positive CAT Scans in an Asymptomatic Group of Patients. Spine 9(6):549-551, 1984.

91. White A and Gordon S: Idiopathic Low Back Pain. Spine 7:141-149, 1982.

92. White A and Panjabi M: Clinical Biomechanics of the Spine, 2nd edition. Lippincott, Philadelphia PA 1990.

93. Witt I, et al: A Comparative Analysis of X-ray Findings of the Lumbar Spine in Patients With and Without Lumbar Pain. Spine 9:298-299, 1984.

94. Wyke B: The Neurological Basis of Thoracic Spinal Pain. Rheumatology and Physical Medicine 10:356-367, 1970.

CHAPTER 6

TREATMENT OF THE SPINE BY PROBLEM

INTRODUCTION

In Chapter 5, treatment of the spine by diagnosis was discussed. This treatment philosophy is founded on the assumption that all spinal signs and symptoms can be traced to distinct pathological processes. A diagnosis is made and the pathological entity is treated with a regime designed to resolve the pathology. The approach of treating the spine by diagnosis is ideal and often works well; however, clinical experience has shown there are situations in which this approach is not successful.

Every clinician is confronted with those patients who have a clear-cut diagnosis for which a particular treatment regime should work; however, for one reason or another, the patient does not respond as expected. Also a clinician sometimes finds a patient who presents with signs and symptoms that do not fit any particular diagnosis. If the clinician's only approach was to treat by diagnosis, he or she would often be frustrated, and many patients would not be helped.

Many patients who do not present with a clear pathological entity do present with easily identifiable problems such as pain, decreased soft tissue or joint mobility, abnormal posture and muscle weakness. When treatment is directed toward resolution of these problems, the signs and symptoms often disappear. In retrospect, one could conclude that the pathology (whatever it was) was properly treated by addressing the problems. This chapter is devoted to discussing some of these problems and how to treat them.

When the particular musculoskeletal pathology cannot be clearly diagnosed, the clinician must at least

make sure the patient's signs and symptoms are musculoskeletal in nature before embarking on a treatment plan. Certain occurrences are clues the patient's complaints are not musculoskeletal. When the following circumstances are observed, the therapist should consult with the patient's physician before attempting treatment.

1. Symptoms increase with rest and during the night.

2. Symptoms are not associated with movement or body position.

3. Symptoms cover large, non-specific areas, or an unusual area not normally associated with musculoskeletal pathology.

4. Symptoms migrate from one joint to another.

5. The patient has a history of serious illness, especially cancer, or symptoms of serious illness such as fever, weight loss, etc.

6. The patient does not respond at all or as expected to a short trial of conservative treatment.

In this chapter, ten specific problems, a summary of their subjective and objective findings and their suggested treatments will be discussed:

Problem #1: Pain, Muscle Guarding, Spasm and Inflammation

Problem #2: Soft Tissue Hypomobility and General Stiffness

Problem #3: Joint Hypermobility (Joint Instability)

Problem #4: Poor Posture

Problem #5: Poor Body Mechanics

Problem #6: Poor Ergonomic Conditions

Problem #7: Poor Physical Condition

Problem #8: Poor Health Habits

Problem #9: Poor Mental Condition

Problem #10: Abnormal Function

PROBLEM #1:
PAIN, MUSCLE GUARDING, SPASM AND INFLAMMATION

Mechanical injuries and/or inflammatory processes often cause pain, muscle guarding, muscle spasm and other symptoms. Regardless of their underlying cause, treatment of these symptoms may be necessary to promote healing. As discussed in Chapter 3, Principles of Spinal Evaluation and Treatment, a complete evaluation may not be possible the first day the therapist examines the patient. The pain and muscle guarding may be severe enough to interfere with a thorough evaluation. It is quite acceptable for the therapist to begin treating the symptoms before the underlying pathology is determined, as long as the therapist reassesses the patient's condition as soon as the initial symptoms are under control.

Sometimes, the patient's symptoms are relieved entirely before the therapist ever finds the true source of the symptoms. This is acceptable as well. It is not always necessary for the therapist to know whether the pain is coming from the joint capsule, ligaments, disc or muscle, as long as the patient improves and normal posture, mobility, strength and function are restored.

Findings

The patient's main complaint will be of pain, sometimes of an incapacitating nature. A positive weight shift test is indicative of spasm or guarding. Palpable tension or nodules in the paraspinals or interscapular muscles is often seen. Inflammation will sometimes cause the skin to be warm to the touch. Cold, clammy skin is sometimes seen when the patient is experiencing acute symptoms. A unilateral difference in tissue tension and temperature is often palpated.

Treatment

Immobilization and rest for short periods may be necessary to help the patient avoid activities that injure healing tissue; aggravate the pain, guarding or inflammation; or which inhibit the healing process. Immobilization and rest may take the form of bed rest; activity restrictions; positions of comfort; supportive braces; and corsets or cervical collars.

Attitudes have changed considerably in the past few years about the benefits and dangers of bedrest and immobilization. We no longer require prolonged bedrest after childbirth and surgery or strict immobilization for several weeks with certain fractures. All of this has changed because we now realize excessive bedrest and immobilization delays healing while promoting depression, weakness, and deconditioning . On the other hand, exercise and activity generally promote healing, strength and a positive mental outlook. Only in the past few years have practitioners begun to see these benefits for their back patients; many still have that lesson to learn. Recent attitudes are encouraging, however, because many respected sources[4, 11, 21] are now advocating the use of bedrest only in cases of severe symptoms, and then for no more than two days at a time without reassessment. Even when bedrest is prescribed, most patients should get out of bed and move about frequently (every two to four hours).

Modality therapies and medications have long been used for relief of pain and muscle spasm. The various forms of heat and cold are usually effective. Ice should be used initially in the case of acute trauma. Electrotherapy and massage are often useful to promote healing. Modalities reducing edema, promoting circulation and stimulating cellular activity all speed the healing of irritated tissue and promote relaxation of muscle guarding and spasm.

When the possibility of disruption of healing tissue is no longer an issue, joint or soft tissue mobilization often relieves pain effectively. The techniques employed usually consist of gentle traction and/or graded movement in the pain free range.

Soft tissue techniques used can consist of myofascial release, muscle energy techniques, or other soft tissue mobilization or stretching techniques. Techniques involving the active participation of the patient and incorporating functional movements are preferred to those that are entirely passive. [8, 25, 26]

PROBLEM #2:
SOFT TISSUE HYPOMOBILITY AND GENERAL STIFFNESS

Adaptive Muscle Shortening

Any skeletal muscle has a given number of sarcomeres at its normal resting length. The muscle can adaptively add or subtract sarcomeres at the musculotendinous junction, thus increasing or decreasing length according to the stresses placed on it. This is a normal, non-pathological response that begins shortly after the new position is introduced. For example, the biceps will adaptively shorten when the elbow is casted for a fracture (sarcomere subtraction). Additionally, within one to two weeks, the collagen fibers of the connective tissue will adaptively shorten and thicken. Following cast removal, the biceps must lengthen (add sarcomeres) and the collagen fibers must be stretched for the biceps to regain normal resting length.[26]

Similarly, postural and structural changes that can lead to adaptive changes in the muscle often occur in response to injury, working position or habits. For example, one usually sees the forward head, slumped posture develop secondary to cervical injuries or in relation to an occupation requiring prolonged sitting. The muscles in the upper back, chest and neck soon adapt to the new posture. Another example is adaptive shortening of the lumbar spinal muscles secondary to hyperlordosis or sway back. Adaptive shortening of muscles may also occur if normal range of joint mobility is lost. Thus, the physical therapist must always take into account the possibility of adaptive muscle shortening when treating patients with postural changes or restricted joint motion.

Adaptive Changes of the Intervertebral Joint Complex Related to Joint Hypomobility

When many therapists speak of joint hypomobility, they tend to forget the entire joint complex is involved. Hypomobility involves adaptive changes in muscular, ligamentous and joint tissue.[8, 16, 25, 26] For this reason, adaptive muscular or soft tissue changes and joint hypomobility should really be thought of as the same condition or a continuation of a progressive condition.

Joint hypomobility is a disorder generally involving the entire spinal segment and is the result of prolonged immobilization, usually secondary to injury, poor posture or inactivity. The facet joint capsule, the disc, the supporting ligaments or any combination of the above may be the primary site of restriction. Joint hypomobility may be due to molecular binding of the collagen fibers within the joint capsule, adhesions or scarring of the surrounding soft tissue following injury[6] (Fig 6-1). It may result following acute sprain if normal mobility and posture are not restored as healing occurs. Hypomobility may occur during and following episodes of disc herniation when certain movements are restricted and/or when scar tissue is laid down to repair the annular defect, or may simply be the result of prolonged poor posture, faulty working positions and general inactivity.

When joint hypomobility occurs over time as the result of habitual activities and postures, the joint(s) may be normal or hypermobile in one or more directions, but hypomobile in another direction. A classic example would be a person whose occupation involves standing stooped at a bench all day. The person's thoracic spine may flex quite well, because he or she is used to rounding the shoulders and flexing the spine at work. Over time, however, the joints of the thoracic spine may lose their ability to extend, especially if the person is relatively sedentary at home. In general, joint hypomobility can lead to early degenerative change, or predispose the patient to further injury.

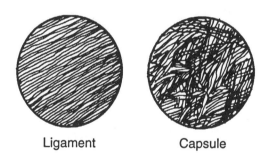

Ligament   Capsule

Figure 6-1. Collagen fibers are arranged in parallel in ligaments and irregularly in joint capsules. The irregular arrangement allows greater mobility. Tissue mobility is soon lost if joints are immobilized because the collagen fibers bind together easily.

William Kirkaldy-Willis[17] describes degenerative changes that occur in the entire intervertebral joint complex, including the muscle, synovium, articular cartilage, capsule and disc. Posterior joint changes produce a reaction on the disc and vice versa. For example, synovitis and a minor facet joint sprain may result in protective guarding, which leads to hypomobility, which in turn produces degenerative changes in the annulus of the disc. As the dysfunction becomes more severe, radial tears in the annulus may form, and a disc bulge can occur. Of course, the adaptive muscular changes described above occur as well.

Findings

As discussed above, muscular length and strength imbalances are often seen in combination with joint hypomobility. For example, in the case of cervical joint hypomobility, interscapular muscles may be stretched and weak, while suboccipital muscles, scalenes and pectoralis muscles are tight. Palpable muscle changes such as areas of ropiness or trigger points may be felt. Mobility tests will reveal a limitation of active and passive movement at the involved segments.

Joint hypomobility may be specific to one or two segments, or may be general, throughout an entire spinal area. The involved levels will be tender to palpation. The tenderness may involve only the interspinous space and facet joints, or it may involve the surrounding soft tissue as well. Pain may be referred and is usually unilateral. As with all joint problems, pain is associated with movement and is noticed especially at the end of available range. Lab findings and routine x-rays will initially be normal. Prolonged segmental hypomobility may lead to degeneration of both the disc and the facets, with pathology becoming evident on x-ray.[17] As with other soft tissue problems, there will be no true neurological signs.

Treatment

Treatment of adaptive changes of the intervertebral joint complex should be directed specifically to the tissues that have undergone the adaptive changes. As discussed above, these changes can involve the muscle tissue, noncontractile tissue, or both.

Treatment of adaptive muscle length changes is most effectively accomplished by emphasizing normal physiological function (active exercises) rather than passive stretching or other techniques.[8, 25, 26] Some of the soft tissue mobilization techniques available, such as myofascial release, can be very useful. However, such techniques should be considered adjunctive to more active forms of therapy. A thorough evaluation is the key to choosing appropriate treatment techniques.

When treating adaptive muscle shortening, one should concurrently treat the joint hypomobility and any structural or postural changes that may be present. It is important to get the patient on an active exercise program as soon as possible in the treatment program.

Emphasis on return to activities of daily living such as walking, work and general fitness exercise is very important. Active exercises can be done in short arcs of motion or isometrically if the patient's primary disorder is aggravated by exercising through the entire range of motion. At any rate, muscles need to be exercised functionally as soon as the condition of the primary disorder allows.

When the patient presents with joint hypomobility, joint mobilization should be used. The earlier mobilization is instituted, the more beneficial it can be, provided it is done without aggravating any concomitant soft tissue injury. Mobilization can take many forms. When one thinks of mobilization, the manual therapist, osteopath or chiropractor comes to mind. Exercise, traction and posture correction are also forms of mobilization, however. Ultrasound loosens stiff soft tissue and can be beneficial when used in combination with mobilization. Ice is often helpful following mobilization to prevent mild inflammation or soreness caused by the mobilization. Ultrasound or other modalities alone are not beneficial, but when combined with exercise and mobilization they are effective adjuncts to treatment. Modalities can be overdone, and caution should be used in applying multiple modalities for pain relief, especially after the first few sessions. The patient must be educated that hypomobility is the main cause of the problem, and restoration of mobility must be the treatment focus.

Methods used to restore mobility can be general or specific. Exercise and traction tend to be more general, whereas some of the mobilization techniques discussed in Chapter 9, Mobilization Techniques, can be more specific. The key to successful treatment is a thorough evaluation, as the therapist must know exactly what type of mobilization technique or exercise program to prescribe.

PROBLEM #3: JOINT HYPERMOBILITY (JOINT INSTABILITY)

Joint hypermobility usually involves the entire spinal segment and may be the result of postural problems, congenital defects, severe trauma such as whiplash, over treatment by manipulation or excessive stretching related to certain sports (gymnastics, dancing). Spondylolisthesis is sometimes hypermobile. Sacroiliac hypermobility often develops with pregnancy. Joint hypermobility, like hypomobility, can also occur as the result of tissue healing following a sprain injury. If the ligaments or joint capsule are over stretched or torn, instability may result.

Sometimes joint hypermobility develops at the spinal segment above or below a hypomobile or fused joint. Although some manual therapists teach that a stiff joint is always accompanied by a hypermobile joint, in our experience the tendency for this to happen is overstated. Joint hypermobility adjacent to a stiff or fused joint only occurs when the patient resumes a relatively active lifestyle that would normally cause significant movement in the stiff area. In such a case, the stiff joint does not move normally as it should. Because the patient is very active, the adjacent joints move more to compensate for the stiff joint's lack of movement. However, many patient's who have experienced significant spinal injury or surgery naturally self-limit their activities, so the above phenomenon does not occur. In fact, such patients usually suffer more from general stiffness and weakness because of the tendency toward a more sedentary occupation or lifestyle.

Compensatory joint hypermobility is more likely to occur in the cervical spine than in the thoracic and lumbar spine because of the tendency for even sedentary patients to achieve functional motion of the cervical spine after injury. For example, a patient may have a stiff mid and lower cervical spine yet develop hypermobility of the upper cervical spine because it is necessary to regain full rotation mobility to drive a car comfortably. On the other hand, a sedentary patient with a stiff lower lumbar spine may not notice the stiffness because he or she is not challenged with activities of daily living requiring full mobility. That patient will therefore never develop a compensatory hypermobility.

Joint hypermobility can lead to early degenerative change, or predispose the patient to further injury. It can also be a source of pain by itself because of the chronic stress placed on the joint capsule and surrounding soft tissue when the joint is at end range for prolonged periods.

Findings

Patients with joint hypermobility complain of general soreness in the spine with or without referred pain down one or both extremities. They generally cannot maintain positions for more than a few minutes without pain and they feel a need to change positions frequently. Pain usually worsens following increased physical activity. They will often describe a "slipping" sensation or feeling of instability associated with movement.

If joint hypermobility is present, the mobility exam will reveal increased active and passive movement at the involved levels. Mobility x-rays may help reveal an unstable joint. The patient will not have any true neurological signs unless the condition is so severe that the bony structure is impinging on a nerve root.

There is evidence that joint hypermobility can lead to joint/disc degeneration due to changes in biomechanical stresses and the increased stress and wear and tear placed on the joint during activity.[9, 16, 24]

Treatment

Patient education and exercise are the keys to treatment of the patient with joint hypermobility. Strengthening exercises for the muscles around a hypermobile joint can give support to the joint. The stabilization exercises described in Chapter 12, Exercise, are particularly helpful. The patient must learn corrective posture, and should be taught to avoid positions or activities that place the joint(s) at extremes of range of motion. Spinal orthoses are helpful, especially in an acute phase of discomfort. Patient compliance with the long term use of corsets or supports is often poor. Furthermore, back supports promoting inactivity should be discouraged because strengthening and stabilization should be emphasized. A more active back support is more practical for prolonged use, and since it encourages activity, it is not contraindicated (see Figures 11-14 and 11-16 in Chapter 11, Spinal Orthoses). The patient must be taught that using a back support does not replace proper exercise and posture principles.

PROBLEM #4:
POOR POSTURE

Poor posture contributes to many types of spinal disorders. In many cases, postural correction will be a primary treatment consideration. True postural strain syndromes fall into three categories: l) lumbar flexion; 2) lumbar extension; and 3) forward head syndrome.

Lumbar Flexion Syndrome

Findings

The lumbar flexion syndrome (flat back) is characterized by the patient who slumps with a flattened lumbar spine while sitting or standing. Working postures often contribute to this disorder. Consider, for example, the secretary who slumps over the desk, or the bench worker who stands slightly bent forward at his or her work. Tight hamstring muscles may also contribute to this syndrome.

Pain is intermittent and only comes on after being in a flexed postural position for a time. Sitting usually hurts more than standing. Coming to the standing position after prolonged sitting is especially painful and difficult. Changing posture or position usually brings relief. Ligaments maintained under prolonged tension will adaptively lengthen. Thus, the ligaments stabilizing the spine in flexion (posterior longitudinal ligament, supraspinous and interspinous ligaments) are all subject to stretch. If once stretched beyond normal resting lengths, support for the facet joints and disc is lessened. Pain arising from the ligaments or posterior annulus is often bilateral and may refer symptoms to the extremities. Patients with lumbar flexion syndrome are usually pain free after resting at night. Bilateral backache is the chief complaint but leg ache may also be present. Initially, full mobility is present but prolonged maintenance of these postures will eventually lead to a loss of lumbar extension. This situation often leads to disc herniation because of increased intradiscal pressure resulting from the flexed posture and the tendency for flexion to displace the nucleus posteriorly.[15, 18, 22]

Treatment

Treatment consists of avoiding prolonged sitting and standing unless maintaining a lumbar lordosis. A lumbar pillow or roll placed against the lumbar spine will help maintain the lumbar lordosis while sitting (Fig 6-2). Hamstring stretching and lumbar stretching and strengthening exercises are often necessary to maintain full range of motion in extension and to strengthen the back muscles. If the poor posture is work related, it may be necessary to raise the work area so the patient can stand or sit with a normal lordosis as he or she works. Since one cannot always eliminate all stressful postural positions from daily routines, it is essential the stressful positions be interrupted or changed frequently when they are a necessary part of the patient's daily activities.

Lumbar Extension Syndrome

Findings

The lumbar extension syndrome (hyperlordosis) is characterized by the complaint of a dull backache that comes on after prolonged standing. Standing usually hurts more than sitting. The pain often covers a large non-specific area. There is often a leg ache in one or both legs. The patient actually slumps into lumbar extension while standing by "hanging" on the anterior hip ligaments (Fig 6-3). He or she will often have tight hip flexor muscles and weak abdominal muscles. A large, protruding abdomen, as with obesity or pregnancy, adds to the strain. In cases of prolonged excessive lordosis, adaptive shortening of the posterior spinal musculature and ligaments occurs and flexion may become restricted. As with other postural problems, the patient will get relief by changing the

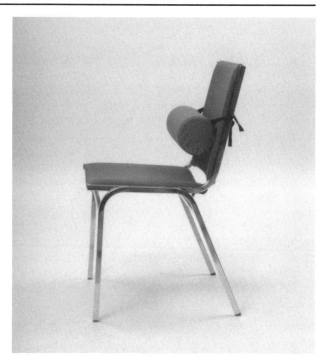

Figure 6-2. Lumbar roll to encourage normal sitting posture.

poor postural position. Rest and recumbency will relieve and the patient is usually asymptomatic in the morning with a gradual return of symptoms during the day. This patient is often younger and hypermobile. The level of physical fitness seen in this type of patient may vary from very athletic to very sedentary. The pregnant woman often suffers from this syndrome.

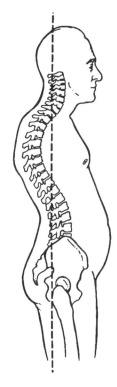

Figure 6-3. Lumbar extension syndrome (hyperlordosis).

Treatment

Treatment consists of postural correction, exercises to stretch the hip flexor muscles and the posterior aspects of the spinal segment and abdominal muscle strengthening. Severe cases may require a corrective support. If prolonged standing is necessary, resting one foot on a small stool may be helpful. Frequently changing the stressful postural position is essential when it cannot be eliminated from the patient's daily activities.

In either the flexion or extension syndrome, it is the extreme, often prolonged posture that creates difficulty. It is a sad fact that many medical practitioners have prescribed the routine use of one set of exercises (i.e., Williams's flexion) or one often ineffective method of postural correction (i.e., pelvic tilt) to treat essentially opposite postural syndromes. If one is to avoid this type of "cookbook" approach, it is essential that the problem first be properly assessed and those principles of treatment applicable to the situation be knowledgeably applied.

Forward Head Syndrome

As previously discussed, it is often difficult to determine the exact pathological process involved when treating a patient with spinal pain. This is especially true with cervical and upper thoracic problems. Postural change is often the only objective evidence one has to base treatment upon. Clinical experience teaches that almost every patient seen with neck pain has poor posture and it is usually some degree of the forward head posture syndrome. Experience also teaches that when poor posture is corrected with patient education and exercise, the patient usually has symptom relief. In this case, the treatment is correct and the patient gets well, yet the therapist never knows what the exact pathology was. As previously mentioned, there is nothing wrong with this approach to treatment. In fact, it may be the only reasonable approach available in some cases.

Findings

In the forward head postural syndrome, the upper cervical spine is extended while the lower cervical and upper thoracic spine is relatively flexed. Additionally, forward head posture is usually accompanied by rounded shoulders; slumped sitting; weakness of upper back muscles; tightness of anterior chest and upper cervical muscles; and abduction of the scapulae (Fig 6-4).

When the head is held in the forward position, there is considerably more weight and tension exerted at the base of the cervical spine. Normally, the bony structures of the neck should act as a weight bearing column and simply transfer the weight of the head to the base of the cervical spine. In the forward head posture, however, the neck acts as a lever arm, causing a torque force at the base of the cervical spine.

Treatment

Treatment of forward head postural syndrome depends on its cause. There are four instances when the forward head posture is seen:

1. The forward head posture may result secondary to or concurrent with either the lumbar flexion or the lumbar extension syndromes.

When forward head posture results as a secondary or concurrent response to lumbar postural problems, treatment of the primary lumbar problem, appropriate spinal strengthening and general physical fitness exercises are all indicated.

2. The forward head posture may result from the development of joint or muscular tightness in the upper cervical spine due to muscular tension or poor ergonomic factors. Because of muscular tension or awkward positions, the upper cervical spine tilts more and more into extension. As this occurs, the lower cervical and upper thoracic spine is flexed to keep the eyes level. Squinting and shoulder elevation often accompany this syndrome.

Treatment in this case consists of mobilization and stretching (traction) of the upper cervical spine and postural training. Relaxation and biofeedback training may be necessary, as many patients do not realize they are "tensing up" and inadvertently causing the suboccipital muscle tightness. If awkward working positions are contributing to the muscular tension, the ergonomic or body mechanics factors need to be addressed as well.

3. The forward head posture may result from weakness of the lower cervical, upper thoracic and

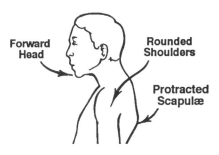

Figure 6-4. Forward head posture.

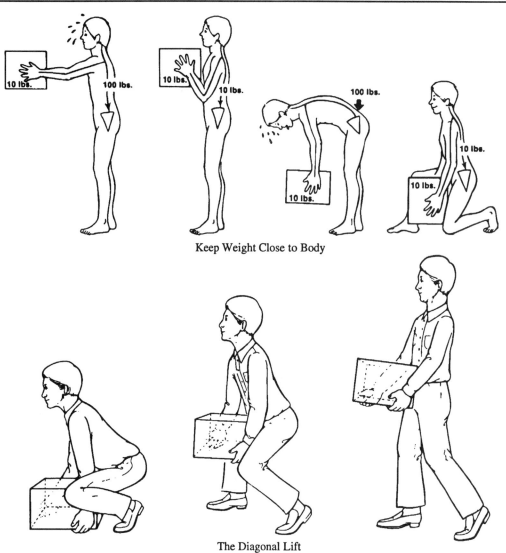

Keep Weight Close to Body

The Diagonal Lift
Squat, Head Up, Back Arched, Feet Spread, One Foot Ahead As You Lift

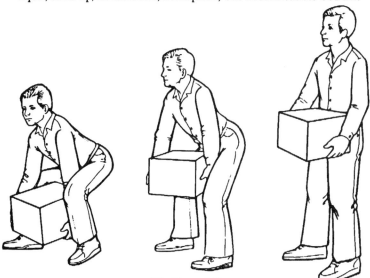

The Power Lift
Partial Squat, Head Up, Back Arched, Feet Spread, One Foot Ahead As You Lift

Figure 6-5. Examples of proper and improper body mechanics.

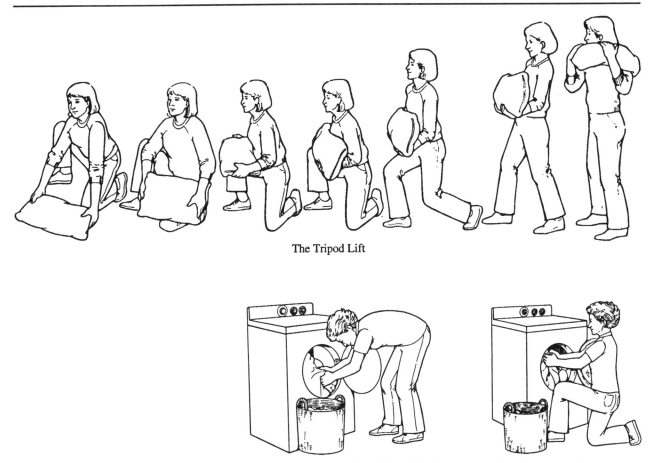

The Tripod Lift

Kneel When Working in a Low Position

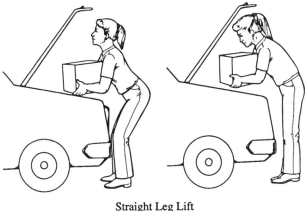

Straight Leg Lift
Bend at the Hips, Not the Back

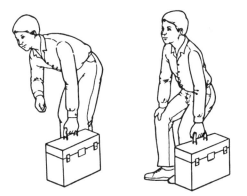

Partial Squat Lift

Figure 6-5 (cont.). Examples of proper and improper body mechanics.

interscapular stabilizing muscles, and tightness of the anterior chest/suboccipital muscles.

Treatment for this problem consists of spinal and interscapular muscle strengthening exercises, anterior chest/suboccipital muscle relaxation and stretching exercises, and postural training.

4. Forward head posture may result from a chronic problem secondary to acute cervical sprain or strain. Because of pain in the acute and sub-acute stages of cervical sprain or strain, the patient is likely to let the cervical spine slump into flexion. If the patient attempts to sit or stand straight with the head held erect, the injured muscles and joints become painful. In time, the muscles become weak and the joints of the lower cervical spine lose extension mobility. At the same time, the upper cervical spine extends to keep the head and eyes level. By the time the precipitating injury has healed, the patient is fixed in the new posture.

Chronic forward head posture causes a strain on the ligaments and muscles in the posterior lower cervical and upper thoracic spine. This syndrome is characterized by generalized, non-specific pain in the neck and upper back, headaches and occasional referred pain into the upper extremities. The upper trapezius, levator scapulæ and rhomboid major muscles are most often involved. A constant state of muscle guarding, spasm, ligamentous stress and generalized inflammation will often cause the patient to believe the original injury has never healed even though many months or years have passed.

Treatment in this case must be directed toward: 1) restoring any loss of flexion mobility in the upper cervical spine and extension mobility in the lower cervical and upper thoracic spine; 2) strengthening the muscles of the posterior cervical, upper thoracic and interscapular areas; 3) stretching the anterior shoulder and chest muscles if they have become adaptively shortened due to the postural changes; and 4) making the patient aware of the correct posture he or she must achieve if treatment is to be successful.

The contributing causes of forward head postural syndrome may not be as clearly defined and specific as outlined above. It is common to see several of these factors involved and it is often difficult to determine which occurred first. Therefore, treatment may need to be directed at more than one area if success is to be expected. Exercises to correct the forward head posture; stretch the anterior shoulder and chest muscles; and strengthen the back, neck and shoulder girdle muscles play a key part in treating the forward head syndrome

regardless of the underlying cause. These exercises are described and pictured in Chapter 12, Exercise.

PROBLEM #5:
POOR BODY MECHANICS

Poor use of body mechanics directly affects other problems a patient may have. For example, constantly bending at the waist when performing functional activities can overstretch spinal ligaments and muscles and contribute to abnormal muscle recruitment and abnormal disc mechanics. Theoretically, this would predispose one to injury. After an episode of back or neck pain, use of improper body mechanics inhibits the normal healing process and can contribute to the development of abnormal posture syndromes, and joint hyper- or hypomobilities. These facts are true whether or not the patient has a labor intensive occupation. For this reason, teaching proper body mechanics cannot be overlooked with any spinal patient.

There is controversy over the definition of proper body mechanics. For lifting, some clinicians promote an anteriorly tilted pelvis with a lordotic lumbar position, while others teach a posterior pelvic tilt. Most clinicians are now teaching a neutral lumbar position. Most clinicians generally agree body mechanics training should be individualized, since what is considered optimal in a normal individual may change in the presence of pathology (Fig 6-5).

When considering whether the use of good body mechanics "comes naturally," one only needs to look to children for the answer (Fig 6-6). The toddler who is just discovering how his or her body moves uses good body mechanics quite easily. His or her spinal range of motion is equal and fluid in flexion, extension, rotation and sidebending. Hip mobility is excellent. All muscles work in harmony to keep him or her from toppling over. The child bends naturally from the hips rather than the low back. Sitting posture is enviable. The child does not begin to break these good habits until later, when he or she develops a more sedentary or specialized lifestyle. When the child begins to attend school, the spine begins to flex more than it extends. The child's legs do not get as much exercise, so he or she begins to bend over because bending expends less energy than squatting. When the child reaches adulthood, he or she may choose an occupation and hobbies that do not promote spinal balance. When considering all of these factors, it is no wonder many humans learn to use their bodies incorrectly. It can easily be argued that, at least initially, good body mechanics do come naturally!

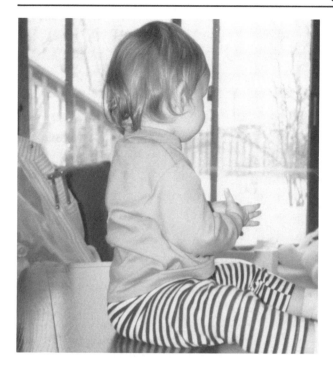
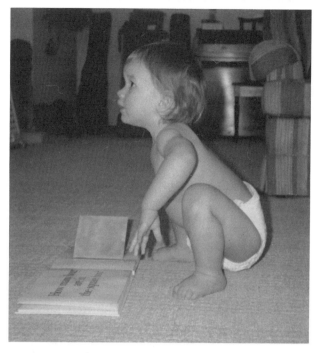

Figure 6-6. A toddler naturally uses good posture and body mechanics techniques.

Treatment

The physical therapist must be skilled at evaluating each patient's individual circumstances. An individual body mechanics training program must be designed for each patient. Techniques for lifting, bending and reaching should be taught to all patients, since nearly everyone must perform these activities to some extent during an average day. The patient should be quizzed about other significant activities. Often, a patient will not realize a simple activity that does not cause pain can be problematic. For example, a patient may think lifting is the main issue when repetitive and prolonged bending is just as important (Fig 6-7). Body mechanics training should begin the first day of treatment, as any treatment performed in the clinic can be counteracted by the harmful effects of poor body mechanics at home.

PROBLEM #6:
POOR ERGONOMIC CONDITIONS

The significant injury recurrence rates observed after some patients return to work indicates ergonomic factors cannot be ignored. Worker behaviors and/or work station or job design problems often need to be addressed to completely resolve the patient's musculoskeletal problems. As discussed in Chapter 4, Evaluation of the Spine, the physical therapist's initial evaluation must include a detailed discussion of the patient's work and home activities, both of which can be direct or indirect causes of the patient's problem.

The therapist should teach the patient basic ergonomic principles so the patient can conduct his or her own "common sense" ergonomic evaluation. The patient and therapist can discuss and demonstrate problem-solving techniques or changes in the work place. In some cases, the physical therapist should perform a job site evaluation to help the patient and the employer develop a solution to more complex problems.

Please note that employer cooperation varies with individual circumstances. Sometimes, the therapist must be very tactful when approaching a change. Likewise, the therapist should be sensitive to the fact that the employer may not be able to make a change because of logistic or economic considerations. The employer is sometimes more motivated to make a positive change for a patient who is off work with a workers' compensation claim, to get that patient back to work. The employer may not be as motivated to make a change in a non-workers' compensation case because, until recently, there was little incentive to do so. However, with the recent enactment of the Americans with Disabilities Act (1992), more employers will become aware of the need to accommodate disabled individuals by changing their work environment.

PROBLEM #7:
POOR PHYSICAL CONDITION

Sometimes it is difficult to find objective problems in the person complaining of spinal pain. This is particularly true of patients complaining of intermittent, non-severe episodes of pain. The patient's joints may move fairly symmetrically, and no particular muscle group seems to be involved. However, the patient is generally in poor physical condition and leads a fairly sedentary lifestyle. The patient initially may have had a significant injury, after which the pre-injury physical condition was not restored. With such a patient, improvement of general physical fitness is the key. More and more evidence is linking general physical fitness to neck and back fitness. For example, a study by Cady, et. al., found firefighters who were fit had significantly fewer episodes of back pain than those who were unfit.[7] Other similar studies can be found in the literature.[1,2,3,5,13,23] Lack of fitness is often seen in conjunction with poor posture, joint hypomobility and poor use of body mechanics. All of these items should be addressed, but simply improving general physical fitness may simultaneously improve the other factors.

Treatment

One of the bigger challenges the therapist faces is encouraging patients to change their lifestyles. The patient must often begin exercise in the clinic because a positive, supportive environment may help motivate the slow starter. Ultimately, however, the patient must take responsibility for self-management of his or her condition. While verbally encouraging self-responsibility, the therapist must avoid inadvertently giving the patient a mixed message. The therapist should avoid the following:

1) Overusing modalities for pain relief. The therapist absolutely must convince the patient that the exercise, posture and lifestyle changes are helping — not the ultrasound and massage!

2) Under-explaining the role of physical fitness. The therapist must be a cheerleader. Quoting statistics and studies about exercise, such as the firefighter study above, can often be helpful.

3) Giving the patient too many exercises to perform. The therapist should become skilled at determining how much each patient is willing to participate in his or her own recovery. If the patient is only willing to invest five minutes per day, it will not help to give him or her a 20 minute exercise program. The therapist should let the patient know that he or she will only be asked to perform those exercises essential to having a healthy back.

4) Giving the patient a pre-printed exercise sheet. When a patient is given a standard handout of exercises titled, "Exercises for Back Patients," he or she does not feel that they have been designed specially for him. This does not mean standard exercise diagrams cannot be used, but it should be clear to the patient that the therapist designed a special exercise program specific to his or her problem.

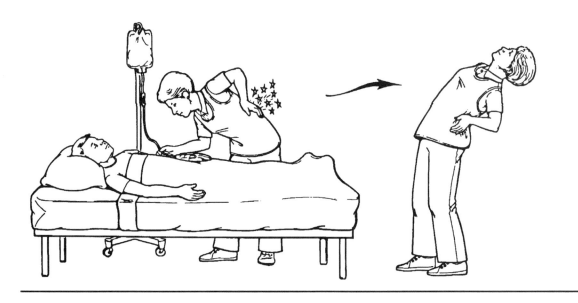

Figure 6-7. Avoiding or interrupting prolonged or repetitive positions is as important as using proper lifting techniques.

5) Using special equipment not available to the patient elsewhere. If the common sense principles explained in this book are followed, the patient should not need specialized equipment to rehabilitate a spinal problem. The therapist should use equipment such as freeweights, mats and elastic tubing, and should emphasize performing ærobic activities that can be performed at home, such as walking. Persistence, not high technology, is the key.

PROBLEM #8:
POOR HEALTH HABITS

There is considerable evidence now that unhealthy living habits contribute to back pain. Deyo and Bass[10] demonstrated a significant relationship between body weight, smoking and decreased physical activity and the occurrence of low back pain. McFadden[18] also has shown adverse effects of cigarette smoking. We know general health habits such as diet and rest have considerable effect on illness, specifically on healing disease and injury.[10, 12, 15, 19] The exact effect an unhealthy lifestyle has on an existing back injury has not been thoroughly studied scientifically. However, one could conclude from the evidence that practicing healthy lifestyle habits is an important etiological factor for prevention and treatment of back pain.

PROBLEM #9:
POOR MENTAL CONDITION

The role of mental fitness and its effect on back injuries cannot be ignored. Stress, emotional problems, chemical dependency and lack of job satisfaction are just a few of the many factors that can influence a patient's response to symptoms and treatment.[4, 20]

Treatment

Treating psychological problems is not within the scope of a physical therapist's training. However, the therapist must be aware that the existence of psychosocial problems will influence the effects of treatment. Some physical therapists make the mistake of continuing to treat a psychosocial problem as though it is purely physical in nature. Such treatment is not helpful to the patient and can be harmful because it prevents the patient from addressing the other issues. As physical therapists, our role is to treat physical problems. Improving the patient's symptoms and general physical condition can relieve stress. Teaching self-management techniques can impart a feeling of confidence and control in a patient who feels that he or she has lost it. However, when we have done all we can from a physical perspective, we should not be afraid to admit we do not have all the answers and refer the patient to appropriate sources or to his or her primary physician.

PROBLEM #10:
ABNORMAL FUNCTION

Treatment to restore active function is the most important part of practicing orthopædic physical therapy. All other treatment goals, such as relieving pain or reducing abnormal anatomy and physiology, are important because these things interfere with normal function. Treating these other factors often improves function naturally, because as the patient feels and moves better, his or her function normalizes. In some cases, however, physical therapists and other medical practitioners are unable to relieve pain and restore normal anatomy and physiology. Every experienced clinician has met patients who simply cannot be "cured" with current medical techniques. The goal of treatment for these patients is restoration of function. Regardless of the patient's level of pain or disability, function can almost always be improved.

Treatment

Patient education is the key to restoring function. The patient must understand and accept the goals of treatment, even when they fall short of his or her initial expectations. Often it is hard for a patient to accept that functional improvement - not pain relief - is the only realistic goal. Exercise is also essential. Exercises chosen for the patient should be those which are directly related to restoration of function. Some of the exercise and functional restoration techniques go beyond the scope of this text. Work hardening and chronic pain programs are often necessary because they address more factors than a physical therapist alone can address. These factors often include psychosocial issues, vocational issues and family issues. Functional restoration is discussed in greater detail in Chapter 13, Spinal Rehabilitation.

SUMMARY

The philosophy of treating a patient's identifiable problems can often be very successful, even if a particular pathological entity is never identified as the source of the patient's problems. Even when a definitive diagnosis is made, patients do not all respond the same to treatments that usually work for a particular diagnosis. The therapist should never hesitate to use a common sense approach when treating a patient's musculoskeletal disorder. An overly analytical "cookbook" approach can never be superior to an approach using sound thinking and good clinical decision making.

REFERENCES

1. Anderson C: Physical Ability Testing as a Means to Reduce Injuries in Grocery Warehouses. International Joul of Retail and Distribution Management 19(7):33-35, Nov/Dec 1991.

2. Anderson C: Preplacement Screening: Survival of the Fittest. Risk Management 44-46, Nov 1987.

3. Biering-Sorenson F: Physical Measurements as Risk Indicators for Low Back Trouble Over a One-Year Period. Spine 9:106-119, 1984.

4. Bigos S, et al: Back Injuries in Industry: A Retrospective Study III: Employee Related Factors. Spine 11:252-256, 1986.

5. Boyer M and Vaccaro B: The Benefits of Physically Active Workforce: An Organizational Perspective. Occupational Medicine 5:691-706, 1990.

6. Burkart S: Personal Communications. Physical Therapy Department, University of West Virginia, Morgantown WV 1983.

7. Cady L et al: Strength and Fitness and Subsequent Back Injuries in Firefighters. Joul of Occ Med 21:269-272, 1979.

8. Cummings G: Proceedings of the Ninth Annual Dogwood Conference. Dogwood Institute, Alpharetta GA 1984.

9. Cyriax J: Diagnosis of Soft Tissue Lesions. Textbook of Orthopædic Medicine, Vol 1, 8th edition. Bailliere-Tindall, London 1982.

10. Deyo R and Bass J: Lifestyle and Low Back Pain: The Influence of Smoking and Obesity. Spine 14:501-506, 1989.

11. Deyo R, Diehl A, Rosenthal M: How Many Days Of Bed Rest For Acute Low Back Pain? N Engl J Med 315:1064-1070, 1986.

12. Frymoyer J and Cats-Baril W: Predictors of Low Back Pain Disability. Clin Orthop and Rel Res 221:89-98, 1987.

13. Gilliam T: A Two Year Prospectus: Pre-Employment Physical Capability Testing Study (Unpublished). Injury Reduction Technology, Inc., 110 Streetsboro St W, Suite 2A, Hudson, OH 44236.

14. Kapandji I: Spine. Vol 3 of The Physiology of the Joints, 2nd edition. Churchill-Livingstone, London-New York 1974.

15. Kelsey J: An Epidemiological Study of Acute Herniated Lumbar Intervertebral Discs. Rheumatol Rehabil 14:144, 1975.

16. Kirkaldy-Willis W: The Three Phases of the Spectrum of Degenerative Disease. In Managing Low Back Pain. WH Kirkaldy-Willis and C Burton, eds. Churchill Livingston, New York NY 1992.

17. McFadden J: Cigarette Smoking May Adversely Affect Chemonucleolysis. Orthopædic News 8(2), Mar/Apr 1986.

18. McKenzie R: The Lumbar Spine. Spinal Publications, Waikanae New Zealand 1981.

19. Nachemson A: Exercise, Fitness and Back Pain. In Exercise, Fitness and Health: A Consensus of Current Knowledge. C Bouchard, et al, eds. Human Kinetics Books, Champaign IL 1990.

20. Quazi M: Body and Spirit. Occupational Health and Safety (July 1992) 34-38, 52 and 57.

21. Quebec Task Force Study: Scientific Approach to the Assessment and Management of Activity Related Spinal Disorders. Spine 12:7S, 1987.

22. Schnebel B, et al: A Digitizing Technique for the Study of Movement of Intradiscal Dye in Response to Flexion and Extension of the Lumbar Spine. Spine 13(3):309-312, 1988.

23. Schonfeld B, et al: An Occupational Performance Test Validation Program for Fire Fighters at the Kennedy Space Center. Joul of Occ Med 32:638-643, 1988.

24. Sheon R, et al: The Hypermobility Syndrome. Postgrad Med 71:199-209, 1982.

25. Tabary J, et al: Experimental Rapid Sarcomere Loss in Concomittant Hypoextensibility. Muscle Nerve 4:198-203, 1981.

26. Tabary J, et al: Physiological and Structure Changes in the Cat's Soleus Muscle Due to Immobilization by Plaster Casts. Joul Physiol 224:231-244, 1972.

CHAPTER 7

EVALUATION AND TREATMENT OF PELVIC GIRDLE DYSFUNCTIONS

by Allyn L. Woerman, MMSc PT

INTRODUCTION

This chapter will focus on evaluation and treatment techniques for the most common pelvic girdle dysfunctions. The reader should have an understanding of the basic biomechanical principles and terminology discussed in Chapter 2, Basic Spinal Biomechanics.

To evaluate pelvic girdle dysfunctions properly, the hip joint and the lumbar spine, especially the L5 and L4 segments, must also be assessed. Dysfunction in any of these joints may lead to dysfunction in the others. The influence of the entire kinetic chain on the function of these joints should not be underestimated. Biomechanical problems such as a pronated foot, genu varus/valgus knees, anteverted/retroverted hips, etc., will influence the entire chain.

The treatment techniques described in this chapter are primarily osteopathic in nature and use muscle energy techniques popularized by Fred Mitchell, Sr., DO. The definitive text for this evaluation and treatment scheme is An Evaluation and Treatment Manual of Osteopathic Muscle Energy Procedures.[10]

A muscle energy technique (MET) is a manipulative treatment procedure that uses a voluntary contraction of the patient's muscle against a distinctly controlled counterforce. The contraction is performed from a precise position and in a specific direction. MET's are considered to be active techniques. They require direct positioning (where the motion restriction barrier is engaged but not stressed). MET's may be used to lengthen shortened muscles, strengthen weakened muscles, reduce localized edema, and mobilize restricted joints.[10,15,4,13]

Evaluation of the sacroiliac joints and pelvic complex by the osteopathic system of positional assessment uses a common sense approach that correlates comparable signs. This means that a given dysfunctional lesion will reflect a fairly consistent pattern of findings. When considered together, these findings yield an assessment of the affected segment in three-dimensional space and in relation to adjoining segments. The therapist simply collects the raw data using palpatory and observational skills, correlates the data to a set of signs and symptoms, and formulates an assessment. The therapist then applies a specific technique to the affected segment based on that assessment. It should be kept in mind that each test viewed by itself does not make an assessment. It is only when all the data are collected and correlated that the therapist can make the correct assessment.

SIGNS OF PELVIC GIRDLE DYSFUNCTIONS

The symptoms of pelvic girdle dysfunctions vary.[5,7,10,13,14,15] The pain may be sharp or dull, aching or throbbing, and so forth. The pain is often unilateral and local to the sacroiliac joint (sulcus) itself, but may be referred distally (usually posterolaterally and not below the knee) possibly due to multiple levels of innervation.[12] There are no associated neurological signs with pelvic girdle dysfunction. A straight leg raise test may be positive but only for pain in the joint or the gluteal region and usually in the higher arc above 60°. The pain is usually aggravated by walking and stair climbing and the patient may limp (with Trendelenburg or similar gait pattern). Pain intensity usually does not increase with prolonged sitting; however, when the condition is acute, the patient may sit shifted onto the opposite ischium. The patient often maintains lumbar lordosis or a flat back posture in forward bending, recruiting motion around the acetabula, and may complain of lumbar pain with forward bending. Ipsilateral tension over the erector spinæ muscles may be noted. The therapist may see a slight swelling over the dorsal aspect of the sacrum. Pain may often be present on the non-blocked side (i.e., the dysfunctional side may be non-painful but causing the opposite side to become hypermobile and painful). Finally, sacroiliac pain is more common in females than in the general population.[3]

DIFFERENTIATION OF STRUCTURAL ASYMMETRY

Structural asymmetry is very common, particularly in the lumbosacral spine. If the relative position of comparable anatomic parts (right and left PSIS's, inferior lateral angles of the sacrum, etc.) remains constant through the full flexion-extension range of motion, then the asymmetry is probably due to *structural variation* of the anatomic part and may not be treatable. However, if the relative position of comparable anatomic parts changes in the full flexion-extension range of motion, then the perceived asymmetry is probably due to *functional alteration* of the parts. These are the treatable pelvic dysfunctions.

The therapist must be able to palpate various anatomical landmarks accurately and consistently and be able to relate their relative positions to one another in three-dimensional space. Only then is the therapist able to assess the patient and to test, re-test and evaluate the effects of treatment. The following landmarks are the keys to accurate assessment: iliac crests, anterior superior iliac spines (ASIS), posterior superior iliac spines (PSIS), ischial tuberosities, greater trochanters, medial malleoli, pubic tubercles, sacral inferior lateral angles (ILA), sacral sulci, sacrotuberous and sacrospinous ligaments, piriformis, and tensor fascia latæ.

SUBJECTIVE EXAMINATION OF THE PELVIS

The reader is referred to the Subjective Examination section in Chapter 4, Evaluation of the Spine, for a thorough discussion of important questions to ask the patient with back and leg pain. Additional questions that have particular significance for a suspected pelvic girdle problem are:

1. Have you had a sudden sharp jolt to the leg, e.g., after unexpectedly stepping off a curb? (This is a very common mechanism for innominate rotations, shears, and upslips.)

2. Have you recently fallen directly onto your buttocks? (This is a very common mechanism for innominate rotations, shears, and sacral flexion lesions.)

3. How is the pain affected by sitting, standing, walking, or maintaining a sustained posture? (If pain increases with sitting, then a discogenic etiology is more suspect, especially with radicular pain; if pain increases with standing, then the sacroiliac joint may be implicated, especially if the patient stands unilaterally a great deal; if the pain increases with walking, then the sacroiliac joint is very much implicated, and a sacral torsion is quite likely.)

4. Have you recently experienced a sudden trunk flexion with rotation, e.g., chopping wood or shoveling snow? (This is a common mechanism for sacroiliac joint strain.)

OBJECTIVE EXAMINATION OF THE PELVIS

Evaluation of the sacroiliac joint and pelvis begins the moment the patient enters the office. Observation of gait, and the patient's ability to sit down, stand and bend will give valuable clues about whether the patient's problem is primarily lumbar in nature or from the pelvic girdle. The following outline of clinical testing procedures and their meaning is categorized according to patient position and follows a sequence that will minimize patient position changes.

The assumption is that the reader is performing a comprehensive spinal evaluation. The components of the Objective Examination as listed here are adjunctive to the examination described in Chapter 4, <u>Evaluation of the Spine</u>.

Standing Position

Posture

Make sure the feet are hip width apart and the knees are fully extended. Observe the patient from the anterior, posterior, and lateral aspects for the general postural conditions (i.e., scoliosis, kyphosis, lordosis, protracted shoulders, forward head, slope of waist, distances of arms from sides).

Iliac Crest Height

Iliac crest height is best observed by using the radial borders of the index fingers and the web spaces of the hands to push the soft tissue up and medially out of the way, and then pushing down on each crest with equal pressure (Fig 7-1). The clinician's eyes must be in the same plane as his or her hands to assess whether or one side is more caudad or cephalad than the other. This method quite accurately and precisely detects leg length discrepancies.[2] If an asymmetry is found, a lift of appropriate dimension should be placed under the short side before any of the other standing position motion tests are executed. The lift can provide pelvic balance and muscle tone symmetry before testing motion. Placing a lift under the foot is appropriate

whether the asymmetry is due to a structural or functional leg length discrepancy.

Posterior Superior Iliac Spine Position

In the standing position, localization of the PSIS's is very important. An assessment should be made about the relative superoinferior and mediolateral relationships. This may be done with the ulnar borders of the thumbs or the tips of the index fingers by hooking them under the inferior aspect to the posterior spine. The clinician must be at eye level with the PSIS's to make an accurate assessment (Fig 7-2).

Anterior Superior Iliac Spine Position

As with the PSIS, the relative superoinferior and mediolateral relationships of the ASIS's must be assessed. This may be done from behind the patient with the clinician's arms extended (Fig 7-3) or from the front by visual inspection and palpation with the thumb (Fig 7-4).

Trochanteric Levels

Trochanteric levels are palpated using the same method as for the iliac crests, with the radial borders of the index fingers and the web spaces resting on the tops of the greater trochanters (Fig 7-5). Levelness here and unlevelness at the iliacs indicate pelvic dysfunctions producing an apparent leg length discrepancy. Unlevelness here indicates a structural leg length discrepancy below the femoral neck level.

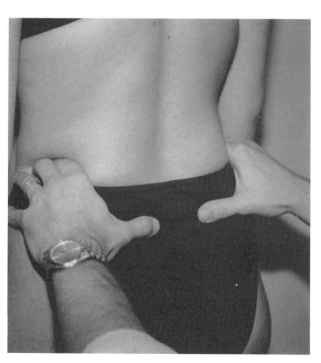

Figure 7-1. Checking iliac crest height.

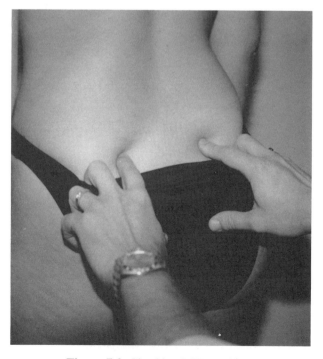

Figure 7-2. Checking PSIS position.

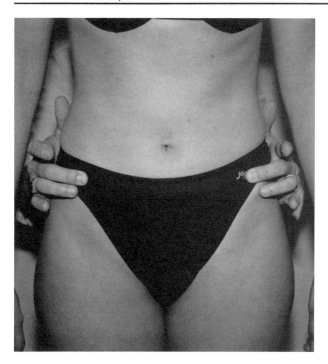

Figure 7-3. Checking ASIS position from behind the patient.

Gait

Observe the patient's gait pattern. Frequently, a pelvic girdle dysfunction produces a Trendelenburg gait or a gluteus maximus gait. The patient may sidebend the trunk away from the affected side, walk with difficulty or may limp.

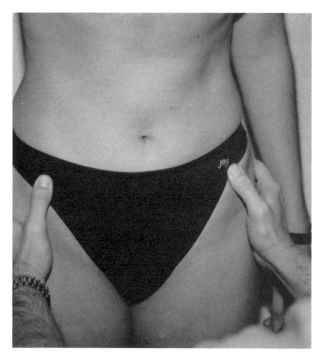

Figure 7-4. Checking ASIS position from in front of the patient.

Standing Flexion Test

The standing flexion test of iliosacral motion is used to help the therapist determine the type of dysfunction and the side of involvement. For example, if the standing flexion test is positive on the left, it tells the clinician that a left-sided iliosacral problem may be present (see further discussion under Sitting Flexion Test).

The standing flexion test is accomplished by localizing the PSIS's, and noting their relative positions. The patient is asked to bend forward as if to touch the toes. The head and neck should be flexed and the arms should hang loose from the shoulders. As the patient bends forward, the examiner should note the cranial movement of the PSIS's (Fig 7-6). If asymmetrical motion exists, the side that moves first and/or the farthest cranially is the blocked (positive) side. The standing flexion test may be thought of as iliosacral motion recruited from the top down.

Gillet's Test (Sacral Fixation Test)

Like the standing flexion test, Gillet's test is also a test of iliosacral motion, but recruitment is from the bottom up. The PSIS's are localized again. The patient is asked to stand first on one leg and then on the other while pulling the opposite knee toward the chest (Fig 7-7). If asymmetry is found, the PSIS on the unblocked side will move farther inferiorly. The blocked side will move very little. An alternate method of assessment

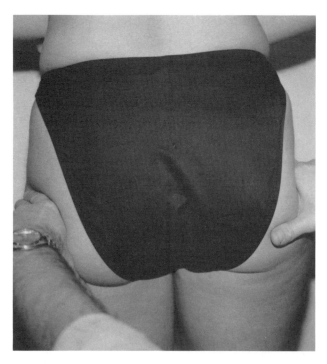

Figure 7-5. Checking greater trochanter height.

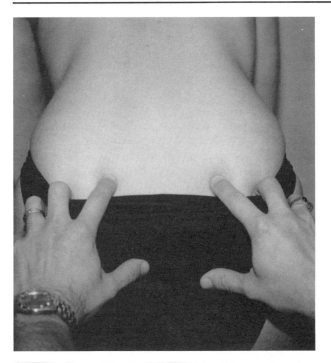

Figure 7-6. The standing flexion test of iliosacral motion. The side that moves superiorly first or farthest is the positive (blocked) side.

uses the S2 spinous process as a fixed reference point for the relative PSIS movement as the patient alternately pulls the knees to the chest. Hip flexion must reach at least 90°. [7,8,9]

Active Lumbar Movements

Since lumbar lesions often occur along with iliosacral and sacroiliac dysfunctions, restrictions of lumbar movements must be assessed as well. When a pelvic girdle dysfunction exists, sidebending the lumbar spine toward the affected side will often exacerbate pain (Fig 7-8). Pain on backward bending may indicate a pelvic girdle lesion as well (Fig 7-9).

Sitting Position

The sitting position fixes the innominates to a chair or table and eliminates the influence of the hamstrings on the pelvis. This allows for sacral movement within the innominates when testing motion. Additionally, active trunk rotation can best be tested since hip and pelvic motions are stabilized. The clinician should also note the posture of the patient in this position; the patient with sacroiliac joint dysfunction often tends to sit on the unaffected buttock. The sitting position also facilitates the neurological examination.

Iliac Crest Height

Iliac crest height is observed in the sitting position to eliminate the influence of the lower extremities on symmetry. If crest height is uneven in the sitting position, structural variation in the innominate bones is a likely cause. Other possible causes of uneven crest height in the sitting position may be shortening or

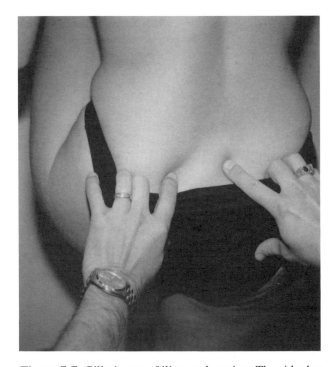

Figure 7-7. Gillet's test of iliosacral motion. The side that moves farthest inferiorly is the negative (unblocked) side.

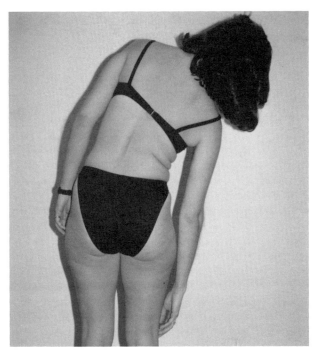

Figure 7-8. Active lumbar sidebending.

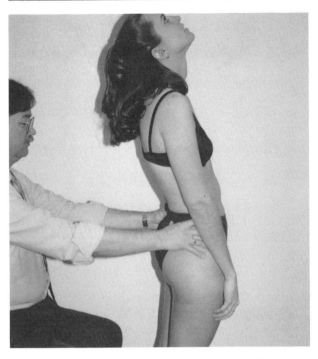

Figure 7-9. Active lumbar backward bending.

spasm of the quadratus lumborum, or a structural scoliosis. If asymmetry is present, a lift of appropriate size should be placed under the ischial tuberosity of the short side before performing the sitting flexion test.

Neurological Examination

The therapist tests the following:

1. Muscle stretch reflexes (deep tendon reflexes)

2. Lower extremity sensation

3. Lower extremity muscle strength.

Sitting Flexion Test

The sitting flexion test of sacroiliac motion is used to help the therapist determine the type of dysfunction and the side of involvement. For example, if the sitting flexion test is positive on the left, it tells the clinician that a left-sided sacroiliac problem may be present.

The therapist must again localize the PSIS's. The patient is asked to cross the arms across the chest and pass the elbows between the knees as if to touch the floor. The patient's feet should be in contact with the floor, or resting on a stool if seated on the edge of an examination table (Fig 7-10). The PSIS on the involved side will move first and/or farther cranially (i.e., the blocked joint moves solidly as one, while the sacrum

on the unblocked side is free to move through its small range of motion with the lumbar spine).

If a blockage is detected in this test, and it is more positive (greater) than a restriction noted in the standing flexion test, then a sacroiliac dysfunction is implied. If the two PSIS's move symmetrically in the seated test position, yet a positive standing flexion test or Gillet's test was noted, then an iliosacral dysfunction is implied. If the standing flexion test and the sitting flexion test are both equally positive, then a soft tissue lesion is suspected.

Supine Position

Straight Leg Raising

The straight leg raising test is a common clinical test used to evaluate low back pain. It is perhaps one of the more commonly misinterpreted clinical tests as well.[11] The test applies stress to the sacroiliac joint in the higher ranges of the arc and can indicate the presence of a unilateral dysfunction of the joint. It could also indicate a coexisting lumbar problem. The following guidelines can help interpret the results of the straight leg raising test:

0 - 30°: hip pathology or severely inflamed nerve root

30 - 50°: sciatic nerve involvement

50 - 70°: probable hamstring involvement

70 - 90°: sacroiliac joint is stressed.

The patient is supine on the examining table. The clinician lifts one of the patient's legs by supporting the heel while palpating the opposite ASIS (Fig 7-11). The leg is raised until the clinician can detect pelvic motion under the fingertips of the palpating hand. This determines the hamstring length in the leg being raised.[6] The other side is then tested similarly.

Long Sitting Leg Length Test

A positive long sitting leg length test indicates an abnormal mechanical relationship of the innominates moving on the sacrum (an iliosacral dysfunction) and helps determine the presence of either an anterior innominate or a posterior innominate by a change in the relative length of the legs during the test.

Malleolar levelness is assessed as depicted in Figure 7-12. The patient is then asked to perform a sit-up (with the clinician's assistance), keeping the legs straight (Fig 7-13). The clinician observes any change

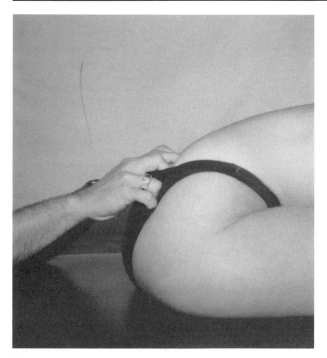

Figure 7-10. The sitting flexion test of sacroiliac motion. The side that moves superiorly first or farthest is the positive (blocked) side.

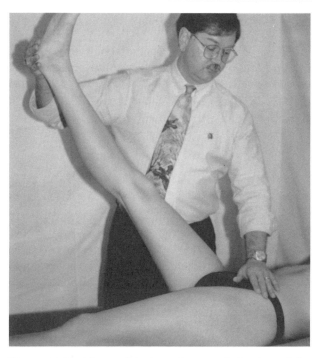

Figure 7-11. The straight leg raise test. Palpation of the opposite ASIS is done to detect pelvic motion when the hamstrings are maximally stretched.

between the malleoli. The presence of a posterior innominate will make the leg in question (same side as the positive standing flexion test) appear to lengthen from a position of relative shortness. This occurs

because, in the supine position, the posterior rotation of the innominate moves the acetabulum and the leg in a superior direction and carries the leg along with it. Thus, the leg appears shortened.

Just the opposite occurs in the anterior innominate. When the long sitting leg length test is performed, the leg in question will appear to shorten from a position of relative elongation.[1] These mechanisms are shown in Figure 7-14.

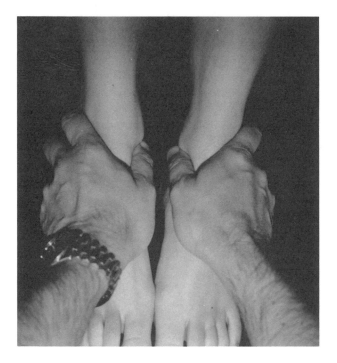

Figure 7-12. Assessing malleoli levelness with the patient lying supine.

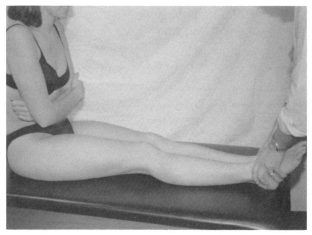

Figure 7-13. Reassessing malleoli levelness after the patient assumes the long sitting position.

Pelvic Rocking

The pelvic rocking test simply involves assessing the end-feel for the relative ease or resistance to passive overpressure for each innominate. The clinician places his or her hand on the ASIS's and gently springs the innominates alternately several times to assess the end-feel to this motion. A harder end-feel indicates a probable movement restriction on that side.

Compression-Distraction Tests

Compression-distraction tests determine the presence of joint irritability, hypermobility, or serious disease such as ankylosing spondylitis, Paget's disease, or infection. The clinician may leave his or her hands on the ASIS's as in the pelvic rocking test or may cross them to opposite ASIS's (Fig 7-15). The clinician then applies pressure down onto them to take up any slack and gives a sudden, sharp spring to the ASIS's. This action compresses the sacroiliac joints posteriorly and gaps the joints anteriorly. The clinician then moves his or her hands to the iliac wings laterally and repeats the same maneuver (Fig 7-16). In doing so, the clinician compresses the anterior and distracts the posterior sacroiliac joints. Pain as a result of either of these maneuvers is a positive sign.

FABERE (Patrick's) Test

The FABERE test can be used to differentiate between hip and sacroiliac joint pain. The hip is **F**lexed, **AB**ducted, and **E**xternally **R**otated, and the lateral malleolus is allowed to rest upon the opposite thigh above the knee. The opposite ASIS is stabilized, and pressure is applied to the other externally rotated leg at the knee (Fig 7-17). Pain located in the groin or anterior thigh is more indicative of hip joint pathology. Pain over the trochanteric region indicates hip capsular problems. Pain in the sacroiliac joint indicates sacroiliac joint involvement.

Piriformis Tightness

Piriformis muscle tightness is easily checked by flexing the hip and knee to 90° and then passively rotating the hip into internal rotation through the lower leg (Fig 7-18). Relative end-feel and range of motion can be assessed.

Pubic Tubercle Position

The pubic tubercles are assessed for their relative superior-inferior and anteroposterior relationships. If they are unlevel, the positive side is correlated to the side of the positive standing flexion or Gillet's test. To avoid embarrassment and unnecessary probing in this

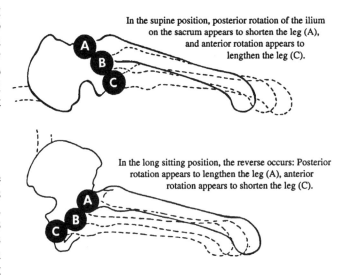

In the supine position, posterior rotation of the ilium on the sacrum appears to shorten the leg (A), and anterior rotation appears to lengthen the leg (C).

In the long sitting position, the reverse occurs: Posterior rotation appears to lengthen the leg (A), anterior rotation appears to shorten the leg (C).

Figure 7-14. Interpreting the results of the long sitting leg length test.

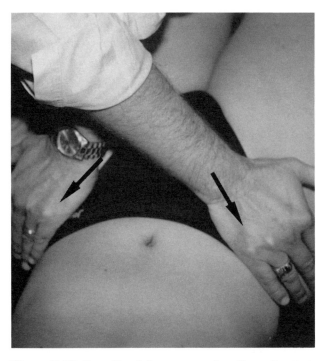

Figure 7-15. Sacroiliac joint compression-distraction test. This maneuver compresses the SI joint posteriorly and gaps the joint anteriorly.

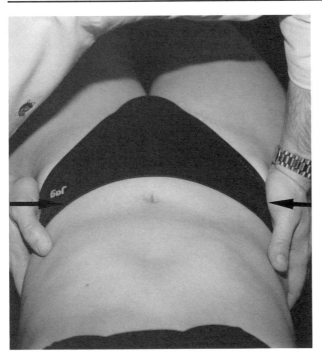

Figure 7-16. Sacroiliac joint compression-distraction test. This technique can be done with the patient in sidelying if more force is required.

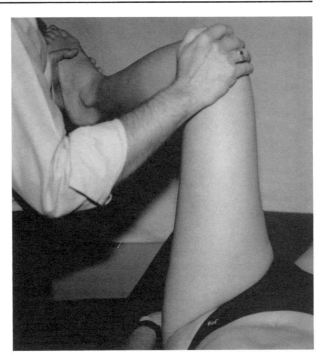

Figure 7-18. Checking for piriformis tightness in the supine position.

region, it is recommended that the clinician slide the heel of his hand down the abdomen until contact is made with the pubic bone (Fig 7-19). The tubercles may then be easily located with the fingertips (Fig 7-20). In most men and some women, because of the strength of the abdominal muscles, it sometimes helps to ask the patient to flex the knees a little to relax the muscles. Palpation is further facilitated by asking the patient to take a breath; upon exhalation, the clinician slides his or her fingers over the top and presses down upon the tubercles.

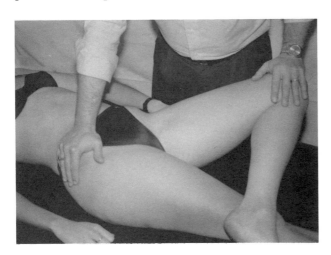

Figure 7-17. FABERE (Patrick's) test. The clinician presses down on the patient's knee while stabilizing the opposite ASIS.

Anterior Superior Iliac Spine Position

The ASIS's must be assessed for any change from the standing position. To assess the superoinferior and mediolateral relationships, the clinician places his or her thumbs under the lip of the ASIS and observes the patient. To determine the anteroposterior relationship of the ASIS's, the clinician places the fingertips on the tips of the ASIS's and sights along the plane of the abdomen. The umbilicus also becomes a reference point for mediolateral positioning. A tape measure may be used from the umbilicus to the inside border of the ASIS to determine the presence of an iliac inflare or outflare (Fig 7-21).

Prone Position

Palpation

Depth and Tenderness of Sacral Sulci (Medial PSIS)

The depths of the sacral sulci are best determined if the clinician uses the tips of the long fingers while curling his or her fingers around the posterior aspects of the iliac crests (Fig 7-22). The clinician assesses not only the relative depth of each sulcus but the quality of the ligaments, by palpating for tightness, tenderness and swelling. If a sacroiliac joint problem exists, tenderness in the sulcus can be quite localized. If one side is found to be deeper than the other, this could indicate a sacral torsion or an innominate rotation.

POSITIVE STANDING FLEXION TEST/GILLET'S TEST

Probable Iliosacral Involvement

RESULTS

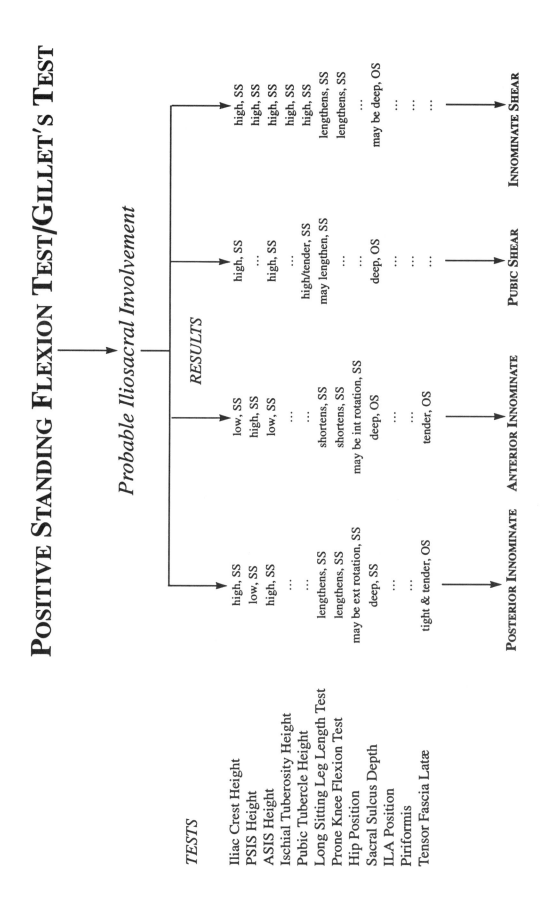

TESTS	POSTERIOR INNOMINATE	ANTERIOR INNOMINATE	PUBIC SHEAR	INNOMINATE SHEAR
Iliac Crest Height	high, SS	low, SS	high, SS	high, SS
PSIS Height	low, SS	high, SS	...	high, SS
ASIS Height	high, SS	low, SS	high, SS	high, SS
Ischial Tuberosity Height	...	...	...	high, SS
Pubic Tubercle Height	...	...	high/tender, SS	high, SS
Long Sitting Leg Length Test	lengthens, SS	shortens, SS	may lengthen, SS	lengthens, SS
Prone Knee Flexion Test	lengthens, SS	shortens, SS	...	lengthens, SS
Hip Position	may be ext rotation, SS	may be int rotation, SS	...	...
Sacral Sulcus Depth	deep, SS	deep, OS	deep, OS	may be deep, OS
ILA Position	...	...	...	...
Piriformis	...	...		
Tensor Fascia Latæ	tight & tender, OS	tender, OS		

SS = *same side as positive Standing Flexion Test/Gillet's Test*
OS = *opposite side as positive Standing Flexion Test/Gillet's Test*

TABLE A. Summary of iliosacral dysfunctions.

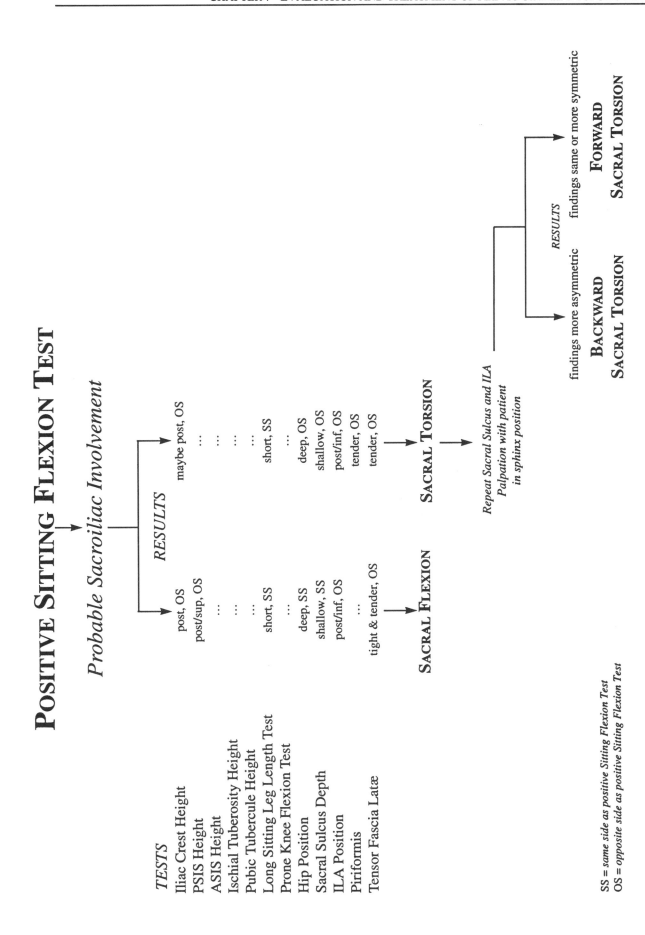

POSITIVE SITTING FLEXION TEST

Probable Sacroiliac Involvement

TESTS

	RESULTS	
Iliac Crest Height	post, OS	maybe post, OS
PSIS Height	post/sup, OS	⋮
ASIS Height	⋮	⋮
Ischial Tuberosity Height	⋮	⋮
Pubic Tubercule Height	⋮	⋮
Long Sitting Leg Length Test	short, SS	short, SS
Prone Knee Flexion Test	⋮	⋮
Hip Position	deep, SS	deep, OS
Sacral Sulcus Depth	shallow, SS	shallow, OS
ILA Position	post/inf, OS	post/inf, OS
Piriformis	⋮	tender, OS
Tensor Fascia Latæ	tight & tender, OS	tender, OS
	SACRAL FLEXION	**SACRAL TORSION**

Repeat Sacral Sulcus and ILA Palpation with patient in sphinx position

RESULTS	
findings more asymmetric	findings same or more symmetric
BACKWARD SACRAL TORSION	**FORWARD SACRAL TORSION**

TABLE B. Summary of sacroiliac dysfunctions

SS = *same side as positive Sitting Flexion Test*
OS = *opposite side as positive Sitting Flexion Test*

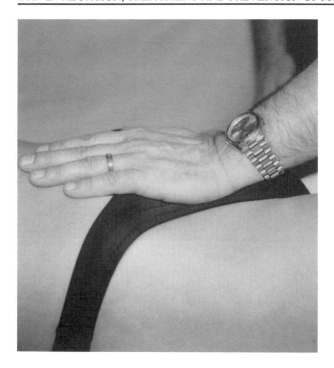

Figure 7-19. Locating the pubic tubercles by sliding the heel of the hand down the abdomen.

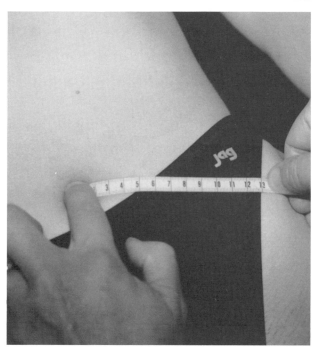

Figure 7-21. Measuring the distance from the umbilicus to the ASIS to check for iliac inflare or outflare.

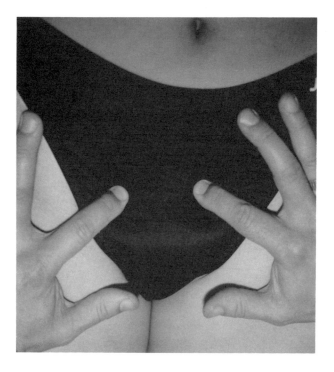

Figure 7-20. Assessing pubic tubercle height with the fingertips.

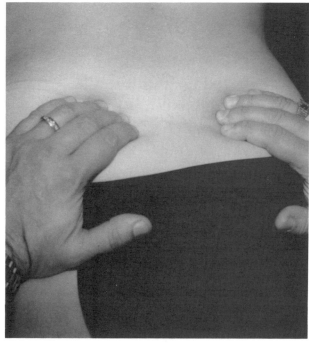

Figure 7-22. Assessing the depth of the sacral sulci.

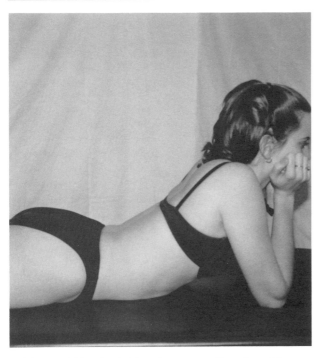

Figure 7-23. The Sphinx (prone on elbows) position.

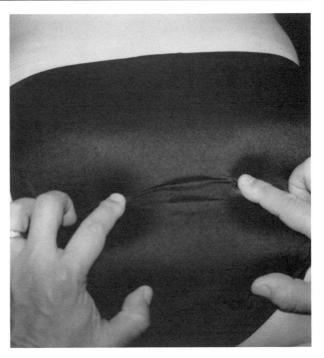

Figure 7-24. Assessing the position of the sacral ILA's.

The depth of the sacral sulci is then reassessed with the patient in the Sphinx position (prone on elbows or press-up position) (Fig 7-23). The clinician notes whether any difference found in sulci depth becomes more pronounced or less pronounced in the Sphinx position. This distinction helps determine whether a possible sacral torsion is backward or forward.

Inferior Lateral Angles

The ILA's are compared as to their relative caudad/cephalad and anteroposterior positions (Fig 7-24). If one side is found to be more caudad or posterior, then a sacroiliac lesion is implicated. If the ILA's are level but a deep sacral sulcus was found, the lesion may be in one of the innominates.

The position of the ILA's is reassessed with the patient in the Sphinx position. The clinician notes whether any differences found in ILA position become more pronounced or less pronounced in the Sphinx position. If a sacral torsion is present, this distinction will determine whether the sacral torsion is backward or forward.

Symmetry of the Sacrotuberous and Sacrospinous Ligaments

These ligaments must be palpated through the gluteal mass (Fig 7-25). The clinician must assess changes in tension and springiness from one side to the other. If such changes are noted, they are due to positional changes of the ilium.

Piriformis Tightness

The piriformis was tested in the supine position while on stretch. It is now tested while not on stretch by having the patient flex the knees to 90° and internally rotate the hips (Fig 7-26). This position also tests the short rotators of the hip.

Ischial Tuberosities

The clinician checks for the relative anteroposterior and cephalad/caudad relationships of the ischial tuberosities by using the thumbs to push soft tissue out of the way (Fig 7-27). A change in the anteroposterior relationship may indicate an innominate rotation. A change in the cephalad/caudad relationship may indicate an ilium upslip or downslip.

Rotation of L4 and L5

To test for rotation of L4 and L5, the clinician uses the thumbs to palpate the transverse processes bilaterally at each level and compares their relative levelness (Fig 7-28). The test is repeated with the patient's lumbar spine in both flexion and extension. This is easily accomplished by the patient assuming the sphinx position for testing extension or assuming the prayer position for testing flexion (Fig 7-29). If unlevelness is seen, the segment is rotated in the

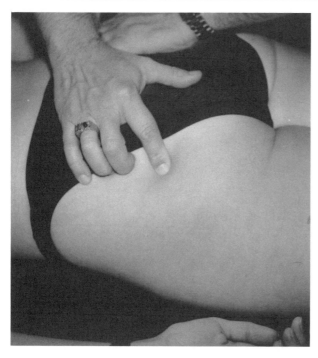

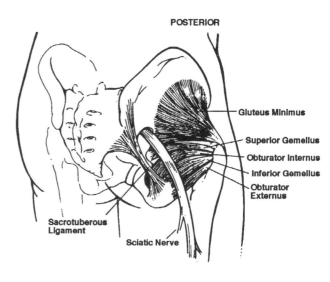

Figure 7-25. Locating the sacrotuberous ligament.

direction of the most posterior transverse process. Rotation of the lower lumbar segments may indicate a compensated curve (Type I) or non-compensated problem (Type II) in response to a pelvic girdle dysfunction.

Sacral Mobility Test

To test the passive mobility of the sacrum within the innominates, the clinician palpates the sacral sulci while applying posteroanterior pressure on the sacrum (Fig 7-30). Hypermobility or hypomobility can be assessed by the relative amount of movement between the PSIS and the dorsal aspect of the sacrum.

Lumbar Spring Test

The standard spring test is applied to the lumbar spine to help rule out the possibility of a lumbar lesion (Fig 7-31).

Prone Leg Length Test

The clinician stands at the foot of the examination table and holds the patient's feet in a symmetrical position with thumbs placed transversely across the soles of the feet just forward of the heel pad. Sighting through the plane of the heel with eyes perpendicular to the malleoli (Fig 7-32), the clinician assesses the relative length of the legs in the prone position (the short side may not be the same as in the supine or standing position). If one leg appears short, it is the positive side. The knees are then simultaneously flexed

to 90° (Fig 7-33). Care must be taken to maintain the feet in the neutral position and to bring the feet up in the midline. Deviation to either side will cause a false impression (Fig 7-34). If the leg still appears short, an anterior innominate is suspected. If the leg that seemed short now appears longer, a posterior innominate should be suspected.

Sacral Provocation Tests

Sacral provocation tests should be done only when the above series of tests has not provided a clear picture of the dysfunction. These tests should not be performed if the previous tests have demonstrated a

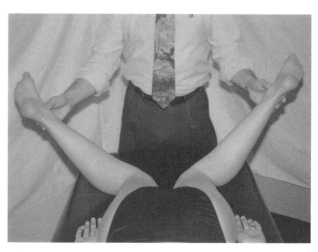

Figure 7-26. Checking for piriformis tightness in the prone position.

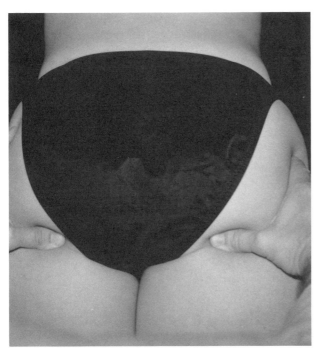

Figure 7-27. Checking the positions of the ischial tuberosities.

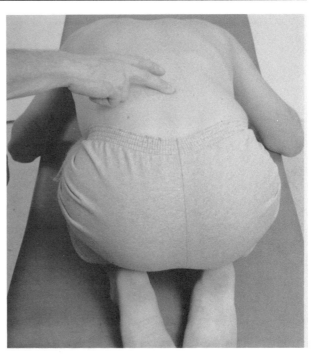

Figure 7-29. The prayer position.

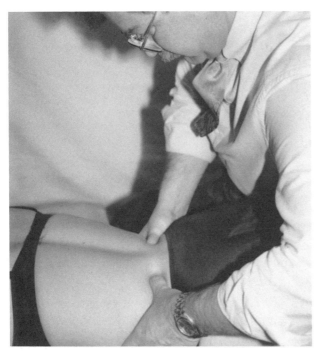

Figure 7-28. Testing for rotation of L4 and L5 in prone. This can also be done in standing.

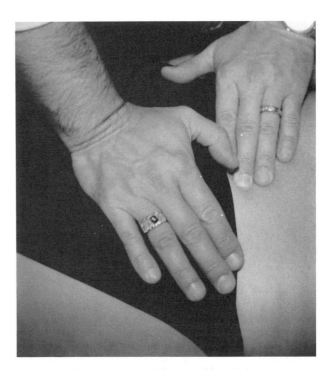

Figure 7-30. A sacral mobility test. The clinician palpates the sacral sulcus while pressing downward on the inferior sacrum.

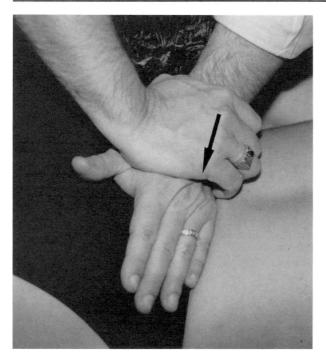

Figure 7-31. The lumbar spring test.

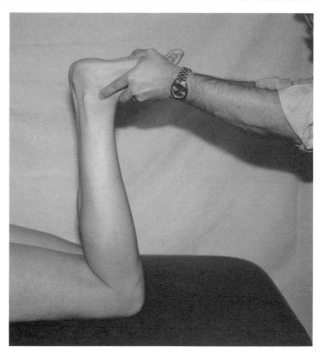

Figure 7-33. Assessing leg length in prone – rechecking leg length after the knees are bent to 90°.

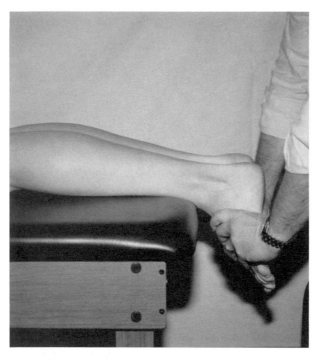

Figure 7-32. Assessing leg length in prone – starting position.

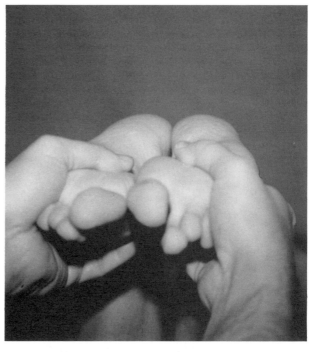

Figure 7-34. Assessing leg length in prone – when the knees are bent, care must be taken to maintain a midline position to avoid the false impression of asymmetry.

hypermobility. They are performed in a manner similar to the sacral mobility test (Fig 7-30). In chronic sacroiliac joint pain, provocation should increase symptoms due to adaptive shortening of the soft tissues.

Sacral provocation tests include:

1. Anteroposterior pressure on the sacrum at its base (this encourages sacral flexion)

2. Anteroposterior pressure on the sacrum at its apex (this encourages sacral extension)

3. Anteroposterior pressure on each side of the sacrum just medially to the PSIS's (this encourages motion about the vertical axis)

4. Cephalad pressure on the sacrum applied near the apex (note pain or movement abnormalities)

5. Cephalad pressure on the sacrum applied near the base (note pain or movement abnormalities)

6. If a sulcus is found to be deep, pressure is applied on the opposite ILA to see if the sulcus becomes more shallow (this encourages torsional movement about the oblique axis)

Sidelying Position

Tensor Fascia Latæ

Length of the tensor fascia latæ is assessed in sidelying. The patient's uppermost hip is extended then adducted (Fig 7-35). Restriction or symptom reproduction in extension and adduction (Ober's sign) indicates a tight tensor fascia latæ.

PHYSICAL FINDINGS AND ASSESSMENT OF PELVIC GIRDLE DYSFUNCTIONS

Physical findings for the major pelvic girdle dysfunctions are summarized in Tables A and B. The physical findings are correlated to the results of the standing and sitting flexion tests. The standing and sitting flexion tests are important because they help determine whether the dysfunction is iliosacral or sacroiliac (Gillet's test is an alternative to the standing flexion test):

• If the standing flexion test is positive, an iliosacral lesion is implicated.

• If the sitting flexion test is positive, a sacroiliac lesion is implicated.

• If both the standing and sitting flexion tests are positive, the patient likely has a combination lesion (multiple lesions) or soft tissue restriction.

• In both the standing and sitting flexion tests, the side that moves first and/or farthest is the restricted side.

Note: Combination or multiple lesions are more common than simple isolated lesions. For simplicity, the findings for each lesion in the following section are presented as though they occur singularly without another dysfunction present. In reality, the patient often presents with findings that do not clearly fit with any of the diagnostic entities.

In the case where two or more findings conflict, the clinician should place more emphasis on the tests that were the most positive, and/or correlate more readily with other objective and subjective findings (i.e., if the standing flexion test is more positive than the sitting flexion test, the restriction is more likely to be iliosacral, and vice versa).

Iliosacral Lesions (Positive Standing Flexion or Gillet's Test)

Iliosacral lesions can involve the following: 1) Posterior innominates, 2) Anterior innominates, 3) Pubic shears, and 4) Iliac subluxations (upslips).

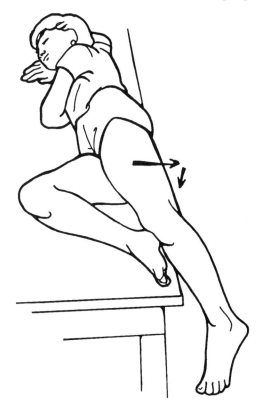

Figure 7-35. Testing for tensor fascia latæ tightness (Ober's sign).

Posterior Innominate

The posterior innominate is a unilateral iliosacral dysfunction. It is by far the most common pelvic dysfunction, particularly on the left. The main findings for a left posterior innominate are summarized in Table A.

Other findings: sacroiliac ligament may be tense; decreased lumbar lordosis; sacral sulcus and/or unilateral buttock pain

Anterior Innominate

The anterior innominate is also a unilateral iliosacral dysfunction. It is essentially the reverse of the posterior innominate and occurs more commonly on the right. The main findings for an anterior innominate are summarized in Table A.

Other findings: possibly increased lumbar lordosis; possible complaint of cervical or lumbar symptoms

Pubic Shear

Dysfunctions of the pubic symphysis are probably the most commonly overlooked lesions of the pelvis. The lesions that usually occur at this joint are shear lesions in a superior or an inferior direction. Anterior and posterior shears are rare and are usually the result of trauma. The main findings for a superior pubis are summarized in Table A.

Other findings: almost all of these lesions occur simultaneously with the posterior innominate or upslip.

Innominate Shear (Upslip)

Once considered uncommon, vertical shear lesions of an entire innominate have been shown to occur more frequently than originally thought.[30] The main findings for a superior shear are summarized in Table A.

Sacroiliac Lesions (Positive Sitting Flexion Test)

Sacroiliac lesions can involve the following: 1) Sacral Torsions, and 2) Sacral Flexions.

Sacral Torsion

Assessment and terminology of sacral torsions can be confusing. First, the clinician must decide whether a sacral torsion is present. Then he or she must determine whether the torsion is a forward torsion or a backward torsion. This is done by retesting the position of the sacral sulci with the patient in an extended (Sphinx) position. Finally, the torsion must be named. The findings for a sacral torsion are summarized in Table B.

Naming the Sacral Torsion

Forward torsions are always right on a right oblique axis or left on a left oblique axis. Backward torsions are always right on a left oblique axis or left on a right oblique axis. The axis of involvement is the same as the side of the shallow sacral sulcus. Most sacral torsions occur around the left oblique axis. More discussion about naming and visualizing sacral torsions is found in Chapter 2, Basic Spinal Biomechanics.

Sacral Flexion

Unilateral sacral flexion occurs primarily around the middle transverse axis of the sacroiliac joint. It might be thought of as failure of one side of the sacrum to counternutate from a fully nutated position. When this occurs, a sidebending component is present, driving the sacrum down the long arm of the joint. Findings for a unilateral sacral flexion are summarized in Table B.

TREATMENT OF PELVIC GIRDLE DYSFUNCTIONS

If the clinician finds multiple lesions, they should all be treated, but in this suggested order:

a. Pubic lesions

b. Nonadapting (Type II) lumbar compensations

c. Sacroiliac lesions

d. Iliosacral lesions

This treatment order takes advantage of the axes of motion, so that unlocking a restriction in one area helps unlock the restriction in another. A very common combination of lumbopelvic dysfunctions consists of left superior pubic shear, left-on-left forward sacral torsion, and left posterior innominate. The lumbar spine is usually adaptive (Type I) in response to these dysfunctions and does not need correction.

Muscle Energy Techniques

As discussed previously, a muscle energy technique (MET) is any manipulative treatment that uses a voluntary contraction of the patient's muscles against a distinctly controlled counterforce from a precise position and in a specific direction. MET's may be used to lengthen shortened muscles, strengthen weakened muscles, reduce localized edema, and mobilize restricted joints. [10,15,4,13] The focus of this section will be on the use of MET's to mobilize joint restrictions.

Iliosacral Lesions

Posterior Innominate

The main features of a posterior innominate were summarized in Table A.

Muscular correction of this positional fault uses muscles that can rotate the innominate in an anterior direction. In this case, the rectus femoris is the major mover:

1. The patient is supine with the involved leg hanging freely over the edge of the treatment table as described previously. The hip is extended and the knee is flexed.

2. The opposite hip and knee are flexed up toward the patient's chest until the freely hanging leg begins to come up. The patient is instructed to hold the flexed knee and hip in that position with her hands. The clinician may assist with a hand, arm, or shoulder.

3. The clinician places the other hand on the anterior supracondylar area of the freely hanging knee and gently pushes down to take up the slack (Fig 7-36).

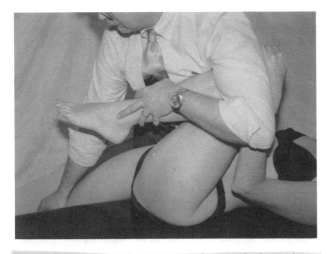

Figure 7-36. Position for treatment of a posterior innominate by muscle energy technique. (R) LE contraction for ant. rot. of ilium.

4. The patient is then instructed to push the freely hanging leg up against the clinician's hand with a submaximal force, holding it constant for 7 - 10 seconds while breathing in a relaxed, smooth manner.

It is important for the clinician to give unyielding resistance to the contraction.

5. As the patient relaxes the contraction, the clinician takes up the slack by pushing down on the freely hanging leg and helps the patient pull the flexed hip and knee up to the new barrier. The contraction is then again executed in the new position. This procedure is repeated three or four times.

6. The patient is now re-examined for any changes produced by these efforts, usually by the long sitting leg length test. Treatment is repeated if necessary.

The patient can be instructed in a modification of this technique for home use simply hanging the uninvolved leg from the edge of his or her bed or other raised surface and bringing the opposite hip and knee to the chest. The patient should then hold that position for 2 - 3 minutes and perform slow, relaxed breathing, taking up any slack occurring from the stretch. The breathing techniques used for both the anterior and the posterior innominate procedures take advantage of rotatory motion of the innominate around the superior transverse (respiratory) axis of the sacroiliac joints.

Anterior Innominate

The main features of an anterior innominate were summarized in Table A.

Muscular correction of this positional fault uses muscles that can rotate the innominate in a posterior direction. In this case, the major mover is the gluteus maximus. The technique is as follows:

1. The patient is supine with the opposite leg hanging freely from the edge of the treatment table, supported at approximately the level of the ischium.

2. The hip and knee are flexed on the involved side until the freely hanging leg begins to come up.

3. The clinician may then stabilize the flexed knee with his or her shoulder or instruct the patient to hold the leg in that fixed position with his or her own hands (Fig 7-37).

4. The patient is then instructed push the knee on the involved side against her own hands or the clinician's shoulder with a submaximal sustained contraction (isometric). Note that the hip is not allowed to move into extension at any time, only flexion.

5. As with other MET's, the forces generated are submaximal, the contraction is held for 7 - 10 seconds, the slack is taken up to the new barrier, and the

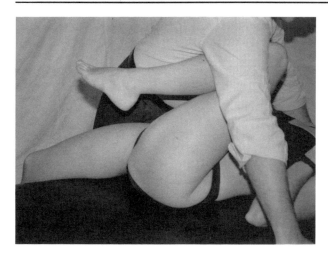

Figure 7-37. Position for treatment of an anterior innominate by muscle energy technique.

technique is repeated three or four times until all slack is taken up.

6. The patient is now re-examined for any change, usually by the long sitting leg length test or the standing flexion test. The treatment is repeated if necessary.

The patient can perform this treatment as a home program two to three times per day for the next several days. It should be noted that this technique is a powerful rotator for the innominate and can be easily overdone unless specific guidelines are given.

Superior Pubic Shear

The main features of a superior pubic shear were summarized in Table A.

Muscular correction of this very common pelvic dysfunction uses the combined forces of the rectus femoris and the hip adductor group to effect the mobilization:

1. The patient is supine with the leg on the involved side hanging freely from the edge of the table.

2. The clinician stands on the same side as the lesion.

3. The lower portion of the freely hanging leg is passively extended at the knee and is held in this position, supported between the legs of the clinician.

4. The clinician then reaches across the patient and places one hand on the ASIS opposite the side of involvement to stabilize it.

5. With the other hand, the clinician gently presses down on the supracondylar areas of the freely hanging leg and takes up the available slack at the hip. The clinician does this maintaining the position of the knee in passive extension between his or her own legs (Fig 7-38).

6. The patient is then instructed, "Squeeze your thigh toward the table and push your leg up against my hand." The clinician offers unyielding resistance to the upward contraction, and the table offers unyielding resistance to adduction. The knee must be maintained in passive extension as the patient tries to raise the leg.

7. As with other MET's, the forces generated are submaximal, the contraction is held for 7 - 10 seconds, the slack is taken up to the new barrier, and the technique is repeated three or four times until all slack is taken up. Stabilization of the opposite ASIS is particularly important during this test.

8. The patient is re-examined and treatment is repeated as needed.

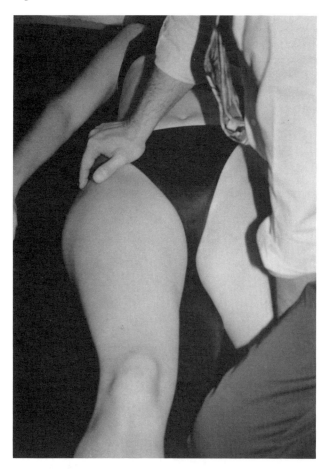

Figure 7-38. Position for treatment of a superior pubic shear by muscle energy technique. The clinician's left leg is maintaining the position of the patient's left leg in passive extension and abduction.

Combined Treatment for Superior and Inferior Pubic Shear

This technique is a powerful mover of the pubic symphysis. It first employs the hip abductors to "gap" the joint and then the hip adductors to "reset" the joint in its normal position.

1. The patient is supine with his or her knees flexed and together.

2. The clinician stands at either side of the table.

3. The clinician places his or her hands on the outsides of the patient's knees and instructs the patient, "Push your legs apart," (abduct the knees) (Fig 7-39). This is done with maximal force, and the clinician resists this effort by pushing against the lateral aspects of the patient's knees. This isometric contraction is held for 7 - 10 seconds. The patient is then instructed to relax.

4. The patient is then instructed to allow his or her legs to "fall apart" (abduct the knees). The clinician guides this action so that the feet are held together and the legs abduct 30 - 45°. Step 3 is now repeated in this new position, with the patient giving a maximal contraction into abduction while the clinician resists this effort (Fig 7-40).

5. As the patient relaxes the contraction, the clinician quickly places his or her forearm between the patient's knees (the clinician's hand and elbow make contact with the medial aspects of the patient's knees), and the patient is instructed, "Squeeze your knees together against my hand" (adduct the knees). This is also done with a maximal contraction (Fig 7-41).

6. The contraction is held for a few seconds and then relaxed. It may need to be repeated once or twice more before repositioning the patient on the table to retest. Treatment may be repeated if necessary. Many times an audible "pop" is heard during this treatment. This represents a separation of the pubic symphysis, allowing it to "reset" itself. This technique can be used separately or in combination with the specific pubic subluxation technique previous described.

Superior Innominate Shear (Upslip)

The main features of an iliac upslip were summarized in Table A.

This is a direct action thrust technique but applies principles of "close-packed" versus "loose-packed" joint mechanics to effect the mobilization.

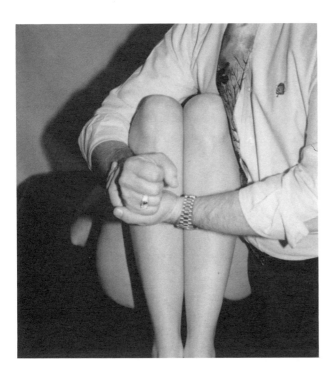

Figure 7-39. Starting position for treatment of a pubic shear by muscle energy technique. The patient tries to abduct the hips as the clinician holds her knees together.

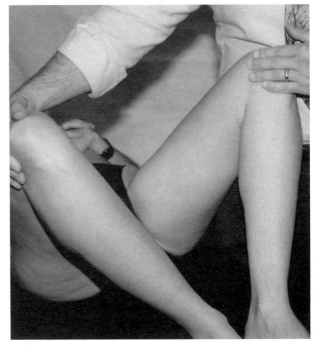

Figure 7-40. Second position for treatment of a pubic shear by muscle energy technique. The clinician repositions the hips into more abduction before the patient repeats resisted abduction.

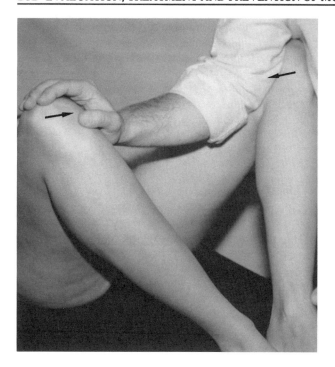

Figure 7-41. Final position for treatment of a pubic shear by muscle energy technique. The clinician quickly places his forearm between the patient's knees and asks her to squeeze the knees together.

1. The patient lies prone, and the clinician stands at the foot of the treatment table on the side of the lesion.

2. The clinician grasps the patient's distal lower leg above the ankle and raises the entire leg into approximately 30° of hip and lumbar extension, hip abduction of 30°, and hip internal rotation. This approximates the closed-packed position of the hip as much as possible.

3. The clinician then instructs the patient to grasp the top table edge with his hands. The clinician the proceeds to take up the slack by distracting the leg along its long axis until tightness is perceived along the kinetic chain (Fig 7-42).

4. The clinician now instructs the patient, "Take a deep breath and cough." Timing is important. As the patient coughs, the clinician gives a quick, caudad tug on the leg.

5. The patient is then retested and treatment is repeated if necessary.

By employing the closed-packed position of the hip, the effect of the distraction is applied to the

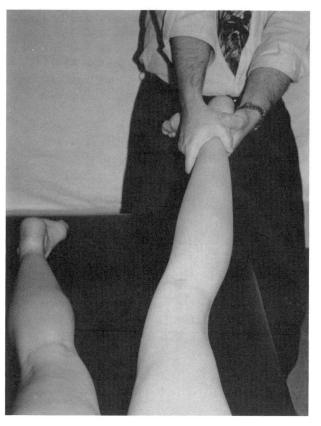

Figure 7-42. Position for treatment of a superior iliac subluxation (upslip) by direct action thrust technique. The leg is extended 30°, abducted 30° and internally rotated to approximate the closed-packed position of the hip.

innominate instead of the hip. Mobilization of the hip is done supine in the loose-packed position.

Sacroiliac Lesions

Forward Sacral Torsion (Left-on-Left or Right on Right)

The main features of a forward sacral torsion were summarized in Table B.

Muscular correction of forward sacral torsion uses the piriformis muscles to move the sacrum on one of its oblique axes. In a left-on-left forward torsion, the right piriformis is holding the sacrum so that it cannot move normally on its left oblique axis. The right oblique axis is free to move. In the following description of treatment for a left-on-left forward torsion, the right internal rotators contract, causing reciprocal inhibition of the right piriformis. This allows the sacrum to move on the left oblique axis. At the same time, the left piriformis contracts, which moves the sacrum into its correct position.

1. The patient lies on the side corresponding to the axis of involvement. Therefore, a patient with a left-on-left torsion would lie on the left side.

2. The clinician stands at the side of the table, facing the patient.

3. The patient should be as close to the edge of the table as possible. The downside arm should rest behind the trunk (the hand may be used to stabilize the patient by gripping the edge of the treatment table behind the patient). The topside arm hangs over the edge of the table closest to the clinician as the trunk of the patient is rotated forward and the chest approximates the table (Fig 7-43).

4. The clinician's cephalad hand palpates the lumbosacral junction while the caudad hand flexes the patient's knees and hips approximately 70 - 90° or until the clinician can appreciate motion occurring at the lumbosacral junction. This is best achieved by grasping both legs together at the ankles and moving the hips passively into flexion. The patient's knees should be resting in the hollow of the clinician's hip as the clinician translates his or her body laterally toward the patient's head to flex the patient's hips (Fig 7-44).

5. The clinician now moves his or her hand from the lumbosacral junction and places it on the patient's shoulder near the edge of the treatment table. The patient is instructed, "Take a deep breath," and as he or she exhales, "Reach toward the floor." As the patient does this, the clinician assists by pressing downward on the patient's shoulder to help take up the slack. This is repeated two or three times until all the slack is gone.

6. The clinician now returns that hand to the lumbosacral junction and, using the hand holding the ankles, lowers the ankles toward the floor until resistance is met and/or motion is felt at the lumbosacral junction (Fig 7-45).

7. The clinician now instructs the patient, "Lift both ankles toward the ceiling." This causes contraction of the right internal rotators and the left piriformis. This is a submaximal contraction, and the clinician must be sure to give unyielding resistance (hold-relax contraction) to the patient's effort. The contraction is held for 7 - 10 seconds and is then relaxed.

8. As the contraction is relaxed, the clinician takes up the slack by translating his or her body cephalad (to increase flexion) and lowers the ankles toward the floor until resistance is met or motion felt at the lumbosacral junction (to increase sidebending), and the patient reaches toward the floor with the hanging arm (to increase rotation).

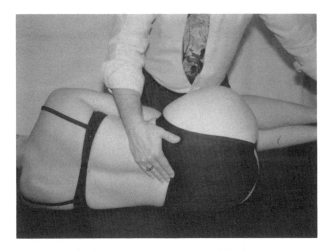

Figure 7-43. Treatment of a left-on-left forward sacral torsion by muscle energy technique – starting position.

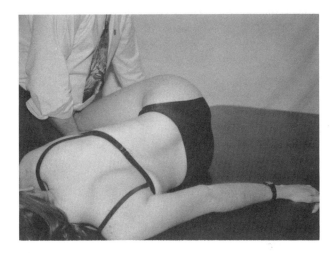

Figure 7-44. Treatment of a left-on-left forward sacral torsion by MET– after flexion of the patient's lumbar spine.

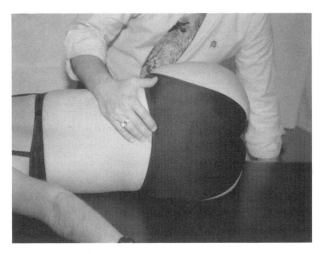

Figure 7-45. Treatment of a left-on-left forward sacral torsion by muscle energy technique – lowering the ankles to left sidebend the lumbar spine until movement is felt at the lumbosacral junction.

9. Steps 7 and 8 are repeated two or three times. Then the patient is retested to check for changes in sacral position. The treatment is repeated if necessary.

In some instances, the edges of the treatment table are uncomfortable to the patient's downside thigh during the contractions in step 7. The clinician must some times support the patient's knees with his or her own thigh or may sit on the treatment table and perform the technique from that position (Fig 7-46).

Backward Sacral Torsion (Left-on-Right or Right-on-Left)

The main features of a backward sacral torsion were summarized in Table B.

Muscular correction of backward sacral torsion uses muscles that will cause the sacrum to move forward on an oblique axis. The technique described uses the gluteus medius, tensor fascia latæ and the gluteus maximus:

1. The patient lies on the side corresponding to the axis of involvement. This means that a patient with a left-on-right torsion would lie on the right side.

2. The patient lies as close to the edge of the table as possible, and the clinician stands at the same edge facing the patient.

3. The clinician grasps the patient's downside arm (usually above the elbow) and pulls it out from under the patient (Fig 7-47). The patient's trunk is now rotated so that the back approximates the table surface. The clinician now somewhat flexes the patient's topmost leg at the hip and knee. The downside leg is allowed to remain straight for the moment.

4. The clinician now palpates the patient's lumbosacral junction with the cephalad hand. With the other hand, the clinician reaches behind the patient's topside flexed knee and passively extends the patient's bottom hip by pushing the leg posteriorly. The clinician does this until motion is perceived at the lumbosacral junction (Fig 7-48).

5. The clinician now repositions his or her hands so that the caudal hand now palpates the lumbosacral junction.

6. The clinician now uses the forearm of his or her caudad arm to stabilize the pelvis and instructs the patient, "Take a deep breath." As the patient exhales, the clinician presses downward on the shoulder, causing greater trunk rotation, and further approximating the trunk to the table surface (Fig 7-49). This maneuver is repeated two or three times to

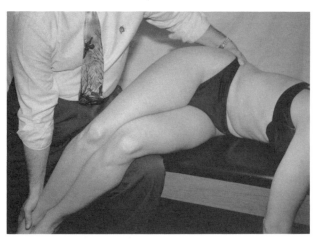

Figure 7-46. Alternate position for treatment of a left-on-left forward sacral torsion.

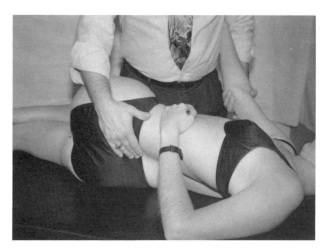

Figure 7-47. Treatment of a left-on-right backward sacral torsion by muscle energy technique – starting position.

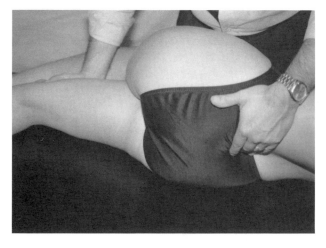

Figure 7-48. Treatment of a left-on-right backward sacral torsion by muscle energy technique – extending the patient's lumbar spine until movement is felt at the lumbosacral junction.

take up all the slack. The clinician must be careful not to allow the pelvis to move and change its alignment.

7. Maintaining trunk rotation and pelvic alignment, the clinician instructs the patient, "Straighten the topside knee and allow the leg to hang freely from the table." Being careful not to change pelvic alignment, the clinician slides the caudad hand down the thigh to the lateral supracondylar area of the patient's knee.

8. The patient is then instructed, "Lift the knee toward the ceiling," while the clinician provides unyielding resistance to the effort. The contraction is held for 7 - 10 seconds and is then relaxed (Fig 7-50).

9. The clinician takes up slack by moving the downside leg back a little (to increase extension), rotating the trunk a little (to increase rotation), and pushing down on the hanging leg until resistance is met (to increase sidebending).

10. Steps 8 and 9 are repeated two or three times, and the patient is then retested to check for positional changes of the sacrum. Treatment is repeated if necessary.

Unilateral Sacral Flexion

The main features of a unilateral sacral flexion were summarized in Table B.

Muscular correction of this sacral positional fault takes advantage of the normal nutation-counternutation movement of the sacrum during respiration. By accentuating the breathing pattern and applying direct pressure, the sacrum can be made to move up the long arm of the joint axis to its normal resting position:

1. The patient lies prone.

2. The clinician stands on the same side as the lesion.

3. With a finger, the clinician palpates the sacral sulcus on the side of the lesion and abducts the patient's hip on the involved side approximately 15°, then internally rotates that hip. This hip position is maintained throughout the procedure (Fig 7-51).

4. Using a straight arm force, the clinician places a constant downward pressure on the ILA on the side of the lesion with the heel of the hand in the direction of the navel (Fig 7-52).

5. Maintaining pressure on the sacrum, the clinician instructs the patient to take in his or her breath in "small sips" (as through a soda straw) until

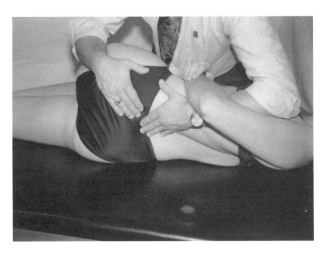

Figure 7-49. Treatment of a left-on-right backward sacral torsion by muscle energy technique – localizing lumbar rotation.

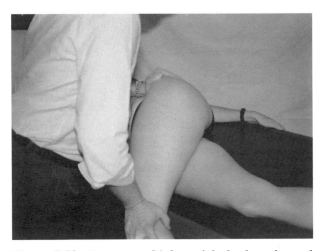

Figure 7-50. Treatment of left-on-right backward sacral torsion by muscle energy technique – stabilizing the final position as patient attempts to raise top leg toward ceiling.

he or she can hold no more air, then hold this breath with lungs maximally filled.

6. After several seconds, the clinician instructs the patient to release this air while the clinician maintains the constant downward pressure on the ILA.

7. Steps 5 and 6 are repeated three or four times, and then the patient is retested for positional changes of the sacrum. Treatment is repeated if necessary.

Self-Treatment Techniques

Posterior Innominate

Self-treatment for a posterior innominate is done by hanging the involved extremity off the edge of a

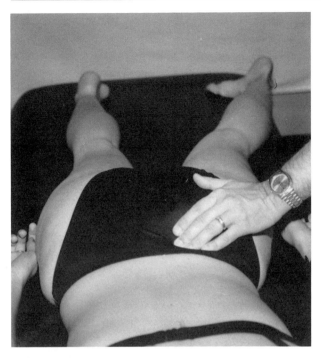

Figure 7-51. Treatment of a left unilateral sacral flexion – palpation of the sacral sulcus with abduction and internal rotation of the hip.

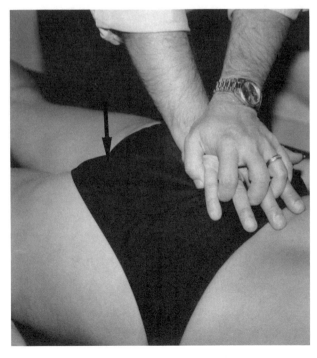

Figure 7-52. Treatment of a left unilateral sacral flexion – exerting downward pressure on the left ILA.

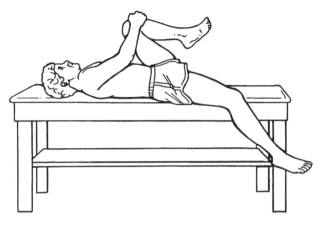

Figure 7-53. Self-treatment for a right posterior innominate.

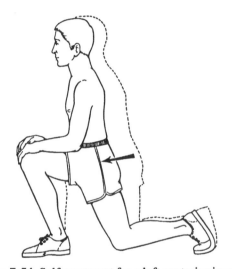

Figure 7-54. Self-treatment for a left posterior innominate.

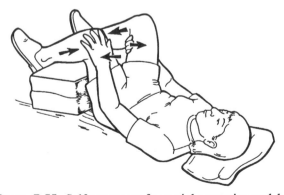

Figure 7-55. Self-treatment for a right anterior and left posterior innominate.

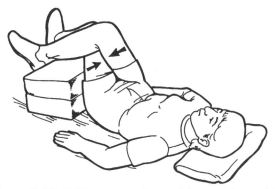

Figure 7-56. Self-treatment for a right anterior and left posterior innominate - alternate technique.

bed or table, while holding the contralateral knee to the chest (Fig 7-53). Ankle weights can be added. The patient should be encouraged to relax completely. An alternate technique involves the half-kneel position shown in Figure 7-54, with the patient kneeling on the involved extremity.

Anterior or Posterior Innominate

Self-treatment for an innominate rotation can consist of contract-relax techniques that are less specific than the muscle energy techniques described earlier. For a right anterior or left posterior innominate, the patient lies supine and places the right hand behind the right knee and the left hand on the right anterior

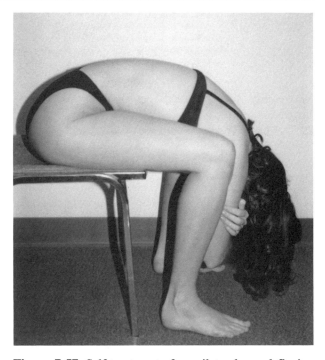

Figure 7-57. Self-treatment of a unilateral sacral flexion lesion.

thigh. The patient performs an isometric contraction of the right hip extenders and the left hip flexors as shown in Figure 7-55. An alternate technique is shown in Figure 7-56.

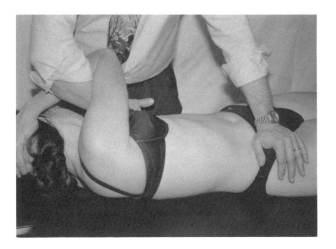

Figure 7-58. Treatment of a right anterior innominate by direct action thrust technique – starting position.

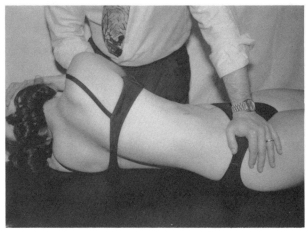

Figure 7-59. Treatment of a right anterior innominate by direct action thrust technique – final position from which the thrust is given.

Unilateral Sacral Flexion

To self-treat a unilateral sacral flexion, the patient is instructed to sit in a chair with the legs abducted. He or she takes a deep breath, holds it, and flexes the trunk between his or her spread knees, passing the elbows between the knees (Fig 7-57). After several seconds, the patient releases the air and straightens the trunk.

Manipulation Techniques

The focus of the techniques presented has been on the "patient-active" muscle energy techniques. A variety of high-velocity thrust mobilizations for the sacroiliac joint exist. They primarily produce rotatory forces on the innominates and are thus more appropriate for the iliosacral lesions. Two particularly effective thrust techniques causing posterior rotation of the innominate are described here:

1. The patient is supine with hands locked behind the head (fingers interlaced).

2. The clinician stands opposite the affected side and makes hand contact with the patient's ASIS on the affected side using the caudad hand.

3. With the cephalad hand, the clinician reaches through the crook of the patient' elbow on the affected side from behind and allows the dorsum of his or her hand to contact the patient's chest (Fig 7-58).

4. Using the dorsum of the hands as a fulcrum against the patient's chest, the clinician rolls the patient's torso toward him or her. The clinician instructs the patient, "Relax, hang on to your head, and let me turn you."

5. The clinician takes up the slack through the pelvis using a stiff arm, applying force down and away.

6. The clinician instructs the patient, "Take in a deep breath and let it out." As the patient does so, the clinician takes up the remainder of the slack through the torso and pelvis and gives a quick thrust to the pelvis through ASIS (Fig 7-59).

The second posterior rotation technique is as follows:

1. The patient is positiioned sidelying with the joint to be mobilized on the top side. One hand is placed on the ASIS and the other is on the ischial tuberosity. The anterior rim of the ilium is pushed posteriorly while the ischial tuberosity is pushed anteriorly, producing a force couple.

2. Additional force may be added to this technique by stabilizing the bottom-side hip in extension and flexing the top-side hip. Even more force can be gained by extending the top-side knee and allowing it to hang over the edge of the treatment table. This tethers the hamstring muscles and helps pull the innominate posteriorly.

Graded passive movements, stretches and thrusts may be used with this technique (Fig 7-60).

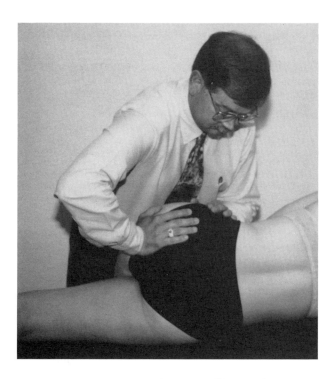

Figure 7-60. Posterior rotation of the ilium on the sacrum.

SUMMARY

The evaluation and treatment of pelvic girdle dysfunctions is an important but complex area of study for the physical therapy clinician. The sacrum's multiple axes pose a particular challenge in understanding the variety of possible disorders. The osteopathic evaluation and treatment scheme presented in this chapter is explained more thoroughly in An Evaluation and Treatment Manual of Osteopathic Muscle Energy Procedures.[10]

REFERENCES

1. Bemis T, Daniel M: Validation of the Long Sit Test on Subjects with Iliosacral Dysfunction. J Orthop Sports Phys Ther 8(7):336, 1987.

2. Binder-MacLeod S, Woerman AL: Leg Length Discrepancy Assessment: Accuracy and Precision in Five Clinical Methods of Evaluation. J Orthop Sports Phys Ther 5:230, 1984.

3. Cyriax J: Diagnosis of Soft Tissue Lesions. Textbook of Orthopaedic Medicine, Vol 1, 7th edition. Bailliere-Tindall, London 1978.

4. Goodridge JP: Muscle Energy Technique: Definition, Explanation, Methods of Procedure. J Am Osteopath Assoc 82(4):249, 1981.

5. Greive G: Common Vertebral Joint Problems. Churchill-Livingstone, New York NY 1981.

6. Kendall F and McCreary E: Muscles: Testing and Function. Williams and Wilkins, Baltimore MD 1983.

7. Kirkaldy-Willis W: Managing Low Back Pain, 2nd edition. Churchill-Livingstone, New York NY 1981.

8. Kirkaldy-Willis WH, Hill RJ: A More Precise Diagnosis for Low-Back Pain. Spine 4(2):102, March-April 1979.

9. Liekens M, Gillets HL: Belgian Chiropractic Research Notes. 10th edition. Brussels, 1973.

10. Mitchell FL Jr, Morgan PS, Pruzzo NA: An Evaluation and Treatment Manual of Osteopathic Muscle Energy Procedures. Mitchell, Moran and Pruzzo Associates, Valley Park MO, 1979.

11. Mooney V and Robertson J: The Facet Syndrome. Clin Orthop and Rel Res 115:149-156, Mar/Apr 1976.

12. Solonen K: The Sacroiliac Joint in the light of Anatomical, Roentgenological and Clinical Studies. Acta Orthop Scand (Suppl 27):1-115, 1957.

13. Somatic Dysfunction: Principles of Manipulative Treatment and Procedures. PE Kimberly, ed. Kirksville College of Osteopathic Medicine, Kirksville MO 1980.

14. Stoddard A: Manual of Osteopathic Technique. Hutchinson, London 1978.

15. Tutorial on Level I Muscle Energy Techniques. Michigan State University College of Osteopathic Medicine, East Lansing MI 1986. Course Notes.

OTHER REFERENCES

1. Caillet R; Low Back Pain Syndrome. 2nd edition. FA Davis, Philadelphia PA 1982.

2. Clemente CD: Anatomy: A Regional Atlas of the Human Body. Lea & Febiger, Philadelphia PA 1975

3. Colachis S, Warden R, et al: Movement of the Sacroiliac Joint in the Adult Male. Arch Phys Med Rehab 44:490, 1963.

4. DiAmbrosia R: Musculoskeletal Disorders. JB Lippincott, Philadelphia PA 1977.

5. Egund N, et al: Movements in the sacroiliac joints demonstrated with roentgen sterophotogrammetry. Acta Radiol (Stockholm) 19:833, 1978

6. Farfan H: Muscular mechanism of the lumbar spine and the position of power and efficiency. Orthop Clin North Am 6(1): 135, 1975

7. Frigerio N, Stowe R and Howe J: Movement of the Sacroiliac Joint. Clin Orthop and Rel Res 100:370, 1974.

8. Fryette HH: Principles of Osteopathic Technique. American Academy of Osteopathy, Carmel CA 1954

9. Gray's Anatomy. R Warwick and P Williams, eds. 35th British edition. WB Saunders Philadelphia PA 1973.

10. Greenman P: Innominate Shear Dysfunction in the Sacroiliac Syndrome. Manual Med 2:114, 1986.

11. Greenman PE: Motion sense. Mich Osteopath J (January 1983) 39

12. Greenman PE: Restricted vertebral motion. Mich Osteopath J (March 1983) 31

13. Greenman PE: The manipulative prescription. Mich Osteopath J. December, 1982

14. Grieve GP: Mobilization of the Spine. 4th edition. Churchill Livingstone, New York NY 1984

15. Hoppenfeld S: Physical Examination of the Spine and Extremities. Appleton-Century- Crofts, Norwalk CT 1976.

16. Janda V: Muscle Function Testing. Butterworths, London, 1983

17. Kaltenborn FM: Mobilization of Extremity Joints: Examination and Basic Treatment Techniques. 3rd edition. Olaf Norlis Bokhandel, Oslo 1980

18. Kapandji I: The Physiology of the Joints. Vol 3 of The Trunk and the Vertebral Column, 2nd edition. Churchill-Livingstone, New York NY 1974.

19. Kessler RM, Hertlig D: Mangement of Common Musculoskeletal Disorders. Harper & Row, Philadelphia PA 1983

20. Koor I: Proprioceptors and somatic dysfunction. J Am Osteopath Assoc 74:638, 1975

21. Kopell HP, Thompson WAL: Peripheral Entrapment Neuropathies. Robert E Krieger, Huntington NY 1976

22. Maitland G: Vertebral Manipulation. Butterworth, London 1977.

23. Mennell J: Back Pain. Little-Brown, Boston MA 1960.

24. Mitchell F: Structural Pelvic Function. AAO Yearbook II: 178, 1965.

25. Nitz PA, Woerman AL: Acute Sacroiliac Joint Strain

in Young Adult Males as Evidenced by Bone Scan. 1988. Preliminary research.

26. Nyberg R: The lumbar and pelvic musculature.1978. Unpublished manuscript.

27. Paris SV: The Spine. Institute of Graduate Health Sciences, Atlanta GA 1979. Course Notes.

28. Pratt WA: The lumbopelvic torsion syndrome. J Am Osteopath Assoc 51 (7): 335, 1952

29. Stratton SA: Muscle Energy Techniques. U.S. Army-Baylor University Program in Physical Therapy, Fort Sam Houston TX 1983-1984. Course Notes.

30. Turek SL: Orthopædics: Principles and Their Applications. 4th edition. JB Lippincott, Philadelphia PA 1984

31. Weisl H: Movements of the sacro-iliac joint. Acta Anat 23:87, 1955

SELECTED READINGS

1. Beal M: The Sacroiliac Problems: Review of Anatomy, Mechanics and Diagnosis. JAOA 81(10):667-679, June 1982.

2. Bourdillon JF: Spinal Manipulation. 3rd edition. Appleton-Century-Crofts, New York NY 1982

3. Bowen V, Cassidy JDL: Macroscopic and Microscopic Anatomy of the Sacroiliac Joint From Embryonic Life until the Eighth Decade. Spine 6(6):620, 1981

4. Erhard R, Bowling R: The Recognition and Management of the Pelvic Component of Low Back and Sciatic Pain. Bull Orthop Sec Am Phys Ther Assoc 2(3):4, Winter 1977

5. Grieve GP: The sacroiliac joint. Physiotherapy 62(12):384, 1976

6. Johnston WL: Hip shift: testing a basic postural dysfunction. J Am Osteopath Assoc 63:923, 1964

7. Retzlaff EW, Berry AH, Haight AS, et al: The piriformis muscle syndrome. J Am Osteopath Assoc 73:799, 1974

8. Stoddard A: Conditions of the Sacroilliac Joint and their Treatment. Physiotherapy 44(4):97, 1958

9. Sutton SE: Postural Imbalance: Examination and Treatment Using Flexion Test. J Am Osteopath Assoc 77:456, 1978

10. Walheim G, Olerud S, Ribbe T: Mobility of the Pubic Symphysis. Acta Orthop Scan 55:203, 1984

11. Weismantel A: Evaluation and Treatment of Sacroiliac Joint Problems. Bull Orthrop Sect Am Phys Ther Assoc 3(1):5, Spring 1978

12. Wilder DG, Pope MH, Frymoyer JW: The Functional Topography Of The Sacroiliac Joint. Spine 5(6):575, 1980

CHAPTER 8

EVALUATION AND MANAGEMENT OF TEMPOROMANDIBULAR DISORDERS

By Steven L. Kraus, PT OCS

INTRODUCTION

Clinicians are faced with daily challenges in the field of orthopædics. One area of the musculoskeletal system that is particularly challenging is the temporomandibular joint (TMJ). Clinicians continuously seek answers pertaining to the evaluation and management of the patient with symptomatic and dysfunctional TMJ. Numbers of textbooks, journal articles and continuing education courses address this topic. Unfortunately, issues surrounding the etiology, terminology, evaluation and management of the TMJ are often clouded by confusion and controversy. For instance, despite all the scientific evidence supporting a particular evaluation and treatment procedure, an equal volume of contradictory material exists. Such confusion mainly occurs because there has been no classification system for the TMJ. The clinician is understandably confused about the signs and symptoms of TMJ involvement and which philosophy of management he or she should follow.

In the following pages, the reader may not find all the answers to his or her questions. I do not presume to address the myriad of references and discussions that abound on the topic of the TMJ. I do believe an examination of the complexity of ideas and data on this subject permits a greater simplicity in our understanding of TMJ. The information that follows is not basic information and is not advanced. It is fundamental enough to help the novice clinician along a stable path, yet informative enough to expand the seasoned clinician's appreciation of TMJ management.

Particular techniques of evaluation and treatment are not the intended substance of this chapter. I will not attempt to integrate clinical decision making concepts. The primary objective is to analyze the essential components of a physical examination that assist sound diagnosis and management of the involved TMJ. A discussion of relevant TMJ anatomy and classification of temporomandibular disorders will help the reader achieve this objective. This chapter contains a common sense approach derived from fundamental principles of physical science. My clinical experience and its concepts are supported, whenever possible, by the scientific literature.

RELEVANT ANATOMY

Osseous Structures

Temporal Bone

The temporal bone forms the roof of the TMJ. Posterior to anterior landmarks on the temporal bone are: (Fig 8-1)

      1. Postglenoid Spine
      2. Mandibular Fossa
      3. Articular Eminence
      4. Articular Crest
      5. Articular Tubercle

The postglenoid spine, or process, is a downward extension of the squamosal portion of the temporal bone. [75] The postglenoid spine forms the posterior

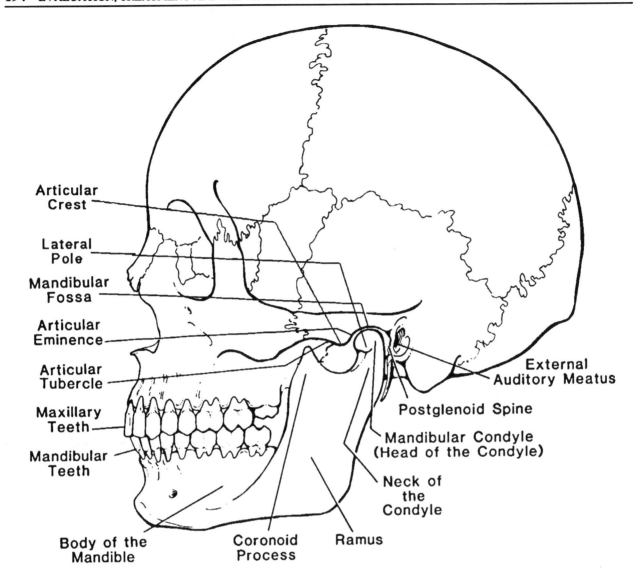

Labels on figure:
- Articular Crest
- Lateral Pole
- Mandibular Fossa
- Articular Eminence
- Articular Tubercle
- Maxillary Teeth
- Mandibular Teeth
- External Auditory Meatus
- Postglenoid Spine
- Mandibular Condyle (Head of the Condyle)
- Neck of the Condyle
- Body of the Mandible
- Coronoid Process
- Ramus

Figure 8-1. Skeletal Anatomy

aspect of the mandibular fossa and is positioned anterior to the external auditory meatus. The postglenoid spine offers attachments for portions of the capsule and posterior attachment tissues.[104] The concave mandibular fossa is occupied by the posterior band of the disc when the teeth are in occlusion or when the mandible is at rest. The mandibular fossa is a non-articular portion of the TMJ.[56] The articular eminence is convex in the anteroposterior direction and concave mediolaterally with a slope of 40° to 60° as measured in a neutral head position.[8] The articular crest is at the anterior end of the slope of the articular eminence before becoming the articular tubercle, which is somewhat concave in the mediolateral direction. The articulating surfaces on the temporal bone are located on the eminence-crest-tubercle areas.[104]

Mandibular Condyle

Each condyle of the mandible has an elliptical shape measuring 20 mm mediolaterally and 10 mm anteroposteriorly (Fig 8-2).[150] The mandibular condyle is a convex surface anterior to posterior and medial to lateral. Considerable variation in the size and shape of the condylar head is seen not only from person to person but from one side to another (Fig 8-3).[150] On the medial and lateral aspects of the condyle are anatomical landmarks called the medial and lateral poles, respectively. The medial pole of the condyle lies posterior and the lateral pole lies anterior to the transverse condylar rotational axis (Fig 8-2).[28] Between the medial and lateral poles of each condyle is the long axis of the condyle. If each long axis is extended

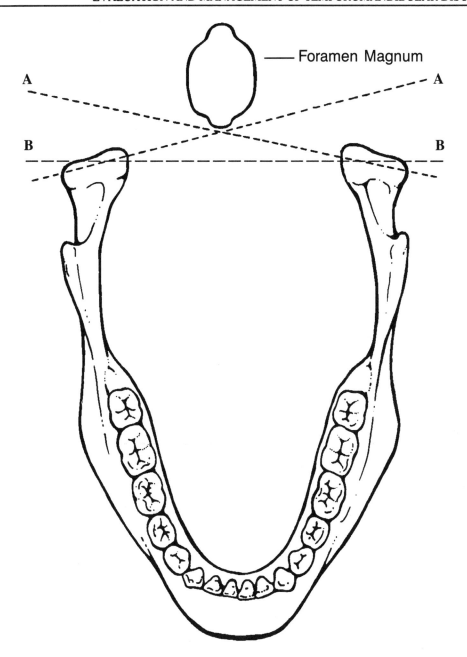

Figure 8-2. If extended, each long axis of the condyle (A) will intersect near the anterior margin of the foramen magnum. The transverse axis of the condyle (B) is anterior to the medial pole and posterior to the lateral pole.

medially, the two axes of the condyles form an obtuse angle varying from 145°-160° (Fig 8-2).[8] The articulating surfaces are located on the anterior/superior/posterior portions of the condyle.[104]

Inferior to the condylar head is the neck. Between the neck and the ramus of the mandible is the projection of the coronoid process. From the ramus starts the body of the mandible. The body of the mandible houses the lower arch of teeth (mandibular teeth) (Fig 8-1).

Clinical Relevance of the Osseous Anatomy

Most articulating joint surfaces in the body are covered by hyaline cartilage. The articulating surfaces of the temporomandibular joint are covered instead by dense fibrous connective tissue that is avascular and aneural.[28] The dense fibrous connective tissue has the same general properties found in hyaline cartilage but tends to be less distensible.[64] The clinical differences between the two types of articular surfaces are that

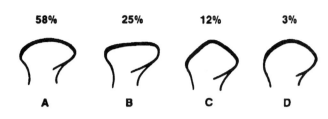

58%   25%   12%   3%

A   B   C   D

Figure 8-3. Four shapes of mandibular condyles when viewed in the frontal plane: A) Convex condyle; B) Flat condyle; C) Angular condyle; and D) Rounded condyle (adapted with permission from Yale[150]).

dense fibrous connective tissue has greater potential to remodel and is less likely to breakdown over time.[136]

Functional activities such as chewing, talking and yawning and parafunctional activities such as clenching and bruxism involve loading the articulating surfaces. Articulation (load bearing) occurs where the dense fibrous connective tissue is the thickest. Dense fibrous connective tissue is located on the articular eminence and crest of the temporal bone, and the anterior/ superior and, to a certain extent, posterior portions of the condyle (Fig 8-4).[104] The TMJ is a load bearing joint.[12] In all treatment techniques and procedures the clinician must remember where load bearing occurs and try not to force loading elsewhere on the temporal bone and condyle. An example of incorrect loading is traction force applied through the mandible. An intraoral appliance that forces incorrect loading when

the opposing surfaces of teeth contact on the appliance is another example.

Specifically, the primary load bearing areas on the temporal bone and condyle are located on the lateral aspect of the eminence and condyle, and include the lateral aspect of the interposed articular disc.[8] Adaptive remolding of the articular surfaces can occur in the TMJ.[104] Regressive remolding normally predominates on the lateral articulating surfaces since this is where most loading occurs. There are limits to the adaptive response of the TMJ to functional, dysfunctional and therapeutic situations.[104] When loading demands exceed adaptive potential, degenerative joint disease (arthrosis) occurs and is seen first in the lateral aspect of most TMJ's.[67, 104]

Excessive force or repetitive loading may strain the disc and collateral ligament laterally and allow the disc to displace not only anteriorly but medially.[8] In the absence of macrotrauma, such excessive loading or repetitive loading is caused by microtrauma. Microtrauma results from daily functional and parafunctional activities such as chewing ice, fingernails, or pencils, etc. The health of the disc and the articulating surfaces is dependent upon the frequency, duration, magnitude, direction and location of such microtrauma.[104] Additional factors that affect the loading of the joint surfaces and disc involve the individual morphological variations of bony and muscular anatomy.

The lateral pole of the condyle, located directly in front of the tragus of the ear, is an important bony

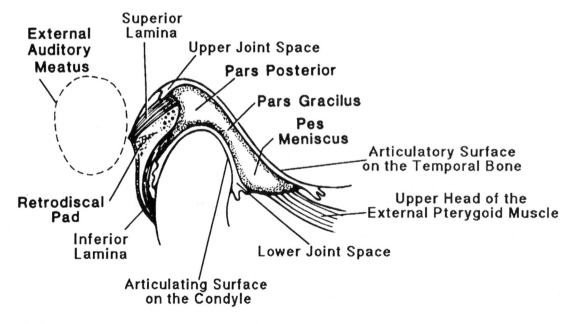

Figure 8-4. A sagittal view of the normal anatomy of the temporomandibular joint (adapted with permission from Mahan[90]).

landmark for the clinician to find for examination and treatment purposes (Fig 8-1). The clinician can easily identify the lateral pole by palpating with the middle or index finger, especially if the patient opens and closes his or her mouth.

A significant clinical feature of osseous anatomy is a row of teeth at one end of the mandibular lever arm (Fig 8-1). The relationship of condyles to teeth provides a unique but unfortunate characteristic of the TMJ. On full closure, when the posterior lower arch of teeth contact the posterior upper arch of teeth, there is a finite, rigid end point of closure. At end range of motion (full closure) the TMJ is therefore unlike any other joint of the body. The occlusion determines the final end point of the condyle to disc to temporal bone relationship when the posterior teeth are together. Because of this special occlusal/TMJ relationship, a great deal of emphasis has been placed on the occlusion as the etiology or key in diagnosing and treating of the TMJ.

In September 1990, the American Academy of Pediatric Dentistry and the University of Texas at San Antonio co-sponsored a working conference about the evaluation and treatment of disorders of the TMJ in children and young adults.[3] Among many interesting conclusions from this conference, a summary statement was made: "At this time, there does not appear to be any scientific basis for believing that malocclusion per se is a predisposing factor for the development of temporomandibular disorders." This conclusion is also echoed in other articles.[83, 134] However, it cannot be denied that in some cases, signs and symptoms of TMJ involvement are improved when the occlusion is treated. Clinical and scientific studies cannot explain why some patients may benefit and other patients may not benefit but may, in fact, become worse from occlusal therapy.[3, 83, 134] Even though occlusion is no longer considered a primary etiology of involvement of the TMJ, malocclusion in the presence of known etiologies may act as an initiating, aggravating, or accelerating variable. Study of the interaction of various etiologies should be the emphasis and the next frontier in TMJ research. For now, the criteria for treating occlusal problems should not differ between patients with TMJ involvement and patients without TMJ involvement.[19]

Intracapsular Structures

Articular Disc

The articular disc (not to be confused with vertebral disc) lies between and articulates with the mandibular condyle and the temporal bone (Fig 8-4). A similar relationship between articulating surfaces and a disc

exists in only the acromioclavicular and sternoclavicular joints and the symphysis pubis (prior to fusion).[140] Weldon Bell clarifies why this structure within the TMJ is a disc rather than a meniscus as it is often identified.[8] Bell states that a meniscus does not divide the joint cavity into separate compartments as the disc of the TMJ does. A meniscus facilitates movement of the bony parts but does not act as a true articular surface.[8] A meniscus is a passive structure. The disc of the TMJ has a contractile tissue and an elastic, non-contractile tissue attaching to it. These tissues let the TMJ move independently of either the condyle or the articular eminence.[75]

The TMJ disc is made of a dense fibrous connective tissue.[104] The disc is avascular and aneural except in the peripheral non-pressure-bearing areas.[149] A firm yet flexible structure, the disc can adapt to incongruities in the shapes of the articulating surfaces. Rees[119] divided the disc into three bands according to thickness: anterior (pes meniscus), intermediate (pars gracilus) and posterior (pars posterior) bands (Fig 8-4). For the purpose of this chapter, I will refer to these poorly demarcated divisions of the disc as bands.

The posterior band is thicker than the anterior band and the intermediate band is the thinnest. With the mouth closed (back teeth together), the normal disc position to the condyle has the posterior band positioned superiorly on the condyle, often referred to as the twelve o'clock position (Fig 8-4);[60] the intermediate band positioned along the articular eminence; and the anterior band lying most anterior to the condyle.

The disc of the TMJ divides the joint into superior and inferior compartments or joint spaces (Fig 8-4). The upper joint space is larger than the lower joint space, extending further anteriorly in the sagittal plane and overlapping the lower joint space in the coronal plane (Fig 8-5). The volumes of the upper and lower joint spaces are 1.2 ml and 0.9 ml, respectively.[10]

The disc has the following attachments:

1. Medial/Lateral

The disc attaches firmly to the medial and lateral poles of the condyle by the medial and lateral (discal-condylar) collateral ligaments (Fig 8-5).[122]

2. Posterior

The disc is contiguous with the posterior attachment* (Fig 8-4).[75, 112] The posterior superior disc attaches to the superior lamina or stratum. The posterior inferior disc attaches to the inferior lamina or stratum.

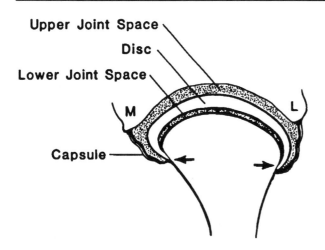

Figure 8-5. A frontal view of the left temporomandibular joint. Arrows depict attachments of the disc and capsule to the medial and lateral poles.

3. Anterior

The disc is attached anteriorly to the capsule and to the superior fibers of the superior lateral pterygoid.[53, 75] Approximately 1/3 of the superior lateral pterygoid has an attachment to the anterior and medial disc/capsule.[53, 75] The remaining portion of the superior lateral pterygoid and the fibers of the inferior lateral pterygoid attach to the medial 1/3 of the neck of the condyle.[75, 112]

* Posterior Attachment (PA)

The term posterior attachment (PA) designates the tissue often referred to as the "bilaminar zone," "retroarticular or retrodiscal pad" and "retrodiscal fat pad."[125] The PA occupies the posterior joint space behind the posterior band of the disc. Scapino states, "The normal PA contains small-caliber, loosely associated collagen fibers, a branching system of elastic fibers, fat deposits, a specialized arterial supply, a large venous plexus, lymphatics, and a profuse nerve supply."[125] For the reader to understand the attachments and functional role the PA has in the dynamics of the disc, the terms bilaminar zone and retrodiscal pad will be used separately to describe distinct anatomical entities.

The bilaminar zone is composed of the superior and inferior lamina with the retrodiscal pad between the two laminæ (Fig 8-4).[119] The superior lamina originates at the posterior superior band of the disc and courses posteriorly to attach in the area of the postglenoid spine.[46] The superior lamina contains loose fibroelastic tissue with a high elastin content. Rees [119] demonstrated 7-10 mm extensibility of the superior lamina in fresh cadaver specimens. The inferior lamina originates from the posterior inferior band of the disc and courses posteriorly around the back of the condyle to attach to the posterior aspect on the condylar neck. The inferior lamina is composed mainly of collagenous fibers with little elastic tissue.

The retrodiscal pad contains many large, blood-filled, endothelium-lined spaces.[51] As the condyle translates forward, the volume of the retrodiscal tissue expands due to venous distention, filling the mandibular fossa.[37] During closure, the retrodiscal pad returns to its smaller size and shape.

Clinical Relevance of the Articular Disc

The anatomical features of the disc create a "self-seating" effect of the disc to the condyle.[100] The self-seating effect of the disc, described by Moffett, is caused by the biconcave shape of the disc created by the thin intermediate band connecting the thick posterior and slightly less thick anterior bands.[100] The self-seating feature, along with the tight medial and lateral collateral ligaments, prevents anterior displacements of the disc to the condyle.[90] Posterior displacements are rare. The disc's shape and attachments allow it to rotate anteriorly and posteriorly on the condyle with ease.[8, 112]

Knowing the disc divides the TMJ into two compartments helps the clinician understand why an arthrogram can be used to diagnose or confirm disc displacement or perforation. Arthrography is an indirect way of visualizing the intracapsular anatomy in a static and dynamic manner. Because the upper joint space is larger in volume than the lower, a water-soluble contrast medium (dye) is injected first into the lower joint space under fluoroscopic visualization (if the dye was injected into the upper joint space first, the dye would obscure the lower joint space). In a normal situation, arthrography would show the dye confined to the lower joint space, providing an outline of the disc's position on the condyle.[10, 51] If a perforation is present, a flow of dye from the inferior to the superior joint space is observed. Under fluoroscopy, a disc displacement would show a characteristic pooling of the dye both in the static and dynamic viewings. The reader is referred to the bibliography for further information on arthrography.[24, 117]

Inflammatory conditions, covered later in this chapter, are further divided into two subcategories of synovitis and capsulitis. Synovitis involves the inner lining of the capsule and the PA. The surfaces of the PA are covered with synovial membrane.[125] In the presence of a significant amount of synovitis, the patient may be unable to bring his or her back teeth together on the side of the involved joint secondary to the amount of swelling in the PA. I believe inflammatory conditions of synovitis and capsulitis are the most common source of the patient's TMJ symptoms.

Capsule

The capsule is composed of fibrous connective tissue.[53] Superiorly, the capsule is attached to the rim of the temporal articular surfaces; inferiorly, the capsule tapers to attach to the condylar neck. The capsule blends medially and laterally with the medial and lateral ligaments of the disc as they attach to the medial and lateral poles. The capsule and the medial and lateral collateral ligaments of the disc form the articular capsule for the lower joint space.[57] At the level of the superior joint space, the capsule has no medial and lateral attachments to the disc (Fig 8- 5).[57] Further laterally, the capsule thickens to become the TMJ ligament. Anteriorly, the capsule blends with the upper and lower head of the external pterygoid and anterior portion of the disc. Posteriorly, the capsule attaches to the PA in the area of the postglenoid spine.[56, 57]

The capsule is lined by a highly vascular, synovial fluid-producing membrane that supplies nutrients to the non-vascularized tissues within the capsule. The capsule is innervated with sensory receptors and nociceptors.

Clinical Relevance of the Capsule

The capsule of the TMJ contains articular mechanoreceptors which provide kinesthetic and perceptional awareness of the mandible. Mechanoreceptor activity of the TMJ also influences motor neuron pool activity, primarily of the muscles that move the TMJ. Conditions such as synovitis/ capsulitis and capsular fibrosis can affect the neurophysiological output of the mechanoreceptors' activity, thereby affecting the kinesthetic and perceptional awareness and muscle tone of the muscles innervated by Cranial Nerve V. Capsular fibrosis also affects the arthrokinematics of the TMJ, often expressed clinically as a restriction in mandibular dynamics. For a review of the effects of capsulitis and capsular fibrosis on mechanoreceptor activity and arthrokinematics of the TMJ, the reader is referred to the bibliography.[74]

Ligaments

Intracapsular ligaments consisting of the medial and lateral collateral ligaments have been discussed. The remaining ligaments are either part of the capsule or are extracapsular.

Temporomandibular Ligament

The temporomandibular ligament is often referred to as the lateral ligament because it is continuous with the capsule and is thus a distinct thickening of the lateral capsule (Fig 8-6).[13] This ligament is composed of two parts, an outer oblique portion and an inner horizontal portion.[112] The outer portion extends from the zygomatic process to run in a posterior and obliquely inferior direction to attach to the posterolateral aspect of the condylar neck (Fig 8-6).[112] The inner horizontal portion extends from the zygomatic process to run in a posterior and horizontal direction to attach to the lateral pole.[112]

Stylomandibular and Sphenomandibular Ligaments

The stylomandibular and sphenomandibular ligaments are extracapsular ligaments (Fig 8-7).[13] The stylomandibular ligament extends from the styloid process of the temporal bone to the posterior aspect of the mandible. The sphenomandibular ligament attaches superiorly to the angular spine of the sphenoid bone and attaches inferiorly on the lingula of the mandibular foramen.[10]

Clinical Relevance of the Ligaments

The temporomandibular ligament reinforces the capsule laterally. The inner (horizontal) portion of this ligament limits posterior movement of the condyle when force is applied to the mandible, thereby protecting the PA from trauma. Some authors state that the arrangements of the outer (oblique) fibers would prevent a separation of the condyle/disc/ temporal fossa and restrain condylar movement on maximum mouth opening, protrusion and lateral excursion.[52, 112, 131] The outer portion of the temporomandibular ligament allows as much as 20- 25 mm of mandibular opening to occur before it becomes tight. Thereafter, the condyle must translate to allow further opening.[112] The reader should recognize that if a patient opens to only 20-25 mm, this movement primarily represents rotation with no translation of the condyle.

Conditions causing capsular fibrosis can produce temporomandibular ligament tightening as the ligament and capsule, in this case, are essentially one and the same. Any treatment of capsular fibrosis will

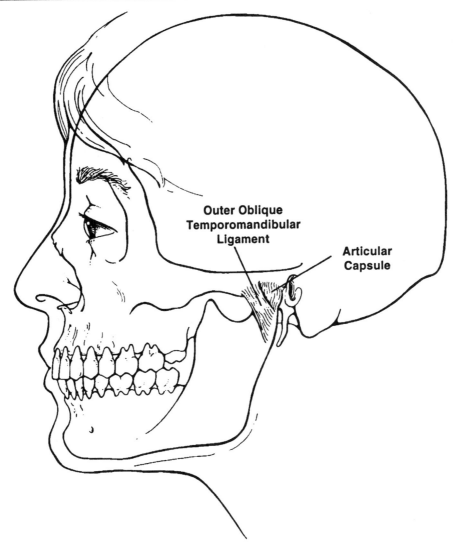

Figure 8-6. A lateral view of the outer oblique temporomandibular ligament and capsular support of the temporomandibular joint.

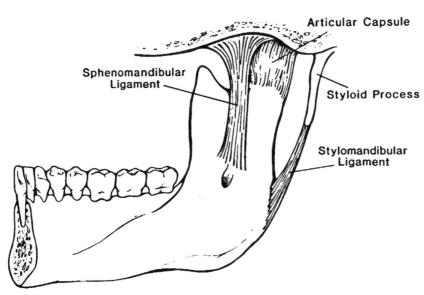

Figure 8-7. A medial view of the ligamentous-capsular support of the temporomandibular joint.

also address tightness of the temporomandibular ligament.

The stylomandibular and sphenomandibular ligaments are not intimately associated with the articulation of the TMJ. They may protect the joint during wide excursive movements.[10, 14] These two ligaments will not be considered as causative factors in TMJ involvement.

Innervation

Innervation of the TMJ is primarily by the auriculotemporal branch of the 3rd division of the trigeminal nerve.[135] The auriculotemporal nerve innervates the PA and the posterior and lateral joint capsule. The most anterior part of the joint is supplied by the masseteric and posterior deep temporal nerves.[135]

Clinical Relevance of Innervation

Anesthetic block to the auriculotemporal nerve can be used as a differential diagnostic tool to determine if the patient's pain is arthrogenous in origin.[8] If the patient's symptoms are myogenous or referred from other adjacent areas, i.e., cervical spine, then the patient's symptoms will not be affected by this block. A successful block would involve patient report of a reduction in preauricular pain. However, a decrease in preauricular pain does not address which TM disorder is the source of the patient's symptoms or what treatment is indicated. The clinician must also be aware the placebo effect may provide a false positive response to this procedure.

OSTEOKINEMATICS AND ARTHROKINEMATICS OF THE TEMPOROMANDIBULAR JOINT

The TMJ is an articulation between the condyle of the mandible and squamous portion of the temporal bone. The TMJ is a true synovial ginglymoarthrodial joint. The TMJ is ginglymoid in that it provides a hinging movement and arthrodial in that it provides for a freely movable gliding motion.[104] There is also an interposed disc between the condyle and temporal bone that can move independently of both of them during active movements of the mandible. The following discussion of mandibular dynamics will be confined to osteokinematic and arthrokinematic movements. Dynamics of disc function are included under arthrokinematics.

Osteokinematics

Osteokinematics pertains to the overall movement of bones, i.e., flexion, extension, rotation, etc., with little reference to their related joints.[87] Functional osteokinematic movements of the mandible are:

Depression

Mandibular depression involves opening the mouth in the sagittal plane. *Functional mandibular depression* describes the patient's ability to actively open his or her mouth to 40 mm, including a 2 mm overbite. The clinician measures this motion by placing a millimeter ruler between the tip of the right or left maxillary and mandibular central incisors (Fig 8-8).

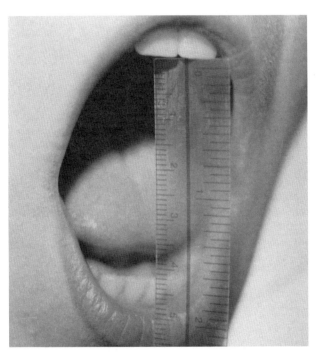

Figure 8-8. Evaluating mandibular depression.

Protrusion

Protrusion describes anterior movement of the mandible in the horizontal plane. *Functional mandibular protrusion* is the patient's ability to actively protrude the mandible so that at least an edge to edge position can be achieved between maxillary and mandibular central incisors. Ideally, the mandibular central incisors should move past the maxillary central incisors by several millimeters (Fig 8-9). No precise measurement is assigned to this movement. It is more an individual functional goal than a rigid unit of measure.

Lateral Excursion

Lateral excursion involves the mandible moving laterally in the horizontal plane. *Functional lateral excursion* denotes the patient's ability to actively

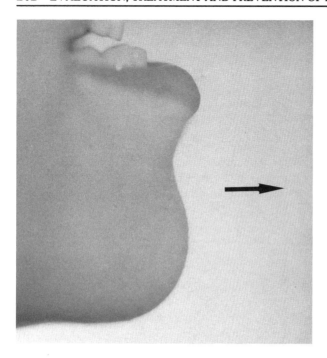

Figure 8-9. Evaluating mandibular protrusion.

move the mandible laterally so that at least the mandibular canine achieves an end to end position in relation to the maxillary canine. Ideally, the mandibular canine should move past the maxillary canine by several millimeters bilaterally (Fig 8-10). Again, no precise measurement will be assigned to this movement for the reason stated above.

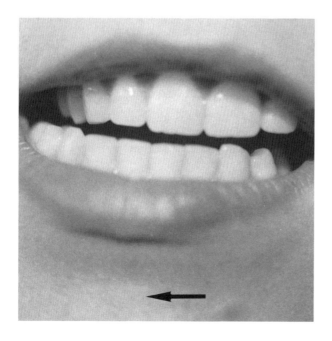

Figure 8-10. Evaluating right mandibular lateral excursion.

General Comments about Osteokinematics

Clinicians often hope to see midline mandibular opening and protrusion versus mandibular deviation or deflection. Deviation is defined as movement of the mandible away from midline during mandibular depression or protrusion, with the mandible returning back to midline by the end of such movement. The "S" curve deviation describes this type of motion. Deflection is defined as the movement of the mandible away from midline during mandibular depression or protrusion but without return to midline. The "C" curve deflection describes this type of motion. To some clinicians, deviation or deflection during opening or protrusive mandibular movements may suggest some degree of TMJ involvement. What must be understood is that mandibular dynamics can be affected by various anomalies of the osseous structures. I would like to see midline depression and protrusion but recognize that good function can occur without midline function. Mandibular deviations and deflections in the presence of functional depression, protrusion and lateral excursions may often be considered insignificant, and require no treatment unless the evaluation was positive for TMJ involvement known to cause mandibular deviations or deflections.

Restricted osteokinematic movements may interfere with the patient's ability to perform functional activities such as chewing, talking, and yawning. Evaluating restricted osteokinematic movements may help differentiate between an arthrogenous and a myogenous involvement and make for a better treatment plan.

The following is a quick screening using osteokinematic movements to differentiate between an arthrogenous and a myogenous involvement:

Instruct the patient to open his or her mouth. If mandibular depression is less than functional opening, either an arthrogenous or myogenous involvement is suggested. Have the patient then move the jaw into protrusion and lateral excursion bilaterally. If these osteokinematic movements are functional, the restriction in mandibular depression would suggest a myogenous cause.

Myogenous involvement that is restricting mandibular depression is often confirmed by palpating the temporalis and masseter muscles and noting any increase in tone or subjective discomfort. Arthrogenous involvement typically restricts the arthrokinematic movement of translation. When translation is limited, the classic osteokinematic restrictions and aberrant movements of the mandible are (Fig 8-11):

1. Mandibular Depression

Less than functional opening with deflection to the side of the involved joint

2. Protrusion

Less than functional protrusion with deflection to the side of the involved joint

3. Lateral Excursion

Normal lateral excursion to the side of the involved joint

Less than functional lateral excursion to the opposite side of the involved joint

Arthrokinematics

Arthrokinematics pertains to movement between two joint surfaces. The disc will be included in this discussion of arthrokinematics.

Condyle to Temporal Bone Relationship

Arthrokinematic movements consist of active and passive accessory movements that must occur to achieve full, pain free movements in diarthrodial joints.[88] The accessory movements of the TMJ are *distraction, compression, rotation, translation, spin and lateral glide*. *Distraction* of the condyle, for example, occurs when biting against resistance (food) placed unilaterally between the upper and lower third molars. Distraction of the condyle occurs on the ipsilateral side of resistance.[55, 128] *Compression* occurs on the contralateral side of resistance in the previous example. Compression of either condyle may also occur during other functional and parafunctional activities secondary to the loading effect of contracting muscles. Accessory movements of *rotation, translation* and *spin* can be appreciated with the following osteokinematic movements of the mandible:

A. Mandibular Depression

Phase I

The first phase of opening involves the accessory movement of rotation of the condyle around the long axis of the condylar heads. Rotation occurs for the first 10-15 mm before mandibular opening enters Phase II.[25] It is described as posterior rotation in relation to the temporal bone.

The dental literature describes condylar rotation during opening as anterior rotation.[115] The orthopædic principle of a convex-concave relation of two opposing joint surfaces states that rotation and translation occur in opposite directions. The TMJ has a convex surface (the condyle) and a relatively concave surface (the articular eminence, which is concave in the mediolateral direction). Since the condyle translates anteriorly, condylar rotation during full opening can be described as posterior rotation. This text will describe condylar rotation during opening as posterior rotation.

Clinically, whether or not condylar rotation is described as anterior or posterior rotation is insignificant. The main point of this discussion is to justify my terminology in this situation.

Phase II

Phase II involves the accessory movement of anterior translation of the condyle. Translation starts between 10-15 mm of mandibular opening in conjunction with continued rotation. Combined rotation and translation let the mandible achieve a functional opening of 40 mm. If condylar translation is severely restricted, a mandibular opening of 20-25 mm can still be achieved via rotation alone. However, 20-25 mm of opening is not functional and significantly limits the patient's use of his or her jaw.

B. Protrusion

Protrusion involves the accessory movement of bilateral anterior condylar translation.

C. Lateral Excursion

Lateral excursion involves the accessory movement of anterior translation on the contralateral side and spin on the ipsilateral side.

Lateral glide is a passive accessory movement that occurs secondary to an external force rather than direct voluntary control. This passive accessory movement is called joint play.[98] Joint play movements are the inherent quality of the joint to "give."[98] A hinge on a door not only allows the door to swing open but can allow minimal up and down movement of the door. This up and down movement of the hinge is analogous to joint play. The joint play movement of lateral glide can occur with any of the other accessory movements at any time during functional and parafunctional activities.

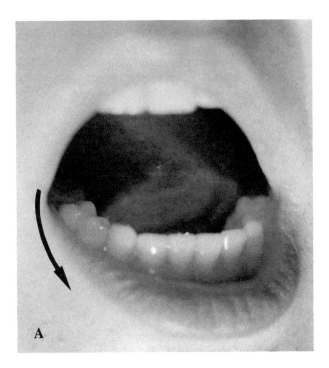 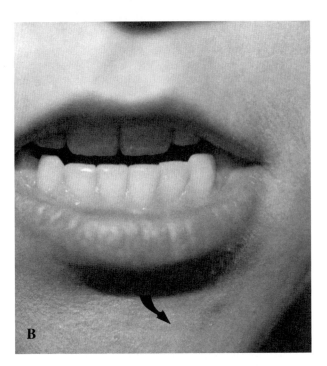

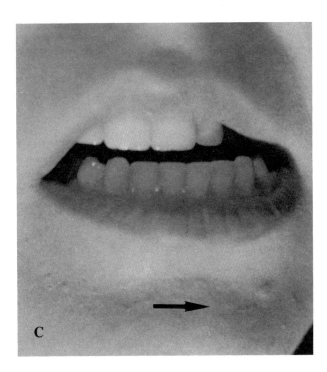 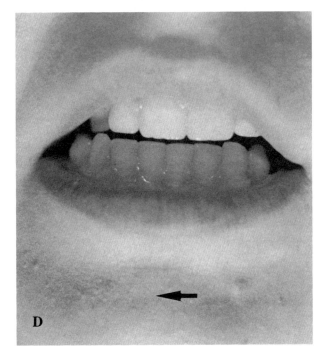

Figure 8-11. Limited and aberrant osteokinematic movements seen when the arthrokinematic movement of translation of the left TMJ is significantly restricted: A) Mandibular depression - less than functional opening with deflection to the left; B) Protrusion - less than functional opening with deflection to the left; C) Left lateral excursion - functional; D) Right lateral excursion - less than functional.

When a capsular or intracapsular arthrogenous problem of the TMJ is present, accessory movements of rotation, spin and compression are seldom restricted.[74] An exception to this occurs where significant joint inflammation or masticatory muscle hyperactivity is present. The primary accessory movements restricted with arthrogenous problems are translation, distraction and lateral glide.[74] Of these three, translation seems to be the primary accessory movement restricted and the more difficult one to regain, regardless of the arthrogenous problem.

Disc to Condyle and Temporal Bone Relationship

A discussion of disc dynamics will be applied to mandibular depression only. Further analysis of disc dynamics during protrusion and lateral excursion will not be addressed in this chapter.

Rotation occurs in the lower joint space between the condyle and the inferior surface of the disc (Fig 8-12).[8, 28, 112] All translation occurs in the upper joint space between the superior portion of the disc and the temporal bone (Fig 8-12).

When the condyle translates anteriorly or posteriorly, the disc moves with it because of the self-seating effect of disc to condyle[100] and the intact medial and lateral collateral ligaments.[90] In addition, the force generated by the condylar head pressing against the thickened anterior band upon initiation of translation literally pushes the disc ahead of the condyle.[112] During closing, the condylar head presses against the thickened posterior band, pushing the disc posteriorly.

During Phase I opening, the condyle simply rotates posteriorly under an essentially stationary disc (Fig 8-13B). First the anterosuperior, then the superior, and finally the posterosuperior aspects of the condyle articulate with the intermediate zone of the disc. At the end of Phase I, the disc is in a more posteriorly rotated position in relation to the condyle when compared to the beginning of opening.

Phase II opening disc dynamics are debated. The disc is anchored posteriorly by the elastic superior stratum and non-elastic inferior stratum. Whether the superior stratum becomes tight as the condyle and disc translate anteriorly[90, 115] or the disc is affected by its own self-seating,[8] the disc is rotated further posteriorly on the condyle during Phase II mandibular depression (Fig 8-13C).[115] The results are:

1. The thinner non-vascularized and non-innervated portion of the intermediate band of the disc is kept between the two compressing joint surfaces.

2. The non-elastic inferior stratum is not stretched.

When the mandible closes from a fully opened position, the disc needs to rotate anteriorly on the condyle. Anteriorly, the disc is attached to the upper head of the external pterygoid muscle. There is debate about what percentage of muscle fibers of the upper head of the external pterygoid attach to the anteromedial portion of the disc.[89, 104, 115, 148] Wilk[147] found "anterior movement of the disc can be produced experimentally in pigs through electrical stimulation of the superior head of the lateral pterygoid. After 14 days the disc was anteriorly placed, but still maintained

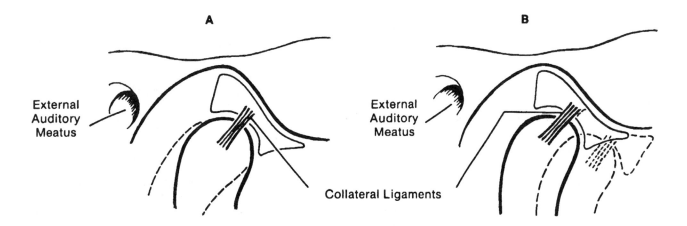

Figure 8-12. A) During Phase I mandibular depression, rotation occurs in the lower joint space; B) During Phase II mandibular depression, rotation continues in the lower joint space with translation occurring in the upper joint space (adapted with permission from W. Bell: Synopsis: Oral and Facial Pain and the Temporomandibular Joint, 1967).

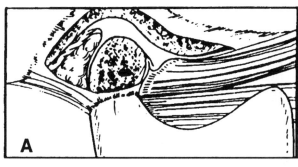

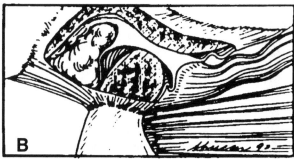

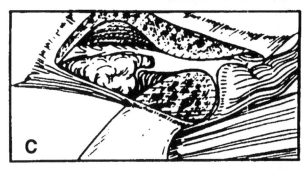

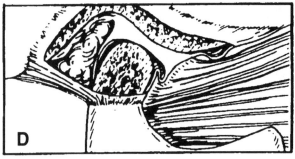

Figure 8-13. The disc and condyle during mandibular opening and closing: A) With the back teeth together; B) During Phase I opening - The condyle rotates posteriorly in the lower joint space as the disc also rotates posteriorly in relation to the condyle; C) At the end of Phase II (full opening) - Anterior translation occurs in the upper joint space with continued rotation in the lower joint space. Tension of the superior lamina influences additional posterior rotation of the disc; D) During closing - Both disc and condyle translate posteriorly while the condyle rotates anteriorly in the lower joint space. Tension in the upper head of the external pterygoid muscle may aid anterior rotation of the disc (adapted with permission from Okeson[112]).

a relationship between the condyle and fossa." The original work of McNamara [94] indicates the superior head of the lateral pterygoid muscle is active during the mandible's closing phase. The disc may therefore be rotated anteriorly during mandibular closing by several factors:

1. Activity of the upper head of the external pterygoid muscle (Fig 8-13D)

2. Relaxation of the superior lamina

3. The self-seating effect of the disc

The complete cycle of opening and closing showing the condyle-disc-temporal bone relationships is demonstrated in Figure 8-13.

CLASSIFICATION OF TEMPOROMANDIBULAR DISORDERS

Dworkin states, "A critical obstacle to our further understanding of temporomandibular disorders is the lack of standardized diagnostic criteria for defining clinical subtypes of TMD."[29] A classification system could establish more meaningful communication among health professionals who are trying to understand the etiology, prevalence, evaluation, treatment and prognosis of TMD. A widely acceptable classification system that focuses on TMD is still in the developmental stages.[111] In addition, there are no specific diagnostic criteria and no reliable, valid operational measurements for identifying the clinical subtypes of TMD.[29] Numerous obstacles must still be overcome before complete acceptance of a classification system exists for TMD.[111] This section of the text will discuss the dilemmas of terminology and clinical research and will identify a TMD classification system consisting of multiple subset diagnostic categories that has developed some acceptance among health professionals.

What's In A Name ?

There still appears to be an attempt to find an all inclusive diagnostic term to describe virtually everything and anything that is symptomatic involving the head, face, jaw and neck. Over the years, erroneous diagnostic terms have been created that have focused upon the TMJ as the source of all symptoms of the head, face, jaw and neck. Treatment, it would follow, has been largely directed towards the TMJ.

The following is a partial list of diagnostic terms that appoint the TMJ as the source of patient signs and symptoms. The date preceding the diagnostic term indicates the period in which each diagnostic term was most common in the literature, not its period of development.

1956 - Costen Syndrome [23]

1959 - TMJ Dysfunction Syndrome [130]

1959 - Temporomandibular Pain Syndrome [127]

1964 - Pain Dysfunction Syndrome [138]

1969 - Myofascial Pain Dysfunction Syndrome (MPDS) [77]

1970 - Internal Derangement [34]

1971 - Occlusomandibular Disturbance [41]

1971 - Myoarthropathy of the TMJ [44]

1975 - Craniocervical - Mandibular Syndrome [40]

1977 - Craniomandibular Disorder (CMD) [97]

1983 - Cranio - Cervical Dysfunction [18]

1984 - Stomatognathic Disorder (SGD) [113]

1984 - Dental Distress Syndrome (DDS) [38, 93]

1992 - Ondontostomatognathic System Syndrome (OSS) [1]

These diagnostic terms obviously broaden to include areas around the TMJ, yet the main focus of the source and treatment of symptoms remains the TMJ. It is as though an all inclusive diagnostic term will justify the numerous symptoms a patient may have and somehow, if the TMJ is treated, resolve them. This form of thinking is not realistic and has blanketed the TMJ with a dark cloud of confusion and controversy. An example of such unrealistic thinking is the notion by some clinicians that the TMJ can disturb the whole body.[1, 93] Dental Distress Syndrome reportedly affects the respiratory system, spinal posture and pathophysiological alterations throughout the total biologic unit.[38] Other symptoms attributed to TMJ involvement are headaches, neck pains and muscular tension. As clinicians, we should be concerned with this overstatement of the symptoms of TMJ. We should also strive to simplify and define criteria relevant to a diagnosis of TMJ involvement. To some clinicians, a malocclusion, muscle tenderness to palpation, and inability to open the mandible in midline or forward

head posture indicates the patient has "TMJ," and treatment focuses upon these often unrelated signs of TM disorders.

Erroneous diagnostic terms and misleading signs and symptoms will lead to wrong thinking and unnecessary and costly treatment that impedes appropriate and necessary treatment. Can we blame the insurance companies for negative positions on TMD reimbursement? Indeed, one can appreciate why some physical therapists, dentists and physicians develop a suspicious attitude toward the patient who claims to have "TMJ." The inappropriate use of diagnostic terms, loose descriptions of the signs and symptoms of TMD and wide variations of suggested treatments will only place TMJ treatment in the category of quackery.[116] This is unfortunate for the patients who *do* have a symptomatic and dysfunctional joint that requires treatment yet often goes unrecognized by ill-informed clinicians.

TMD Classification System

The diagnostic term that will be used in this text to signify involvement of the TMJ will be temporomandibular disorders (TMD's). This term was adopted at The President's Conference on the Diagnosis and Management of Temporomandibular Disorders held in Chicago, 1982.[76] This conference brought together leading authorities on the TMJ. Conference participants focused their attention on many areas pertaining to the TMJ. One focus was to agree on the diagnostic term of TMD's to indicate TMJ involvement.

At the time this was written, nine diagnostic systems for classifying TMD had been reviewed in the literature.[111] The nine taxonomic systems were compared according to stringent evaluation criteria.[111] All nine taxonomic systems do require modifications to achieve higher scientific merit.[111] The subset diagnostic classification system for TMD's used in this chapter will follow the American Academy of Craniomandibular Disorders (AACD) classification system for TMD's.[2] The academy formed a committee of experts whose consensus and evaluation of the research literature arrived at a classification system for TMD's.[111] The AACD classification system was influenced by and follows closely the classification project undertaken by the International Headache Society's Classification and Diagnostic Criteria for Headache Disorders, Cranial Neuralgias and Facial Pain.[15] The International Headache Society lists "Disorders of the Temporomandibular Joint" as one of eight subcategories of the 11 major classifications of pain titled, "Headache or facial pain associated with disorders of the cranium, eyes, ears, nose, sinuses, teeth, mouth or other facial or cranial structures."[15]

The International Headache Society's integration of TMD into a larger framework of face, head and neck pains may stimulate productive developments between medicine, dentistry,[111] physical therapy and third party payers. The following terminology and diagnostic classification criteria for TMD's will therefore adhere to generally agreed upon standards that are integrated with an existing medical diagnostic system.[96] Considerable modification of this and other classification systems will no doubt occur as they are subjected to stringent analysis based on accepted standards for clinical research.[111] When accepted standards for clinical research are not adhered to, clinical dilemmas will emerge.

THE CLINICAL "DILEMMAS"

Comparative Analysis of the TMJ Literature

When reviewing scientific and clinical research on the TMJ, it is clear that the criteria used to establish a "TMJ" patient population in one study are not the criteria used in another study. Therefore, epidemiologic studies, etiologic studies, and studies investigating the success of treatment and prognosis are probably not using homogenous subjects in the patient, control and non-patient groups. Comparable and equivalent studies of the TMJ are essentially nonexistent[152] or at best, very recent.[111] The conclusions from most scientific and clinical research articles must be viewed critically. In the section that follows entitled "Management for TMD's," the reader should appreciate that consistent guidelines for management are not available in the literature and the information represents my opinions.

Clinical Research Considerations

As clinicians, we may tend to be lulled into a state of complacency with respect to the objectivity of our diagnostic tools. We use these diagnostic tools to "objectively" assess the patient's response to a form of treatment. Being objective with our diagnostic tools is extremely important because results that cannot be measured are easily misinterpreted.

The reliability and validity of diagnostic tools, whether they be the clinician's hands or a machine, must be reevaluated constantly. Clinicians should always be concerned about inter- and intra-rater reliability of examination procedures. *Reliability* is concerned with repeatability, or how consistently the test shows the same result. To measure *validity*, one asks, "Does the test measure what it says it measures?" Where reliability and validity are not maintained,

serious questions may be raised about the conclusions of evaluation and treatment.

Once the reliability and validity of a test has been established, the clinician must be concerned about external validity, which requires knowledge of the predictive values of a test.[47, 145] *External validity* is represented by the sensitivity and specificity of a test when applied to groups with known characteristics.[47] *Sensitivity* is the ability of the test and diagnostic criteria to detect patients with disease (true positive). *Specificity* is the ability of the test and diagnostic criteria to detect patients without disease (true negative).[151]

The sensitivity and specificity of a test do not indicate the accuracy of a test when applied to an individual patient. *Predictive values* of a test indicate how accurate the test result is for a particular patient.[47] *Positive predictive value* is the probability that a patient with a positive test result has the disease or attribute being tested.[47] *Negative predictive value* is the probability that a patient with a negative test result does not have the disease or attribute being tested.[47, 81]

The predictive value is an accepted method for evaluating a test's ability to discriminate between a control group and patients with a particular condition.[7] Clinicians must strive to answer the question: "Does the test administered over-diagnose or under-diagnose the condition?" The acceptable level of diagnostic sensitivity and specificity depends on the prevalence and gravity of disease and the cost of errors due to misdiagnosis.[95] Because of the low occurrence of TMD in the population and the zero mortality, one can accept the potential to misclassify someone with TMD as asymptomatic (false negative).[146] On the other hand, the asymptomatic patient who is incorrectly diagnosed as having the disorder (false positive) can be faced with costly, unnecessary and potentially damaging treatments.[146] For patients who have been properly diagnosed as having a TMD, the initial treatment plan should consider the cost, risk, invasiveness and discomfort of the patient.

Clinicians need to use evaluation tools that are reliable, valid and predictive. This text will not examine all the radiographic (MRI, CT, conventional radiographs, etc.) and electrodiagnostic equipment (EMG, sonography, jaw tracking devices, etc.) that are currently used to help diagnose. The reader is referred to the bibliography for the review of these paraclinical evaluative tools.[90, 117, 143, 145]

Before a clinician orders any diagnostic test the following questions should be asked [66]:

1. Will the information provided help establish a diagnosis or rule out other pathology?

2. Will the information change the proposed treatment plan?

3. Will the information help determine how far the disease has progressed and hence predict the clinical course?

At the time of this writing, the only generally agreed upon diagnostic procedures for TMD are [3, 43, 45, 101-103]:

1. Evaluation of the patient's chief complaint by taking a history.

2. Physical examination with basic techniques performed by skilled clinicians.

3. Radiographs when indicated. The panorex is ideally suited because of its low ionizing radiation exposure, minimal expense and availability. If the history and physical examination indicates a significant or life-threatening disease, other radiographic films would be required.[54] The 1982 American Dental Association conference recommended screening radiographs for all patients.[76]

HISTORY AND PHYSICAL EXAMINATION FOR TEMPOROMANDIBULAR DISORDERS

The following subset diagnoses of TMD's will not classify every patient. It is unwise to assume that each patient's TMD will fit neatly into a specific peg hole. Diagnostic criteria (history and clinical findings) for each subset diagnosis of TMD will be highlighted. Even though the diagnostic criteria for TMD's will be similar to the criteria promoted by the International Headache Society,[15] such guidelines are still not fully up to date due to growing scientific research. I will modify and add to the diagnostic criteria based upon my own clinical insight and interpretation of the scientific and clinical literature. Comparison with the original article by the International Headache Society[15] will allow the reader to see the modifications I have

made. I encourage the reader to review the other classification systems to appreciate the differences and similarities.[111] The International Classification of Diseases' code (ICD.9 CM) for each TMD medical diagnosis is listed in parentheses.

Patients frequently present with multiple disorders of the TMJ along with symptomatic and functional involvement of adjacent areas, i.e., muscles of mastication and disorders of the cervical spine. The clinician evaluating TMD should thoroughly understand the evaluation and treatment of other musculoskeletal disorders, so the concepts presented in the chapter can be integrated appropriately. Experience and good clinical decision making permit the clinician to differentiate a multitude of signs and symptoms, make a sound diagnosis and establish the initial treatment plans. The clinician must recognize and exclude intracranial (i.e., tumors) and extracranial (i.e., referred pain from the heart) pathology responsible for head, face and jaw symptoms. If the clinician is unable to exclude such problems in other areas, a referral should be made to the appropriate health professional.

Significant Issues in the History

Because we are discussing a joint disorder, the clinician should listen for a history that would incriminate the temporomandibular joint as the source of the patient's head, facial and jaw symptoms. A TMD is not the only possible cause of symptomatic functional and parafunctional activities (bruxism, clenching, nail biting, pencil chewing, etc.) of the mandible. Clinicians will need to recognize that myogenous involvement of the muscles of the mandible can also contribute to pain and dysfunction during functional or parafunctional activities. A physical examination for myogenous involvement of the muscles of the mandible should be done to differentiate between myogenous or arthrogenous involvement. Clinicians also need to recognize the cervical spine as a major source for symptoms in the head, face and jaw areas.[31] Unless evaluated by a competent medical and physical therapy clinician, the cervical spine must always be considered as a source of such local and cephalic symptoms [70, 80] that mimic various symptoms thought to be associated with TMD's.

1. Cardinal symptoms related to TMD's are:

a. Symptoms located in the preauricular area with or without reference into the temporal or mandibular areas.

b. Symptoms reproduced, increased, or decreased with functional or parafunctional activities of the mandible.

2. Symptoms consist of any one or combination of:

    a. Pain/discomfort.
    b. Joint noises during jaw movements.
    c. Limitation or difficulty in jaw movement.

The onset, frequency, duration and intensity of the symptoms must be obtained to determine irritability and progression of the disorder. The clinician needs to document what the patient does to either increase or decrease symptoms so these specific activities can be reassessed. The patient's positive or negative response to any previous treatment methods should be recorded. The clinician should document any other medical or dental information that may have a bearing on the final interpretation of the examination.[9]

The following are 12 subset diagnostic categories of TMD's. Under each diagnostic category is listed the ICD code, previously used terms, and findings in the history and physical examination that are used to diagnose the specific disorder. The 12 diagnostic categories are grouped into six general conditions of TMD's.

Inflammatory Conditions

Synovitis and Capsulitis (ICD #716.98 and ICD # 727.09)

Previously used terms for synovitis: capsulitis, discitis, retrodiscitis, arthritis. Previously used terms for capsulitis: retrodiscitis, arthritis, arthralgia, contusion

History

1. The symptoms of pain/discomfort are located in the preauricular area with or without reference into the temporal or mandibular areas.

2. The symptoms are produced, increased, or decreased with functional or parafunctional activities of the mandible.

3. Depending on the degree of intracapsular effusion that occurs with synovitis, the patient may state that he or she is unable to bring the back teeth fully together without experiencing pain on the ipsilateral side of the involved joint. Opening may also be limited (less than 40 mm) secondary to pain.

4. The symptoms are decreased or at least not aggravated by resting the mandible from functional or parafunctional activities.

Physical Examination

1. TMJ Palpation

    a. Palpate Lateral to the Lateral Pole (Fig 8-14)

    Using either the index or middle fingers, the clinician palpates lateral to the lateral pole with the patient's back teeth lightly touching. A positive test is an increase or reproduction of symptoms on the side of the involved TMJ.

    If positive, the clinician should suspect capsulitis.

    b. Palpate Posterior and Lateral to the Lateral Pole (Fig 8-15)

    The examiner palpates posterolaterally to the lateral pole with the patient opened to approximately 30 mm. A positive test is an increase or reproduction of symptoms on the side of the involved TMJ. If positive, the clinician should suspect capsulitis.

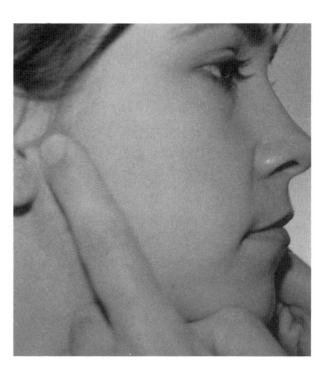

Figure 8-14. Palpation of the lateral pole with the back teeth lightly touching.

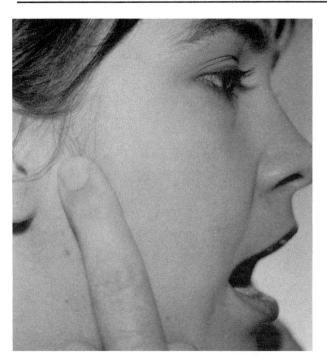

Figure 8-15. Palpation posterior and lateral to the lateral pole with the mouth opened to ≈ 30 mm.

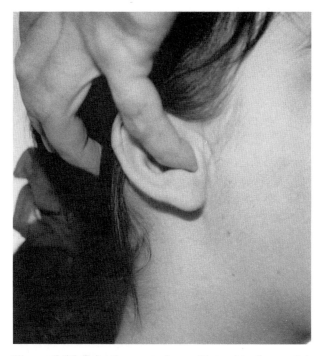

Figure 8-16. Palpation posterior and lateral to the condyle via the external auditory meatus.

c. External Auditory Meatus (EAM) Palpation (Fig 8-16)

With the patient's mouth opened, the examiner places his or her little finger (pad of the finger facing towards the condyle) in the patient's EAM and then applies slight pressure forward with his or her finger as the patient is asked to bring his or her back teeth together. A positive test is an increase or reproduction of the symptoms on the side of the involved TMJ. If positive, the clinician should suspect synovitis.

The clinician will not be concerned about any joint noises that may occur with this test while the clinician's finger is in the patient's EAM, especially if this is the first time the patient expresses hearing any joint noises.

2. TMJ Loading

a. Dynamic Loading and Distraction (forced biting)

This is a selective test involving either loading (compression) or distraction of the TMJ. Hylander [55] and others [128] have shown that biting against resistance (cotton roll) unilaterally placed between the upper and lower third molars will cause distraction of the condyle on the ipsilateral side of the resistance. Compression then is believed to occur on the contralateral side of the resistance (Fig 8-17).[144]

If the test is positive (an increase or reproduction of the symptoms) on the ipsilateral side of the resistance (distraction), the clinician may consider "capsulitis" as the working diagnosis, especially if 1a and 1b above are positive. If only 1c is positive, synovitis would then be suspected with a positive response to this test.

If the test was positive on the contralateral side of the resistance (loading), the clinician may consider synovitis as the working diagnosis. Clinically, I find dynamic loading to be more valid when trying to differentiate between synovitis or capsulitis.

b. Passive Loading (retrusive overpressure)

With the patient's back teeth slightly apart, the examiner grasps the chin with the index and thumb. The clinician applies posterosuperior pressure on the mandible centrally, and to the right and left while

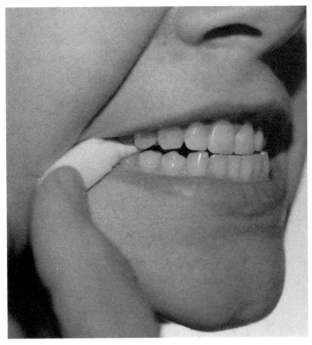

Figure 8-17. Biting against resistance. A cotton roll is placed between the back molars on the right to distract the right condyle and compress the left condyle.

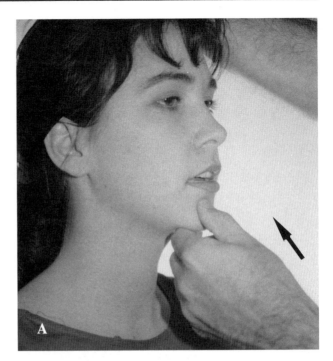

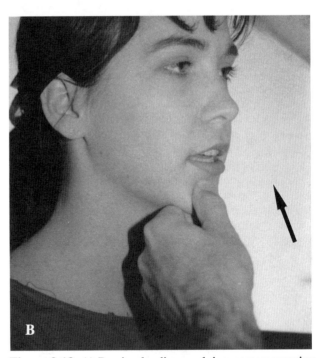

Figure 8-18. A) Passive loading applying posterosuperior pressure on the chin; B) Passive loading applying posterosuperior pressure directed toward the left. Not shown: passive loading applying posterior superior pressure directed toward the right

giving counterforce on the back of the patient's head with the other hand. (Fig 8-18) This test is not selective for either the right or left TMJ. A positive test is an increase or reproduction of the patient's TMJ symptoms. This test can be positive for both synovitis and capsulitis. To avoid a false negative response, the clinician must encourage the patient to relax the mandible prior to the various posterosuperior pressures that are applied.

3. Mandibular Dynamics

The clinician should not rely upon altered or limited mandibular dynamics to render a diagnosis of an inflammatory condition of the TMJ. Because joint effusion and swelling may be minimal, mandibular dynamics may appear normal. However, with significant pain or joint effusion, the clinician may observe the classic osteokinematic restrictions seen when the arthrokinematic movement of translation is restricted (Fig 8-11). Pain/discomfort would be the patient's complaint on the side of the involved joint during the osteokinematic testing.

Capsular Fibrosis
(ICD #716.98)

A subset diagnostic category for capsular fibrosis was not included in this classification system by the

International Headache Society. I will include capsular fibrosis in the category of inflammatory conditions because chronic capsulitis ultimately predisposes a patient to capsular fibrosis.[8, 120] Capsular fibrosis will be considered painless unless force is used during mandibular dynamics that can cause injury or overextension to the capsule.[8] The history and physical examination for an asymptomatic capsular fibrotic condition is given below. If capsular fibrosis is associated with pain, a secondary diagnosis of capsulitis must also be assigned.

History

1. Patient presents with a long-term history of capsulitis.

2. History of prolonged immobilization, i.e., intermaxillary fixation (post orthognathic surgery), or any other factor that restricts full mandibular dynamics over a several week period.

3. History of trauma such as a blow to the mandible, open joint surgery, or microtrauma derived from chronic positional habits such as leaning on the chin.

4. History of arthritides, especially the polyarthritides.

Physical Examination

Osteokinematic movements of the mandible are altered or limited in a way that suggests a decrease in the arthrokinematic movement of translation on the side of the involved joint (Fig 8-11). The degree of limited mandibular mobility and deflection from midline will depend on the extent and location of the capsular fibrosis.

General Comments on Inflammatory Conditions

Differentiation between the two inflammatory conditions (synovitis and capsulitis) of the TMJ is difficult with the current guidelines. Testing procedures (with the exception of the dynamic loading test) are not very selective for synovitis and capsulitis. Instead, the testing procedures are used to determine the degree of irritability of the joint tissues. In the absence of any meaningful altered or limited mandibular dynamics secondary to joint effusion, the physical examination for synovitis and capsulitis will require the patient to respond verbally to the manual testing of palpation and loading. An examination depending exclusively on verbal feedback from the patient means the examination becomes more subjective than objective. When the subjective portion of the examination becomes pivotal, the inexperienced clinician may tend to over-diagnose or under-diagnose the condition of inflammation of the temporomandibular joint.

The key in diagnosing capsular fibrosis is the history. For example, a patient who has had open joint surgery to the TMJ performed several months previously may present with limited mandibular dynamics, suggesting capsular fibrosis.

The dynamic loading procedure involves a strong contraction of the elevator muscles of the mandible. If a masticatory muscle disorder is also present, this test may elicit symptoms stemming from the involved elevator muscles. Differential diagnosis includes a clinical examination to the muscles of mastication. Location of the patient's symptoms also aids the differential diagnosis. For example, pain/discomfort indicated directly in front of the tragus of the ear suggests an arthrogenous problem while pain/discomfort in the area of the temporalis or masseter muscles would suggest a myogenous disorder.

Clinicians express concern about palpation via the external auditory meatus. They worry that the disc could be displaced during this form of examination. I have never experienced this. This is not to say that if the clinician's little finger is incorrectly positioned and if excess pressure is applied, that a disc could not possibly be displaced. If the patient already has a disc displacement with reduction, such pressure in the ear may cause a temporary acute disc displacement without reduction, but this should be no cause for alarm for either the clinician or patient. A majority of patients with disc displacements with reduction experience intermittent acute disc displacements without reduction. In the event a patient experiences an acute disc displacement without reduction, simply have the patient move his or her jaw from side to side. This often will allow the disc to return to a disc displacement with reduction. With a history that suggests disc displacement with reduction, the alert clinician will approach the EAM with a more sensitive finger placement and pressure or simply bypass this portion of the examination.

Osseous Mobility Conditions

Temporomandibular Joint Hypermobility(TJH) (ICD #728.5)

Previously used terms: subluxation, hypertranslation, hyperextension, ligament laxity

History

1. Patient may state, "My jaw feels like it goes out of place." Patient is most likely to be aware of this condition when he or she eats a thick sandwich or yawns.

2. Patient may report joint noises.

3. Patient may state that he or she has had short term episodes where his or her jaw would tend to "catch" in the fully opened position, preventing easy closure of his or her mouth. The patient may have had an intermittent dislocation of the condyle.

Physical Examination

The following are objective findings for TJH listed from most significant to least significant. The clinical examination is done while the patient performs active mandibular depression.

1. If excessive anterior movement of the lateral pole is present, the clinician will palpate a larger than expected indentation behind it (Fig 8-19).

2. If unilateral TJH is present, there will be a deflection of the mandible towards the contralateral side of the involved joint at the end of opening.

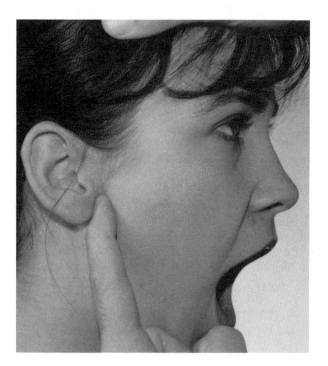

Figure 8-19. Palpation of a hollow behind the condyle, suggesting excessive translation of the condyle.

3. Palpable irregularities, when present, will occur at the end of mandibular depression and at the beginning of mandibular closure. The term "joint noises" implies that the clinician hears the noises. Patients frequently hear noises that are not heard by the clinician. Joint noises may not always be heard by the clinician but are instead easily felt by the clinician's fingers. Thus, the term "palpable irregularities" may be more fitting to use to indicate the presence of joint noises.[48] I believe that if palpable irregularities cannot be felt by the clinician, but are only detected with the use of a stethoscope, then such joint noises may not be significant.

4. Mandibular depression is in excess of 40 mm.

Dislocation (ICD #718.38)

Previously used terms for dislocation: "open lock," subluxation, luxation

History

History and clinical findings are one and the same for a dislocation condition. This condition may not be painful and pain need not be present to diagnose this disorder.

Physical Examination

The patient presents with his or her mouth fully opened, deflected toward the contralateral side of the involved joint with the inability to close his or her mouth (Fig 8-20).

General Comments on Osseous Mobility Conditions of the TMJ

I once considered hypermobility to be present when the condyle translated past the articular crest onto the articular tubercle. Even though the condylar position previously described is still valid for identifying TJH, the condylar position cannot be determined without an x-ray in the open mouth view. To avoid an x-ray, TJH will be determined by an excessive indention behind the lateral pole at the end of mandibular depression as described in the physical examination for TJH.

The excessive indention may be explained by the biomechanics of the condyle during jaw opening.[28] The lateral pole of the condyle moves downward and backward during mandibular depression.[8, 28] If a significant indention behind the condyle is palpated, excessive translation and thus TJH is indicated. During

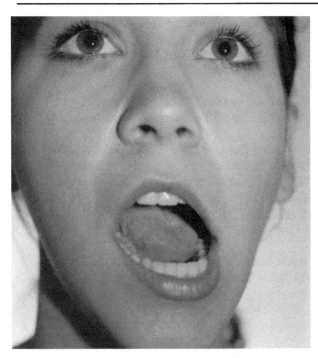

Figure 8-20. A dislocated condyle on the right.

normal translation, only a minimal indention ("dimple") should be palpated.

The subset diagnosis of TJH occurs frequently in both the patient and non-patient population. Because of the high prevalence of TJH, when a person is evaluated for TMD's, TJH will often be diagnosed or be among other subset diagnoses of TMD's. TJH usually is asymptomatic. TJH is symptomatic when an additional diagnosis of synovitis or capsulitis is present. I consider TJH to be a perpetuating factor for the inflammatory conditions of the temporomandibular joint. Therefore, if TJH is present, controlling for hypermobility will become important in the treatment of inflammatory conditions of the TMJ. If TJH is not controlled, the inflammatory condition will be aggravated every time the patient opens wide during daily activities such as yawning,

TJH accompanied by a late opening click and early closing click is often misdiagnosed as a disc displacement with reduction. By observing the guidelines for diagnosing TJH and the criteria for diagnosing of disc displacement with reduction that follow, one may learn to differentiate between these two TM disorders.

With dislocation, the condyle and disc translate well beyond the articular crest onto the tubercle and get stuck in this position. The patient cannot close his or her mouth volitionally. A predisposing factor for dislocation appears to be an articular eminence with a short, steep slope.[8, 112]

Articular Disc Displacement Conditions
Disc Displacement With Reduction (DDWR) (ICD # 718.38)

Previously used terms: internal derangement, anterior disc dislocation with reduction, reciprocal click

History

Patient reports hearing joint noises during mandibular opening and closing. The patient may describe two "pops" or "clicks," one on opening and the second on closing.

Physical Examination

1. Palpation over the lateral poles during opening and closing of the mandible reveals the classic palpable irregularities of the "reciprocal click."[35] Features of the reciprocal click are:

    a. The opening click is the reduction of the disc. The closing click is the disc displacing anterior to the condyle (Fig 8-21).

    b. The reciprocal click occurs at different mandibular positions during opening and closing. The opening click can be felt to occur either early ($\approx$10-20 mm), intermittent ($\approx$20-30 mm), or late (after 30 mm). The closing click occurs towards the very end of closing, i.e. the last 5 mm, just prior to back teeth coming together.

    c. The opening noise is typically the loudest and the closing noise is the softest.

    If a reciprocal click is not present, a DDWR is not present or it simply cannot be detected clinically. There is no need to proceed with tests #2 and #3 below. If a reciprocal click is present, the sole purpose of performing #2 and #3 is to confirm that the reciprocal click is related to a DDWR.

2. With the clinician's fingertips holding under the angle of the mandible bilaterally, the clinician lifts in an anterosuperior direction while the patient opens and closes the mandible several times (Fig 8-22). The following are objectives:

    a. "Preload" the joint to enhance the loudness of the reciprocal click (posterior band having to negotiate a tighter joint space),

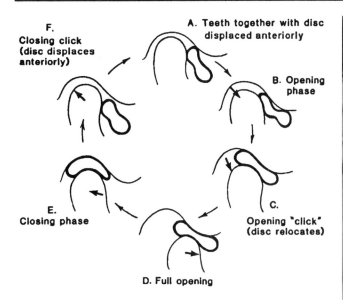

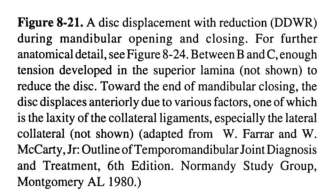

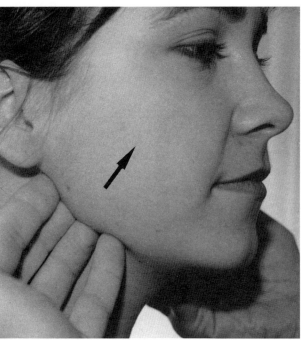

Figure 8-21. A disc displacement with reduction (DDWR) during mandibular opening and closing. For further anatomical detail, see Figure 8-24. Between B and C, enough tension developed in the superior lamina (not shown) to reduce the disc. Toward the end of mandibular closing, the disc displaces anteriorly due to various factors, one of which is the laxity of the collateral ligaments, especially the lateral collateral (not shown) (adapted from W. Farrar and W. McCarty, Jr: Outline of Temporomandibular Joint Diagnosis and Treatment, 6th Edition. Normandy Study Group, Montgomery AL 1980.)

especially the closing click, to confirm the presence of a DDWR.

b. Determine if the patient's pain correlates with joint noises in a consistent manner. Loading the joint during movement to enhance the noises often will increase or reproduce the pain if such pain is related to the DDWR. If the patient reports pain occurring infrequently, i.e., once a month, but has joint noises daily, then the clinician knows the patient's condition is not irritable and the test probably will not reproduce any pain.

Remember, pain does not need to be associated with this condition and is therefore not a primary finding in the diagnosis of this TM disorder.

3. The clinician asks the patient to open wide enough to get the opening click, then close forward to bring the upper and lower anterior

Figure 8-22. Lifting on the ramus in an anterosuperior direction as the patient opens the mouth. Performed to enhance the loudness of the reciprocal click associated with a DDWR.

central incisors together in an end-to-end position (Fig 8-23). From this forward position of the mandible, the patient opens and closes as wide as possible several times while the clinician palpates over the lateral poles. A large percentage of reciprocal clicks will cease to exist. On closing, the condyle is not allowed to go back to its original position and thus the disc cannot displace anterior to the condyle.

Disc Displacement Without Reduction (DDWoR) (ICD # 718.28)

Previously used terms: non-reducing disc, "closed lock," acute anterior disc dislocation without reduction, chronic anterior disc dislocation without reduction

Acute Disc Displacement Without Reduction

History

1. Patient reports that he or she used to have joint noises (reciprocal click) and previous episodes of intermittent "locking" but now joint noises are gone.

2. Patient reports inability to open his or her mouth wide and difficulty performing

functional jaw movements, i.e., difficulty in chewing, talking and yawning.

Physical Examination

1. Mandibular dynamics (Fig 8-11):

   a. Depression:

   Opening is limited to 20-25 mm [27] with deflection toward the side of the involved joint.

   b. Protrusion:

   Limited with deflection towards the side of the involved joint.

   c. Lateral Excursion:

   Limited toward the opposite side of the involved joint.

2. No palpable irregularities will be present with this condition.

Chronic Disc Displacement Without Reduction

History

Patient reports a history similar to a DDWR that eventually progressed to an acute DDWoR. At examination time, the patient no longer feels limitation in the use of the jaw but instead describes hearing joint noises such as crepitus with jaw movement.

Physical Examination

1. Mandibular dynamics:

   a. Depression:
   Functional or close to functional depression. Slight deflection to the involved side toward the end of opening.

   b. Protrusion:
   Functional or close to functional protrusion. Slight deflection to the involved side towards the end of protrusion.

   c. Lateral Excursion:
   Functional or close to functional lateral excursion towards the opposite side of the involved joint.

2. Palpable irregularities of crepitus will be present.

General Comments on Articular Disc Displacement Conditions

In any stage of disc displacement, the thick posterior band of the disc is anterior to its normal twelve o'clock position when the mandible is in the closed mouth position. For the disc to displace anteriorly (actually anteromedially) on the condyle, translation must have occurred in the lower joint space.[8, 112, 115] For translation to have occurred in the lower joint space, the medial and lateral collateral ligaments must be elongated (primarily the lateral collateral ligament).[8, 112, 115] This sequela involves elongation of both the inferior and superior laminae and the loss of the self-seating mechanism of the disc due to disc deformation.[142]

During Phase I of opening of a DDWR, the condyle rotates on the PA and against the posterior band of the disc instead of rotating as it should on the thin intermediate zone (Fig 8-24). During Phase II of opening, translation is initially limited because the disc displacement functions as a mechanical obstruction to translation until sufficient tension develops in the superior lamina. Once sufficient tension develops in the superior lamina, the condyle either moves under the posterior band or the posterior band is pulled back over the condyle, resulting in a palpable and possibly audible "click." The opening click signifies the disc returning to its proper position on the condyle (Fig 8-24). The range at which the opening click occurs will no doubt be dependent upon how elongated the superior lamina is and how much "loading" the joint surfaces are experiencing from masticatory muscle hyperactivity.[62]

The closing click occurs as the condyle moves behind the posterior band of the disc, or the posterior band moves anterior to the condyle. Displacement of the disc on closing is due to ligamentous laxity mentioned earlier. The diagnosis of DDWR means the disc has the potential to reduce or relocate itself correctly on the condyle during opening, but this disc position is only temporary. When the patient brings his or her back teeth together, the disc once again displaces anteriorly to the condyle.

Deflections/deviations that frequently accompany DDWR were intentionally not discussed. Aberrant movement of the mandible is not necessary for accurate diagnosis. The palpable irregularity of the "reciprocal click" as described previously makes the diagnosis. A patient with a DDWR does not always present with a consistent and repeatable method of mandibular opening so I do not attach significance to these features.

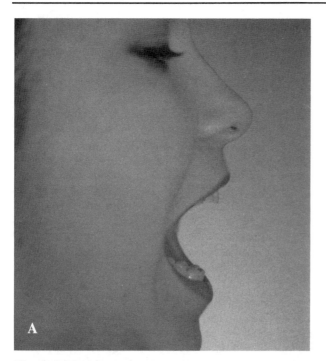
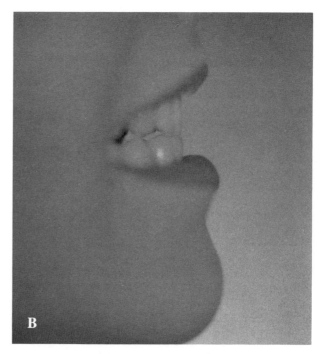

Figure 8-23. Repositioning the mandible anteriorly to temporarily stop the reciprocal click associated with a DDWR. A) The patient opens wide enough to get the opening "click"; and B) The patient closes forward to bring the upper and lower central incisors together in an end to end position. From this forward position, the patient repeats opening and closing of the mandible.

In patients experiencing an acute DDWoR, the disc remains anterior to the condyle throughout the entire phase of opening and closing (Fig 8-25). The disc acts as a mechanical obstruction for condylar translation which causes the limited and altered mandibular dynamics discussed under physical examination (Fig 8-26). Why some patients remain in the category of a DDWR for years while other patients progress within months to an acute DDWoR is not clear.

The key to diagnosing a chronic DDWoR is palpable irregularities of crepitus present throughout the full opening and closing movement of the mandible.[132] Diagnosing a chronic DDWoR based upon history alone is controversial because a chronic DDWoR would involve a DDWR progressing to an acute DDWoR and then on to a chronic DDWoR with crepitus.[61] Chronic DDWoR usually involves the perforation of the posterior attachments [115] which results in crepitus (bone on bone) throughout the full opening and closing movements of the mandible. Because the disc is no longer attached posteriorly to the postglenoid spine, the mandibular dynamics are often seen to be near normal.[32]

Why some patients with disc displacements can have mild to severe pain and others have none poses a very perplexing question.[139] The clinician must decide, in this instance, whether to treat disc position or to treat pain.

Arthritides

Osteoarthritis (ICD #716.98)

Previously used terms: arthritis, osteoarthrosis, degenerative joint disease

History

Refer to history for Inflammatory Conditions

Physical Examination

Similar to the physical examination given for Inflammatory Conditions, except for the following:

1. Osteoarthritis has palpable irregularities of crepitus or multiple joint noises during movements of the mandible.[132] The inflammatory conditions will have no palpable irregularities.

2. Osteoarthritis has radiographic evidence of structural bony change.[50] The inflammatory conditions have no evidence of structural changes.

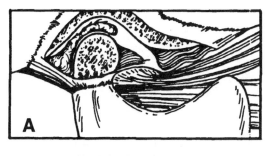

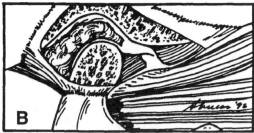

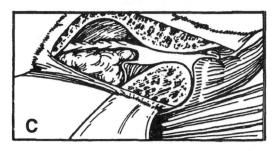

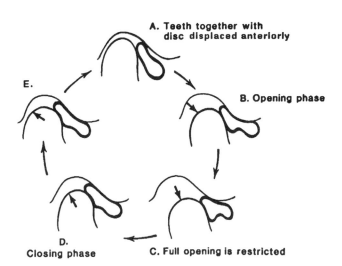

A. Teeth together with
disc displaced anteriorly

E.

B. Opening phase

D.
Closing phase

C. Full opening is restricted

Figure 8-24. Disc displacement with reduction (DDWR) showing detail of pertinent anatomical structures: A) The mouth is closed with the back teeth together; B) Translation of the condyle begins to place tension in the superior lamina; and C) The disc reduces with an audible "click" or palpable irregularity occurring (adapted from Okeson[112]).

Figure 8-25. Acute disc displacement without reduction (DDWoR). For further anatomical detail, see Figure 8-26. The range of condylar translation is limited because of the displaced disc (adapted from W. Farrar and W. McCarty, Jr: Outline of Temporomandibular Joint Diagnosis and Treatment, 6th Edition. Normandy Study Group, Montgomery AL 1980).

Osteoarthrosis
(ICD #715.38)

Previously used terms: osteoarthritis, arthritis, degenerative joint disease, arthrosis deformans

History

1. A number of patients progress to osteoarthrosis without an awareness of any pain at all.[59]

2. Patient's primary complaint is usually joint noises (crepitus).

Physical Examination

1. The key objective finding is palpable irregularities of crepitus present throughout the full opening and closing movements of the mandible.

2. This condition is often the end result of the progression of osteoarthritis. The pain of osteoarthritis tends to recede over an approximately nine month period and the joint is often left with characteristic osseous changes without pain and disability.[59] Even though relatively good function is often seen with this condition,[32] the following may be seen with mandibular dynamics:

   a. Depression:

      Functional or close to functional depression. Slight deflection to the involved side toward the end of opening.

   b. Protrusion:

      Functional or close to functional protrusion. Slight deflection to the involved side toward the end of protrusion.

c. Lateral Excursion:

Functional or close to functional lateral excursion towards the opposite side of the involved joint.

3. Radiographic evidence shows structural bony change.[50, 59]

Polyarthritides (ICD #714.9)

This subset diagnosis is seen infrequently in the standard physical therapy and dental practices. Polyarthritides are caused by a generalized systemic polyarthritic condition. Polyarthritides that can affect the temporomandibular joint are:

Rheumatoid Arthritides

Juvenile Rheumatoid Arthritis

Spondyloarthropathies

Crystal-Induced Diseases

Reiter's Syndrome

Each of the polyarthritides is best diagnosed with serologic tests and managed by a rheumatologist. Physical therapy management relates to secondary complaints and contributing factors. It is beyond the scope of this chapter to cover the history and physical examination of this group of arthritides. I refer the reader to the bibliography for further information on these conditions.[67]

General Comments on Arthritides

Often a patient presents with cephalic and neck symptoms that are accompanied by crepitus during opening and closing movements of the mouth. Unless the patient associates other jaw symptoms with functional or parafunctional jaw movements, the crepitus is rarely an issue. Coincidentally, the patient has an asymptomatic osteoarthritic condition of the TMJ along with some other symptomatic disorder of the head, face, or neck.

Evidence suggests that palpable crepitus is a valid sign of the osteoarthritic changes seen on radiological examination of the TMJ.[16] There is also developing evidence that disc displacements may precede osteoarthritis and osteoarthrosis.[59]

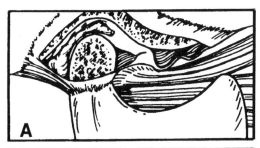
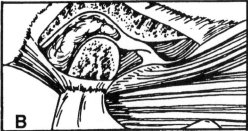
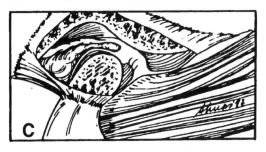

Figure 8-26. Acute disc displacement without reduction (DDWoR) showing detail of pertinent anatomical structures: A) The mouth is closed with the back teeth together; B) Early phase of opening with the condyle functioning on the posterior attachment area; and C) Translation is restricted because the disc acts as a mechanical obstruction (adapted from Okeson[112].)

Ankylosis

Previously used term: arthrokleisis

Fibrous Ankylosis (ICD #718.58)

History

Usually significant trauma or surgery precipitates hemarthrosis that results in fibrous adhesions within the joint.[8]

Physical Examination

Restricted mandibular dynamics are seen with fibrous ankylosis. The degree to which mandibular dynamics are restricted depends on the extent, location, and length of the fibrous adhesions. Classically, the altered and restricted mandibular dynamics are those associated with the restricted arthrokinematic movement of translation (Fig 8-11).

Bony Ankylosis
(ICD #718.58)

History

Bony ankylosis, or ossification, is less common than fibrous ankylosis. Ossification is more likely to occur when an infection has been present.[8]

Physical Examination

Bony ankylosis is often bilateral due to the etiology of infection. If unilateral involvement is seen, the mandibular dynamics would be similar to those observed with fibrous ankylosis. Alterations in mandibular dynamics with bilateral bony ankylosis are as follows:

1. Depression:

    Opening is severely limited to several millimeters.

2. Protrusion:

    Severely limited.

3. Lateral Excursion:

    Severely limited bilaterally.

General Comments on Ankylosis

Ankylosis consists of intracapsular adhesions or actual ossifications that tether the disc-condyle complex to the articular eminence-fossa surface.

Deviation in Form

(ICD #719.68)

Previously used term: Dyscrasia - an abnormal or pathological condition

History

The patient reports joint noises with mandibular movement.

Physical Examination

Palpation reveals a repetitive, nonvariable palpable irregularity or joint noise. The joint noise occurs at the exact same condylar position during mandibular opening or closing.

General Comments on Deviation in Form

Irregular surfaces on the articulating surfaces of the condyle or temporal bone may form "obstacles" for rotation of the disc against the condyle or translation of the disc against the articular eminence.[133, 139] A clicking sound may occur when the disc passes this bony irregularity. The clicking is characterized by the coincidence in the opening and closing path of the mandible.[133, 139]

MANAGEMENT FOR TEMPOROMANDIBULAR DISORDERS

General Comments on Management for TMD's

I have divided treatment of TMD's into seven phases. It is not necessary to administer them in numerical order. The clinician's experience and clinical decision making will help select and progress each phase. This section will not to go into details of specific treatment protocols for TMD's, but will discuss general treatment concepts.

The following factors may also affect selection of treatment:

1. Age of the patient.

2. Chronicity of a TMD complaint.

3. Severity of TMD's interference with the patient's function and life-style.

4. Past treatments that failed where the clinician feels the past treatment did not meet his or her standards of excellence.

5. Past treatments that the clinician feels have been properly executed, but have failed for unknown reasons.

6. Refusal by the patient to consider surgery under any circumstances.

7. The definition of successful treatment differs between clinician and patient.

8. Compliance by the patient is seriously doubted by the clinician.

9. Clinician bias and treatment philosophy.

The disorders for which each treatment phase would be most appropriate are stated. Most disorders will be covered. Since disorders of polyarthritides are not common for the general physical therapy and dental practices, they should be treated symptomatically and patients referred on to a specialist familiar with these disorders.

In the management of TMD's, the clinician should be aware of masticatory muscle disorders (MMD's). The relationship between TMD's and MMD's is unclear. MMD's may play a primary role as a predisposing, precipitating and perpetuating factor to some TMD's.[109, 126] Both disorders can coexist and may not influence each other or the two disorders can coexist and have a significant influence on each other. I believe that once a symptomatic disorder of the TMJ does exist, the presence of an MMD can be a perpetuating factor to the symptomatic TMD.

The International Headache Society [15] lists ten subset diagnoses under masticatory muscle disorders. It is my opinion that the more common MMD's seen clinically fall in the categories of "myofascial pain" and "myositis." With current guidelines for performing an examination for nondiseased/nonneurological muscular involvement, the clinician will have great difficulty differentiating myofascial pain from myositis. For the purpose of this chapter, myofascial pain and myositis will be collectively referred to as masticatory muscle hyperactivity.

Some clinicians promote electromyography (EMG) to diagnose normal and abnormal masticatory muscle activity during rest and during function.[146] However, concerns exist about the reliability, validity, sensitivity and specificity of EMG testing for masticatory muscle hyperactivity.[145, 146] I feel that an adequate history and a physical examination that includes palpation of the muscles of mastication can determine if masticatory muscle hyperactivity is present. Palpation of masseter and temporalis muscles is valuable to decide if masticatory muscle hyperactivity is present (Fig 8-27). Goulet and Clark[43] have shown that muscle palpation tenderness can be performed reliably when additional training in standardization (pressure and duration) is done. *I want to emphasize that in my opinion, proper diagnosis of TMD's may be made without an evaluation of the muscles of mastication.* Like the examination of other areas around the TMJ, masticatory muscle examination is done to establish a differential diagnosis. Knowledge of the degree of masticatory muscle hyperactivity is important clinically in the management of TMD's because the presence of masticatory muscle hyperactivity can be a perpetuating factor to the symptomatic TMD.

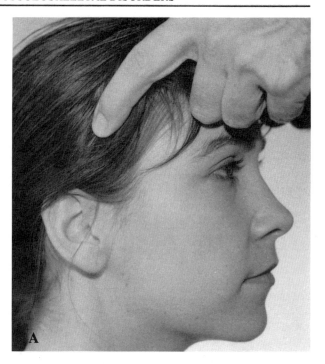

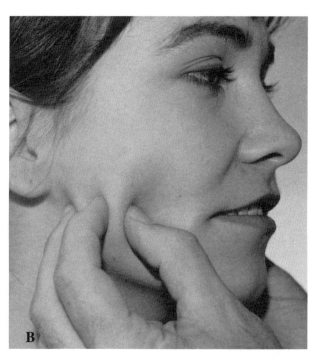

Figure 8-27. Palpation of the temporalis muscle (A) and the masseter muscle (B).

Of the various TMD's previously covered, I believe that inflammatory conditions (synovitis or capsulitis) are the primary source of the patient's pain and discomfort. All other disorders can be asymptomatic or, if they are symptomatic, it is because of the inflammatory conditions. For example, the reader must not assume that a displaced disc, osteoarthritic findings on x-rays or palpable irregularities are causing the patient's pain and discomfort. Instead, the clinician should take the attitude that the patient's symptoms are originating from inflammatory conditions. Inflammation control is the key to decreasing the patient's symptoms. Therefore, Treatment Phases I, II, and III address inflammation control, either directly or indirectly, regardless of the presence of another TM disorder. If masticatory muscle hyperactivity is occurring, this will also need to be controlled due to the possible increase in loading/compression that masticatory muscle hyperactivity precipitates. An increase in masticatory muscle activity can maintain and aggravate an inflammatory condition of the TMJ.

If the inflammatory condition is not resolved after adequate treatment in Phase I, II, or III, the clinician may progress to any one or combination of the remaining phases. Through clinical reasoning, the clinician may conclude that a disc displacement may indeed be the primary etiology of the inflammatory condition and a possible source of masticatory muscle hyperactivity.

Usually, Phases I through VII represent an escalation from a less costly, less risky, less invasive and less uncomfortable approach to a more costly, more risky, more invasive and more uncomfortable approach. However, when the clinician carefully considers the nine factors listed at the beginning of this section, he or she may find that surgery (Phases VI and VII) may be the most appropriate choice of treatment for select patients.

Seven Phases Of Treatment

Phase I

Phase I treatment is initiated for inflammatory conditions of the TMJ. Phase I is divided into Part A and Part B. Part A is directed towards the arthrogenous involvement of inflammation. If masticatory muscle hyperactivity is present, Part B is directed towards such myogenous involvement.

Part A

1. Instruct the patient in habit awareness and control, i.e., biting finger nails or pencils, leaning on the chin, etc.

2. Instruct the patient in a soft food diet.

3. If the TMJ is inflamed and TJH is present, TJH needs to be viewed as a perpetuating factor to

the inflammatory conditions, and needs to be controlled. To control TJH [74]:

   a. Instruct the patient to yawn with tongue up against the palate of his or her mouth to restrict opening.

   b. Instruct the patient on how to control condylar translation:

      Instruct the patient to palpate his or her lateral poles on the involved sides.[74] Have the patient open and close, maintaining the lateral pole underneath his or her palpating finger so that only a "dimple" verses a "hollow" occurs behind the lateral pole.

4. Apply physical modalities as indicated to decrease inflammation (i.e., ultrasound, phonophoresis, iontophoresis, ice or heat over the involved TMJ).

Part B

1. Continue with Phase I, Part A

2. Apply physical modalities to decrease masticatory muscle hyperactivity, i.e., heat, ultrasound, various parameters of electrical stimulation.

3. Increase patient self awareness and management of clenching and bruxism. This will be accomplished through patient education concerning rest position of the tongue (upright postural position of the tongue).[73, 74] The rest position of the tongue will help the patient avoid harmful activities of clenching and bruxism during waking hours.

Phase II

In Phase II, cervical spine disorders are treated to indirectly relieve inflammatory conditions of the TMJ. Non-diseased disorders of the cervical spine involve the muscles, soft tissues, facet joints, peripheral nerves and, to a much lesser extent, nerve roots. In my opinion, the primary non-diseased disorders of the cervical spine are muscle disorders. Muscle disorders of the cervical spine may predispose, precipitate or perpetuate masticatory muscle hyperactivity.[70] Therefore, treatment to the cervical spine would attempt to control masticatory muscle hyperactivity perpetuating the inflammatory condition of the TMJ. It is beyond the scope of this chapter to discuss clinical theories of how the cervical spine can influence masticatory muscle hyperactivity [70] or the treatments rendered to the cervical spine.[36, 70, 71]

Phase III

In Phase III, an intraoral appliance is used to treat inflammatory conditions of the TMJ. Theoretically, a splint may directly or indirectly reduce TMJ loading by decreasing masticatory muscle hyperactivity. A decrease in TMJ loading will help eliminate TMJ inflammation.

These appliances may cover all or part of either the maxillary arch of teeth or mandibular arch of teeth. Most of these splints are made of hard acrylic [17] while others may be made of resilient acrylic or latex rubber.[11] There are a number of intraoral appliances with different names such as stabilization splint, centric related splint, occlusal splint, bite plates, night guards and bite guards.[17, 42] Still other appliances are given names based upon special features of the appliances such as the modified hawley or anterior bite splint,[141] repositioning splint,[17] pivot appliance,[84] hydrostatic appliance,[79] mandibular orthopædic repositioning appliance (MORA),[40] and myo-monitor appliance.[63]

These appliances differ greatly in design such as vertical thickness, extent of tooth coverage, amount of mandibular repositioning. How the dentist establishes an occlusal contact on the appliance, how the appliance influences the trajectory of jaw closure into the appliance, and how the appliance influences the way the teeth disocclude from the appliance during lateral and protrusive movements are additional variables that need to be considered when fabricating an appliance. All of the splints and their individual features are designed to fulfill a particular theory in the treatment of TMD's. Five major theories covering the purposes and objectives of appliance therapy have been described by Clark.[17, 21]

It is beyond the scope of this text to discuss appliance theory. The reader is referred to articles by Clark and others for more detailed discussion.[17, 21, 72, 99, 118] Dr. Messing states, "It is important to understand that splint therapy is a concept, not merely the introduction of a piece of acrylic. It is not a therapy that functions alone, but within the context of other treatment measures..."[99] Even though the current literature states that occlusal splints and biofeedback are "the only proven technologies for treatment of TMD," [78] why splints are therapeutic remains to be answered. Until the validity and predictive value of splint use is scientifically determined, splints for Phase III should be comfortable, aesthetic, retentive, functional and most importantly *reversible and noninvasive* to the occlusion and muscles of the jaw and cervical spine.

Phase IV

In Phase IV, an intraoral appliance called an anterior repositioning appliance (ARA) is used, primarily for DDWR (Fig 8-28). The objective of an ARA is to establish the proper relationship between condyle, disc and temporal bone to let the injured tissues associated with DDWR "heal" (lateral collateral ligament and posterior attachments). To help any tissue heal, it is essential that the appliance be used 24 hours a day.[99]

As the name implies, an ARA repositions the mandible forward. The mandible is positioned as far forward as necessary until the opening and closing clicks do not occur, which supposedly signifies that the disc is recaptured. The term "recaptured" indicates that the disc is in proper position on the condyle during all functional movements of the mandible. Roberts [121] and others [92] suggest an arthrogram or computed tomography (CT) more accurately assesses disc position than the use of clinical findings or plain radiographs alone. So unless these other procedures are done, the clinician may not know if the disc is in proper position even in the absence of the reciprocal click.

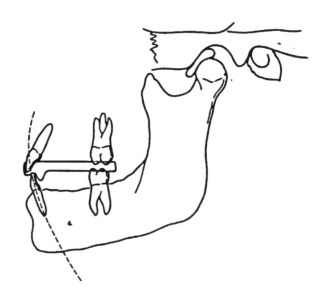

Figure 8-28. An anterior repositioning appliance (ARA) used to maintain a proper disc-condyle relationship. During closing, the ARA will cause the jaw to close forward, preventing the disc from displacing anteriorly (from Razook S: Non Surgical Management of TMJ and Masticatory Muscle Problems. In TMJ Disorders Management of the Craniomandibular Complex, 1st edition. S Kraus, ed. Churchill Livingstone, New York, NY 1988.)

Even though the ARA may be the treatment of choice to recapture the disc, the clicking often returns later, indicating a disc displacement with reduction is once again present and that the ARA failed to permanently recapture the displaced disc.[22, 65, 85, 86, 105] In their literature review, Zamburlin and Austin [152] find anterior repositioning of the mandible is likely to recapture the disc long-term in only one third of the patients. Wabeke and co-workers in their literature review state that after joint sounds are treated, the joint sounds return within a few years 50% of the time.[139] Moloney and Howard's [105] study showed that if an ARA was used in patients who had been experiencing clicking for less than a year, 80% success occurred in reducing clicking. In this same study only 8% of patients who had an extended history of clicking reported an absence of clicking with ARA therapy. No mention was made in this study whether or not an arthrographic, CT or MRI study was done to see if the disc was in proper position in those subjects whose noises ceased following ARA therapy.

The notion that the patient will have increasing pain and limitation of function if the disc is not recaptured is not supported with current studies.[30, 68, 69] Because of the high incidence of asymptomatic displaced discs, a displaced disc may be a variation of the normal.[68, 69] Most joints with long standing disc displacement appear to have a higher prevalence of osteoarthrosis.[61] However, a symptomatic or asymptomatic disc displacement does not reliably progress towards decreased oral function.[30]

ARA's may alter the existing occlusion because they require extended use.[139] Following the use of an ARA, patients are often committed to permanent stabilization of their occlusion with equilibration, prosthodontic, orthodontic or oral surgery (osteotomy) procedures.[139] The risk, of course, is that irreversible and costly procedures will be performed for a condition in which repeated disc displacement may occur. Furthermore, the disc displacement may not have been the cause of the patient's pain/discomfort in the first place. Before initiating the use of an ARA, all pros and cons must be discussed by clinician and patient. Both the patient and clinician must understand that the recapturing of the disc and the absence of clicking may not be realistic goals. Instead, success must be defined as freedom from pain and functional limitations of the TMJ.[105]

Phase V

In Phase V, manual intraoral techniques are used to restore functional mandibular dynamics for an acute DDWoR (Fig 8-29). Manual intraoral techniques for an acute DDWoR consist of any combination of distraction or translation depending on how one wants to influence the displaced disc. Restoration of functional mandibular dynamics via these techniques can occur three different ways:

1. An acute DDWoR returns to its normal position.

When manual intraoral techniques are used to encourage the disc to return to its normal position, the joint space must be sufficiently increased to allow the disc to reposition itself on the condyle. The success of intraoral techniques are often identified by an audible "pop" or "snap" followed by restoration of functional mandibular dynamics. However, the disc will probably not stay repositioned. In particular, once the patient brings his or her back teeth together, the disc will either revert to an acute DDWoR or remain as a DDWR. If the disc reverts to an acute DDWoR, manual intraoral techniques will need to be applied again, and if successful again, an ARA will need to be considered immediately. Recalling the limitations of an ARA as previously noted, the clinician and patient will need to decide if manual reduction of the disc followed by an ARA is sufficiently valuable.

2. An acute DDWoR becomes a DDWR.

If the patient remains with a DDWR, he or she will have functional mandibular dynamics accompanied by clicking. If this is not satisfactory to the patient, an ARA is used with all the pros and cons adequately discussed.

3. An acute DDWoR becomes a chronic DDWoR.

The purpose of manual intraoral techniques is to restore functional mandibular dynamics regardless of disc position.[129] At this point, the physical therapist, patient and dentist/oral surgeon fully agree on the purpose of performing manual intraoral techniques. Studies [125] have shown that the PA, when subject to compressive loading, is capable of remolding and fibrosing. Thus a pseudo-disc may be said to have developed. However, in some patients, remolding of the PA does not occur, occurs but is inadequate, or occurs and is adequate for a time and then fails.[124] In cases where intraoral techniques were unable to restore functional mandibular dynamics and a continuation of arthrogenous pain persists, the clinician would reassess the patient's condition and may elect to move on to Phase VI or Phase VII.

Phase VI

In Phase VI arthroscopy is performed to lyse or lavage the superior joint space to restore translation between the disc and temporal bone. Arthroscopy is

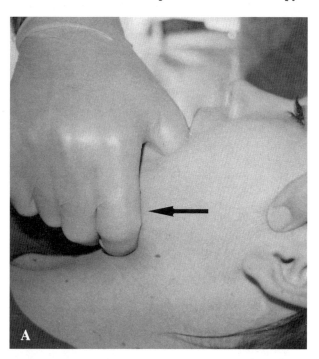

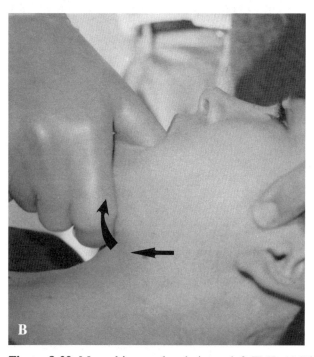

indicated when conservative care has failed to reduce the pain originating from the TMJ and when mandibular function is restricted. This procedure can be used for any of the disc displacement conditions.[58] The success of arthroscopy is not from altering disc position.[107, 110] Montgomery and co-workers [106] compared 48 patients who underwent arthroscopy for disc displacement to 51 patients who underwent arthrotomy to reposition the disc. Follow up examinations were performed at one and 52 weeks after surgery. Both groups were found to have improved significantly (decrease in pain and improvement in function) with a similar pattern of recovery. Radiography revealed the disc position was unchanged or worse in 83% of the arthroscopy group and in 88% of the arthrotomy group. In one study, joint sounds were present in 61% of patients preoperatively and in 78% post arthroscopically.[20] This previous study recommends telling the patient that joint noises may occur or continue to exist following arthroscopy. In summary, relief of pain and improvement in function following arthroscopy appears to have no correlation between joint noises and the repositioning or recapturing of the disc.[39, 110, 114] We can best clarify what is not occurring with TMJ arthroscopy. Unfortunately, reasons for positive outcome remain unclear.

Phase VII

In Phase VII, open joint surgery (arthrotomy) is performed. Indications for an arthrotomy are the same as for arthroscopy in that conservative care has failed

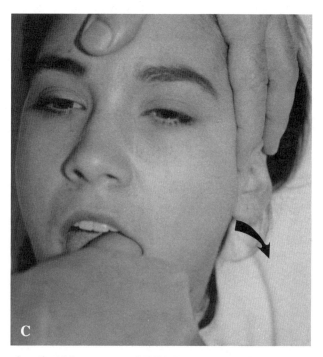

Figure 8-29. Manual intraoral techniques–left TMJ: A) Distraction (used for an acute DDWoR or capsular fibrosis); B) Distraction with translation (used for an acute DDWoR or capsular fibrosis); and C) Lateral glide (used for capsular fibrosis).

to reduce the pain originating from the TMJ and function of the mandible is restricted. Some authors feel that arthrotomy should be performed only when arthroscopy has been tried and has failed, but this point is debated.[4] Arthrotomy can be done for any of the disc displacement conditions. Arthrotomy and arthroscopy are also the interventions of choice for ankylosed conditions. If the degenerative process is advanced, arthrotomy accompanied by reconstructive surgery may be done for arthritides and for any advanced degenerative changes associated with deviation in form. Most arthrotomies for TMD's are for disc displacements and will be the focus of this section. The reader is referred to the bibliography for more details of the various surgical procedures for disc displacements and other disorders of the TMJ.[4, 6]

Surgery for disc displacement includes a variety of options. Surgical options are influenced by the evolving philosophy of the surgeon and long-term results cited in the literature. The more common procedures may include:

1. Disc Plication

   Disc plication involves the repositioning and repair of the discal attachments. The disc is repositioned from an anteromedial position to a posterolateral position.[6, 26]

2. Discectomy

   Only the avascular portion of the disc is removed and often that portion of the disc that is removed is replaced by materials mentioned in #3. If the disc is not replaced, only minimal changes in joint morphology is noted.[49]

3. Autogenous and alloplastic materials are often used to replace the disc [4]

   a. Autogenous materials may include:

      Fascia Lata

      Temporalis Fascia

      Muscle

      Dermis

      Cartilage

   b. Alloplastic materials may include:

      Acrylic

      Silastic Sheeting

      Gore-Tex

Silastic and Gore-Tex replacements have been used as temporary implants. Both are removed after a fibrous capsule has formed and assumed a disc-like function[137].

Replacement of the disc with Proplast-Teflon implants has been discontinued because of condylar destruction and severe erosion of the mandibular fossa resulting in perforation of the middle of the mandibular fossa.[5, 108]

Reasons for surgical success are unclear with disc repositioning. As is the case following arthroscopy, continued displaced discs are common. Montgomery, et al,[106] and Farole [33] showed that anterior positioning of the disc is still evident from radiographic analysis following surgery despite improved condylar translation and disc mobility as well as positive patient response. In a study of 20 temporomandibular joints in 10 patients, MRI's were taken 6 to 23 months post discectomy and replacement by an autogenous dermal graft, most joints showed no return of the repaired disc to its normal position.[82]

The long-term follow up of open joint surgeries for disc displacements indicates that arthrotomy is a successful intervention whether it be a disc repair, discectomy or replacement with autogenous or alloplastic material.[4] Disc position does not appear to be a critical factor. Variables that will influence success center on patient selection, indications for surgery, patient-physician rapport, other adjunctive therapy and reporting criteria.[123]

Following arthrotomy or arthroscopic surgery, post surgical management will be necessary.[91] Post surgical management repeats any one or combination of Phase I, II, and III. These therapeutic measures control for inflammation of the involved joint and masticatory muscle hyperactivity. Capsular fibrosis can also occur and is seen more frequently following arthrotomy than arthroscopic surgery. Treatment for capsular fibrosis involves the use of modalities to the joint capsule followed by manual intraoral techniques (Fig 8-29).[74] Manual intraoral techniques are used to restore restricted arthrokinematic movements secondary to capsular fibrosis. Instructing the patient in a home exercise program to encourage restoration of functional mandibular dynamics will round out the management for post arthrotomy and arthroscopic surgery.[74, 91] Of course, the degree of pre-surgical joint involvement, the type of surgical intervention, and the degree of post surgical masticatory muscle hyperactivity will have to be considered when tailoring a post surgery management program for the individual patient.[74, 91]

Addendum

Dislocation has not been addressed in the seven phases of management. In the event of a dislocated condyle, appropriate sedation through medication or physical modalities is applied if necessary. An intraoral technique of distraction is applied on the side of the involved joint. With the clinician's thumb on the patient's molars, the condyle is distracted from the articular tubercle. Distraction is followed by translating the condyle posteriorly to its normal position along the articular eminence. The clinician may want to wrap his or her thumb with a 4 x 4 gauze in the event the patient has a strong reflex contraction of the elevator muscles. Following reduction of the condyle, symptomatic treatment for inflammation and masticatory muscle hyperactivity may be offered.

SUMMARY

In this chapter, the clinical relevance of osseous anatomy was addressed. A discussion of osteokinematics and arthrokinematics was included to help the clinician understand function and dysfunction between the condyle, disc and temporal bone. This text introduced a classification system that is acceptable to the medical and dental professions. If followed, questions about what "TMJ" is and (more importantly) what "TMJ" is not can be avoided. If the International Headache Society's classification system for TMD's is followed, current and future clinical and scientific research articles will be more meaningful. This statement is made with the understanding that this system is being modified constantly. Adherence to a classification system allows the reader to draw conclusions from homogenous patient populations rather than the hodgepodge of patient populations that presently characterize much of the clinical and scientific research.

Information gathered through history and physical examination will help the clinician identify TMD's. Following the seven phases of management systematically and progressively will help alleviate most symptoms and limitations in mandibular function related to TMD's. The reader should recognize the need for cost effective, conservative, and reversible treatments for most TMD's. As clinicians, we must understand that *dysfunction in the presence of function and in the absence of symptoms is permissible.* If research indicates that the long-term outcome of more costly and irreversible forms of treatment proves no more beneficial than no treatment at all, the clinician must pursue noninvasive options. Conversely, when pain and limitation of jaw function follows appropriate conservative treatment, surgery may prove the most therapeutic method of treatment.

Physical therapy and dentistry are the primary source of treatments for TMD's. It is not within the scope of this text to detail the importance of adjunctive therapies (medications, biofeedback, stress management and psychotherapy, etc.) that are often of great benefit to the patient with TMD. Physical therapy and medical management of cervical spine disorders will help further decrease symptoms and improve function related to the cervical spine. Managing cervical spine related symptoms will help in the differential diagnosis of what symptoms, if any, remain to be associated with TMD's. The other crucial team player in the successful management of TMD's is the patient. Therapeutic outcome will always fall short of the anticipated goals without the patient's cooperation.

Thanks to
My wife, Pattie,
for her love, understanding, and patient support;
to my daughter, Emily Jane,
who gives me such joy and happiness;
and to my parents,
Dottie and Kenneth L. Kraus,
my inspiration

REFERENCES

1. Abdel-Fattah RA: Evaluating TMJ Injuries. Wiley Law Publications, John Wiley & Sons, New York, Chichester, Brisbane, Toronto, Singapore 1992

2. American Academy of Craniomandibular Disorders: Craniomandibular Disorders, Guidelines for Evaluation, Diagnosis and Management. Quintessence Publishing, Lombard IL 1990

3. American Academy of Pediatric Dentistry and University of Texas Health Science Center at San Antonio Dental School: Treatment of Temporomandibular Disorders in Children: Summary Statements and Recommendations. JADA 120:265, 1990

4. Assael LA: Arthrotomy for Internal Derangements. In Temporomandibular Disorders, Diagnosis and Treatment. AS Kaplan, et al, eds. WB Saunders, Philadelphia PA 1991.

5. Baraducci J, Thompson D and Scheffer R: Perforation into the Middle Cranial Fossa as a Sequel to Use of a Proplast-Teflon Implant for TMJ Reconstruction. J Oral Maxillofac Surg 48:496, 1990

6. Bays RA: Arthrotomy and Orthognathic Surgery for TMD. In Temporomandibular Disorders, 2nd edition. S Kraus, ed. Churchill Livingstone, New York NY 1993.

7. Begg CB: Statistical Methods In The Medical Diagnosis. Crit Rev Med Inform 1:1-22, 1986.

8. Bell WE: Temporomandibular Disorders: Classification, Diagnosis, Management, 3rd edition. Year Book Medical Publishers, Chicago IL 1990

9. Benoit P: History and Physical Examination for TMD. In Temporomandibular Disorders, 2nd edition. S Kraus, ed. Churchill Livingstone, New York NY 1993.

10. Blaustein DI and Heffez LB: Arthroscopic Atlas of the Temporomandibular Joint. Lea & Febiger, Philadelphia PA 1990.

11. Block S: The Use of a Resilient Rubber Bite Appliance in Treatment of MPD Syndrome. J Dent Res 57 :A71, 1978.

12. Boyd RL, et al: Temporomandibular Joint Forces Measured at the Condyle of Macaca Arctoides. Am J Orthod Dentofac Orthop 97:472, 1990.

13. Burch JG: Activity of the Accessory Ligaments of the Temporomandibular Joint. J Prosthet Dent 24: 621-628, 1970.

14. Burch JG: The Cranial Attachment of the Sphenomandibular (Tympanomandibular) Ligament. Anat Rec 156: 433-438, 1966.

15. Cephalalgia: An International Journal of Headache. Vol 8, Supplement 7, 1988.

16. Cholitgul W, et al: Clinical and Radiological Findings in Temporomandibular Joints with Disc Perforations. Int J Oral Maxillofac Surg 19:220-225, 1990.

17. Clark G: A Critical Evaluation of Orthopedic Interocclusal Appliance Therapy: Design, Theory, and Overall Effectiveness. JADA 108, March 1984.

18. Clark G: Examining Temporomandibular Disorder Patients For Cranio-Cervical Dysfunction. J Craniomand Prac 2(1):56-63, Dec 83-Feb 84.

19. Clark GT, et al: Guidelines for the Treatment of Temporomandibular Disorders, J Craniomand Disorders: Facial & Oral Pain. 4(2), 1990.

20. Clark GT, Moody DG, Saunders B: Arthroscopic Treatment of Temporomandibular Joint Locking Resulting from Disc Derangement: Two-year Results. J Oral Maxillofac Surg 49:157-164, 1991.

21. Clark GT: Occlusal Therapy: Occlusal Appliances. In The President's Conference on the Examination, Diagnosis and Management of Temporomandibular Disorders. D Laskin, et al, eds. American Dental Association 1982.

22. Clark GT: Treatment of Jaw Clicking with Temporomandibular Repositioning: Analysis of 25 Cases. J Craniomand Pract 2:263-270, 1984.

23. Costen J: Classification and Treatment of Temporomandibular Joint Problems. Ann Otol Rhinol Laryngol 65:35, 1956.

24. Danielson P: Arthrography. In Temporomandibular Disorders, Diagnosis and Treatment. AS Kaplan, et al, eds. WB Saunders, Philadelphia PA 1991.

25. Dawson P: Occlusal Splints. In Evaluation and Treatment of Occlusal Problems. CV Mosby, St Louis MO 1988.

26. Dolwick M, et al: 1984 Criteria for TMJ Meniscus Surgery. American Association of Oral and Maxillofacial Surgeons, 1984.

27. Dolwick MF: Diagnosis and Etiology of Internal Derangements of the Temporomandibular Joint. In The President's Conference on the Examination, Diagnosis and Management of Temporomandibular Disorders. D Laskin, et al, eds. American Dental Association 1982.

28. DuBrul EL: The Craniomandibular Articulation. In Oral Anatomy, 7th edition. H Sicher, ed. CV Mosby, St Louis MO 1980.

29. Dworkin S: Approach To The Problem. J Craniomand Disorders: Facial & Oral Pain 6(4), 1992.

30. Dworkin SF, et al: Epidemiology of Signs and Symptoms in Temporomandibular Disorders: Clinical Signs in Cases and Controls. JADA 120, March 1990.

31. Edmeads J: The Cervical Spine and Headache. Neurology 38:1874-1878, 1988.

32. Eriksson L and Westesson PL: Clinical and Radiological Study of Patients with Anterior Disc Displacement of the Temporomandibular Joint. Swed Dent J 7:55, 1983.

33. Farole A: Correlation of Postoperative TMJ MRI and Patient Clinical Symptoms. J Oral Max Surg 48-8(132), Aug 1990.

34. Farrar W: Diagnosis and Treatment of Painful Temporomandibular Joints. J Prosthet Dent 28:629-636, 1972.

35. Farrar WB and McCarty WL: Inferior Joint Space Arthrography and Characteristics of the Condylar Path in Internal Derangements of the TMJ. J Prosthet Dent 41:548, 1979.

36. Farrell JP: Cervical Passive Mobilization Techniques. In Physical Medicine and Rehabilitation: State of the Art Review. J Saal, ed. 4(2), June 1990.

37. Findlay IA: Mandibular Joint Pressures. J Dent Res 43:140, 1964.

38. Fonder AC: The Dental Physician, 2nd edition. Medical-Dental Arts, 303 2nd St W, Rock Falls, IL 61071, 1984.

39. Gabler MJ, et al: Effect of Arthroscopic Temporomandibular Joint Surgery on Articular Disk Position. J Craniomand Disorders: Facial & Oral Pain 3(4), 1989.

40. Gelb H and Tarte J: A Two-Year Clinical Evaluation of 200 Cases of Chronic Headache: The Craniocervical-Mandibular Syndrome. JADA 91:1230-1236, 1975.

41. Gerber A: Kiefergelenk und Zahnokklusion. Dtsch Zahnaerztl Z 26:119, 1971.

42. Goharian RK and Neff P: Effect of Occlusal Retainers on Temporomandibular Joint and Facial Pain. J Prosth Dent 44(2), August 1980.

43. Goulet JP and Clark GT: Clinical TMJ Examination Methods. CDA Journal, March 1990.

44. Graber G: Neurologische und Psychosomatische aspekte der Myoarthropathien des Kauorgans. ZWR 80:997, 1971.

45. Greene CS: Can Technology Enhance TM Disorder Diagnosis? CDA Journal, March 1990.

46. Griffin CJ and Sharpe CJ: The Structure of the Adult Human Temporomandibular Meniscus. Austral Dent J 5:190-195, 1960.

47. Griner PF, et al: Selection and Interpretation of Diagnostic Tests and Procedures. Ann Intern Med 94:553-600, 1981.

48. Gross A and Gale EN: A Prevalence Study of the Clinical Signs Associated with Mandibular Dysfunction. JADA 107:932-936 Dec 1983.

49. Hall M: Evaluation of Patients 5 Years After Diskectomy for TMJ Pain. In Educational Outlines and Summaries, pp 208. American Association of Oral and Maxillofacial Surgeons, 1988.

50. Hansson TL: Temporomandibular Joint Anatomical Findings Relevant to the Clinician. In Perspectives in Temporomandibular Disorders. GT Clark and WK Solberg, eds. Quintessence Publishing, Chicago IL 1987.

51. Helms CA, et al: Internal Derangements of the Temporomandibular Joint. Radiology Research and Education Foundation, 1983.

52. Hesse JR and Hansson TL: Factors Influencing Joint Mobility in General and in Particular Respect of the Craniomandibular Articulation: A Literature Review. J Craniomand Disorders: Facial & Oral Pain 2(1), 1988.

53. Holmlund A, Hellsing G and Wredmark T: Arthroscopy of the Temporomandibular Joint. Int J Oral Maxillofac Surg 15:715-721, 1986.

54. Howard JA: Imaging Techniques for the Diagnosis and Prognosis of TMD. CDA Journal, March 1990.

55. Hylander WL: An Experimental Analysis of Temporomandibular Joint Reaction Force in Macaques. Am J Phys Anthropol 51:433, 1979.

56. Hylander WL: Functional Anatomy. In Perspectives in Temporomandibular Disorders. BG Sarnet, DM Laskin and CC Thomas, eds. Springfield 1979.

57. Ide Y and Nakazawa K: Anatomical Atlas of the Temporomandibular Joint. Quintessence Publishing, Tokyo 1991.

58. Indresano AT: Arthroscopic Surgery of the TMJ. J Oral Maxillofac Surg 47:439-441, 1989.

59. Irby WB and Zetz MR: Osteoarthritis and Rheumatoid Arthritis Affecting the Temporomandibular Joint. In The President's Conference on the Examination, Diagnosis and Management of Temporomandibular Disorders. D Laskin, et al, eds. American Dental Association 1982.

60. Ireland VE: The Problem of the "Clicking Jaw." Proc R Soc Med 44:363, 1951.

61. Isberg A, Stenstrom B and Isacsson G: Frequency of Joint Bilateral Joint Disc Displacement in Patients with Unilateral Symptoms: A 5 year Follow-Up Of The Asymptomatic Joint. Dentomaxillofac Radiol 20:73-76, 1991.

62. Isberg A, Widmaim SE and Ivarsson: Clinical, Radiographic, and Electromyographic Study of Patients with Internal Derangement of the Temporomandibular Joint. Am J Orthod 88:453, 1985.

63. Jankelson B: The Myo-monitor: Its Use and Abuse. Quint Int 2:47, 1978.

64. Jee W: The Skeletal Tissues. In Histology, Cell and Tissue Biology. L Weiss, ed. Elsevier Biomedical Publishers, New York NY 1988.

65. Jendresen MD, et al: Report of the Committee on Scientific Investigation of the American Academy of Restorative Dentistry. J Prosth Dent 57(6), June 1987.

66. Kaplan AS and Goldman J: General Concepts of Treatment. In Temporomandibular Disorders,

Diagnosis and Treatment. AS Kaplan, ed. WB Saunders, Philadelphia PA 1991.

67. Kaplan, et al, eds.: Temporomandibular Disorders, Diagnosis and Treatment. WB Saunders, Philadelphia PA 1991.

68. Kircos LT, et al: Magnetic Resonance Imaging of the TMJ Disc in Asymptomatic Volunteers. J Oral Maxillofac Surg 45:852-854, 1987.

69. Kozeniauskas JJ and Ralph WJ: Bilateral Arthrographic Evaluation of Unilateral Temporomandibular Joint Pain and Dysfunction. J Prosth Dent 60(1), July 1988.

70. Kraus S: Cervical Spine Influences on the Management of TMD. In Temporomandibular Disorders, 2nd edition. S Kraus, ed. Churchill Livingstone, New York NY 1993.

71. Kraus S: Evaluation and Management of Cervical Spine Dysfunction. Boston MA, December 5-6, 1992. Course Notes.

72. Kraus S: Evaluation and Management of Temporomandibular Disorders. Boston MA, December 5-6, 1992. Course Notes.

73. Kraus S: Influences of the Cervical Spine on the Stomatognathic System. In Orthopædic Physical Therapy, 2nd edition. B Donatelli and M Wooden, eds. Churchill Livingstone, New York NY 1993.

74. Kraus S: Physical Therapy Management of the Temporomandibular Joint. In Temporomandibular Disorders, 2nd edition. S Kraus, ed. Churchill Livingstone, New York NY 1993.

75. Langton D and Eggleton M: Functional Anatomy of the Temporomandibular Joint Complex. An IFORC Publication, Santiago Chile, Sept 1992.

76. Laskin D, et al (eds): The President's Conference on the Examination, Diagnosis and Management of Temporomandibular Disorders. Am Dent Assoc 1982.

77. Laskin D: Etiology of the Pain Dysfunction Syndrome. J Am Dent Assoc 79:147, 1969.

78. Laskin DM and Greene CS: Technological Methods in the Diagnosis and Treatment of Temporomandibular Disorders. Quintessence Int 23:95-102, 1992.

79. Lerman M: The Hydrostatic Appliance: A New Approach to Treatment of the TMJ Pain Dysfunction Syndrome. JADA 89:1343, 1974.

80. Lester J, Windsor R, et al: Medical Management of the Cervical Spine. In Temporomandibular Disorders, 2nd edition. S Kraus, ed. Churchill Livingstone, New York NY 1993.

81. Levitt SR: The Predictive Value of the TMJ Scale In Detecting Psychological Problems and Non-TM Disorders in Patients with Temporomandibular Disorders. J Craniomand Prac 8(3), July 1990.

82. Lieberman JM, et al: Dermal Grafts of the Temporomandibular Joint: Postoperative Appearance on MR Images. Radiology 176:199, 1990.

83. Lipp MJ: Temporomandibular Symptoms and Occlusion: A Review of the Literature & the Concept. NY State J Dent 56(9):58-64, 1990.

84. Lous J: Treatment of TMJ Syndrome by Pivots. J Prosth Dent 40:179, 1978.

85. Lundh H, et al: Anterior Repositioning Splint in the Treatment of Temporomandibular Joints with Reciprocal Clicking: Comparison With A Flat Occlusal Splint And An Untreated Control Group. Oral Surg Oral Med Oral Pathol 60:131-136, 1985.

86. Lundh H, et al: Disc-Repositioning Onlays In The Treatment Of Temporoamandibular Joint Disk Displacement: Comparison With A Flat Occlusal Splint And With No Treatment. Oral Surg Oral Med Oral Pathol 66:155-162, 1988.

87. MacConaill MA: Studies In The Mechanics Of Synovial Joints II. Ir J Med Sc 6:223, 1946.

88. MacConaill MA: The Movements of Bones and Joints. J Bone Joint Surg [Br] 35:290, 1953.

89. Mahan PE, et al: Superior and Inferior Bellies of the Lateral Pterygoid Muscle EMG Activity at Basic Jaw Positions. J Prosthet Dent 50:710, 1983.

90. Mahan PE: The Temporomandibular Joint in Function and Pathofunction. In Temporomandibular Joint Problems. WK Solberg and Clark, eds. Quintessence Publishing, Lombard IL 1980.

91. Mannheimer JS, Keith T and Osborn J: Physical Therapy Protocol Post Arthroscopic, Arthrotomy and Orthognathic Surgery. In Temporomandibular Disorders, 2nd edition. S Kraus, ed. Churchill Livingstone, New York NY 1993.

92. Manzione JV, et al: Direct Sagittal Computed Tomography of the TMJ. AJNR 3:677-679, 1982.

93. May W: Physiologic Functional Position of the Mandible. Basal Facts 3(3):137-148, 1980.

94. McNamara JA, Jr: The Independent Functions of the Two Heads of the Lateral Pterygoid Muscle. Am J Anat 138:197, 1973.

95. McNeil BJ, Keeler E and Adelstein SJ: Primer on Certain Elements of Medical Decision Making. N Engl J Med 293:211-215, 1975.

96. McNeill C: Craniomandibular Disorders. Quintessence Publishing, Chicago IL 1990.

97. McNeill, et al: Craniomandibular (TMJ) Disorders - The State of the Art. J Prosthet Dent 44(4):434-437, 1980.

98. Mennell J: Joint Pain. Little Brown, Boston MA 1964.

99. Messing SG: Splint Therapy. In Temporomandibular Disorders, Diagnosis and Treatment. S Kaplan, et al, eds. WB Saunders, Philadelphia PA 1991.

100. Moffett BC: Histological Aspects of Temporomandibular Joint Derangements. In Diagnosis of Internal Derangements of the Temporomandibular Joint, Vol 1. BC Moffett, ed. University of Washington, Seattle WA 1984.

101. Mohl ND, et al: Devices for the Diagnosis and

Treatment of Temporomandibular Disorders, Part I: Introduction, Scientific Evidence, and Jaw Tracking. J Prosthet Dent 63:198, 1990.

102. Mohl ND, et al: Devices for the Diagnosis and Treatment of Temporomandibular Disorders, Part II: Electromyography and Sonography. J Prosthet Dent 63:332, 1990.

103. Mohl ND, et al: Devices for the Diagnosis and Treatment of Temporomandibular Disorders, Part III: Thermography, Ultrasound, Electrical Stimulation, and Electromyographic Biofeedback. J Prosthet Dent 63:472, 1990.

104. Mohl ND: Functional Anatomy of the Temporomandibular Joint. In The President's Conference on the Examination, Diagnosis and Management of Temporomandibular Disorders. D Laskin, et al, ed. American Dental Association 1982.

105. Moloney F and Howard JA: Internal Derangements of the Temporomandibular Joint III: Anterior Repositioning Splint Therapy. Aust Dent J 31:30-39, 1986.

106. Montgomery M, et al: Meniscal Repositioning and Arthroscopic TMJ Surgeries: Outcome Comparisons. J Dental Research, Special Issue:1004, 1990.

107. Montgomery MT, et al: Arthroscopic TMJ Surgery: Effects on Signs, Symptoms, And Disk Position. J Oral Maxillofacial Surg 47:1263, 1989.

108. Morgan DH: Evaluation of Alloplastic TMJ Implants. J Craniomand Prac 6(3), July 1988.

109. Naeije M and Hansson TL: Electromyographic Screening of Myogenous and Arthrogenous TMJ Dysfunction Patients. J Oral Rehabil 13:433-441, 1986.

110. Nitzan DW, Dolwick MF and Heft MW: Arthroscopic Lavage and Lysis of the Temporomandibular Joint: A Change In Perspective. J Oral Maxillofac Surg 48:798-801, 1990.

111. Ohrbach R: Review of the Literature: Part I - A Current Diagnostic Systems. J Craniomand Disorders: Facial & Oral Pain 6(4), 1992.

112. Okeson JP: The Management of Temporomandibular Disorders and Occlusion, 3rd edition. Mosby-Year Book Publishing Company, St Louis MO 1993.

113. Padamsee M, Tsamtsouris A and Ahlin J: Functional Disorders of the Stomatognathic System: Part I - A Review. J Pedodontics 9:179-187, 1985.

114. Perrott DH, et al: A Prospective Evaluation of the Effectiveness of Temporomandibular Joint Arthroscopy. J Oral Maxillofac Surg 48:1029-1032, 1990.

115. Pertes R and Attanasio R: Internal Derangements. In Temporomandibular Disorders, Diagnosis and Treatment. AS Kaplan, et al, eds. WB Saunders, Philadelphia PA 1991.

116. Questionable Care: JADA 115:679-685, Nov 1987.

117. Benoit P and Razook S : Radiology of the Temporomandibular Joint. In Temporomandibular Disorders, 2nd edition. S Kraus, ed. Churchill Livingstone, New York NY 1993.

118. Razook SJ and Lawrence ES: Nonsurgical Management of Mandibular Disorders. In Temporomandibular Disorders, 2nd edition. S Kraus, ed. Churchill Livingstone, New York NY 1993.

119. Rees LA: The Structure and Function of the Mandibular Joint. Br Dent J 96:125, 1954.

120. Rheumatoid Arthritis. J Am Med Assoc, Section 7 (suppl) 224:687, 1973.

121. Roberts RR, et al: Correlation of Clinical Parameters to the Arthrographic Depiction of TMJ Internal Derangements. Oral Surg Oral Med Oral Pathol 66:32-36, 1986.

122. Saizar P: Centric Relation and Condylar Movement: Anatomic Mechanism. J Prosthet Dent 26:581-591, 1971.

123. Sanders B and Buonocristiani R: Temporomandibular Joint Arthrotomy, Management of Failed Cases. Oral and Maxillofac Surgery Clinics Of North America 1:443, 1989.

124. Scapino RP: Histopathology of the Disc And Posterior Attachment In Disc Displacement Internal Derangements of the TMJ volume of Magnetic Resonance Imaging Of The Temporomandibular Joint. E Palacios, ed. Georg Thieme Verlag, Stuttgart 1990.

125. Scapino RP: The Posterior Attachment: Its Structure, Function, and Appearance in TMJ Imaging Studies: Part 1. J Craniomand Disorders: Facial & Oral Pain. V5(2), 1991.

126. Schiffman EL, et al: The Prevalence and Treatment Needs of Subjects with Temporomandibular Disorders. JADA 120:295-303, 1990.

127. Schwartz L: A Temporomandibular Joint Pain Dysfunction Syndrome. J Chron Dis 3:284, 1956.

128. Scully JJ: Cinefluorographic Studies of the Masticatory Movements of the Human Mandible. University of Illinois, 1959. Thesis.

129. Segami N, Murakami KI and Fukuda M: Arthrographic Evaluation of Disk Position Following Mandibular Manipulation Technique for Internal Derangement with Closed Lock of the Temporomandibular Joint. J Craniomand Disorders: Facial & Oral Pain.4(2), 1990.

130. Shore N: Occlusal Equilibration and Temporomandibular Joint Dysfunction. JP Lippincott, Philadelphia PA 1959.

131. Sicher H: Oral Anatomy, pp183-189, 532. CV Mosby, St Louis MO 1980.

132. Solberg W and Clark G: Temporomandibular Joint Problems. Quintessence Publishing, Chicago IL 1980.

133. Spruijt RJ and Hoogstraten J: The Research on Temporomandibular Joint Clicking: A Methodological Review. J Craniomand Disorders: Facial & Oral Pain 5(1), 1991.

134. Takensoshita Y, Ikebe T, Yamamoto M, et al: Occlusal Contact Area and Temporomandibular Joint Symptoms. Oral Surg Oral Med Oral Pathol 72:388-394, 1991.

135. Thilander B: Innervation of the Temporomandibular Disc in Man. Acta Odontol Scand 22:151, 1964

136. Toller PA: Temporomandibular Arthropathy. Proc R Soc Lond 67:153, 1974.

137. Tucker MR and Burkes J: Temporary Silastic Implantation Following Discectomy in the Primate Temporoamandibular Joint. J Oral Maxillofac Surg 47:1290, 1989.

138. Voss R: Die Behandlung von Beschwerden des Kiefergelenkes mit Aufbisplatten. Dtsch Zahnaerzil Z 19:545, 1964.

139. Wabeke KB, et al: Temporomandibular Joint Clicking: A Literature Overview. J Craniomand Disorders: Facial & Oral Pain 3(3), 1989.

140. Warwick R and Williams PL: Gray's Anatomy, 36th edition. Churchill Livingstone, London 1980.

141. Weinberg L: Treatment Prosthesis in TMJ Dysfunction-Pain Syndrome. J Prosth Dent 39(6), June 1976.

142. Westesson PL, Bronstein SL and Liedberg J: Internal Derangement of the Temporomandibular Joint: Morphologic Description with Correlation to Joint Function. Oral Surg Oral Med Oral Pathol 59:323, 1985.

143. Widmer C: Evaluation of Diagnostic Test for TMD. In Temporomandibular Disorders, 2nd edition. S Kraus, ed. Churchill Livingstone, New York NY 1993.

144. Widmer C: Evaluation of Temporomandibular Disorders. In TMJ Disorders, 1st edition. S Kraus, ed. Churchill Livingstone, New York NY 1988.

145. Widmer C: Review of the Literature, Part I-B: Reliability and Validation of Examination Methods. J Craniomand Disorders: Facial & Oral Pain 6(4), 1992

146. Widmer CG, Lund JP and Feine JS: Evaluation of Diagnostic Tests for TMD. CDA Journal 18(3):53-60, 1990.

147. Wilk R: Anterior Movement of the TMJ Disc Following Lateral Pterygoid Stimulation: Preliminary Observations. Poster 33, at the Scientific Poster Session of the AAOMS, 1990.

148. Wilkinson TM: The Relationship Between the Disk and Lateral Pterygoid Muscle in the Human Temporomandibular Joint. J Prosthet Dent 60:715, 1988.

149. Wong GV, Weinberg S and Symingen JM: Morphology of the Developing Articular Disc of the Human Temporomandibular Joint. J Oral Maxillofac Surg 43:565-569, 1985.

150. Yale SH, Allison BD and Hauptfuehrer JD: An Epidemiological Assessment of Mandibular Condyle Morphology. Oral Surg 21:169, 1966.

151. Yerushalmy J: Statistical Problems in Assessing Methods of Medical Diagnosis, with Special Reference To X-ray Techniques. Public Health Rep 62:1432-1449, 1947.

152. Zamburlini I and Austin D: Long-Term Results of Appliance Therapies In Anterior Disk Displacement with Reduction: A Review of the Literature. J Craniomand Prac 9(4), October 1991.

SECTION 3
Specific Treatment Techniques

CHAPTER 9

JOINT MOBILIZATION

HISTORY

Joint mobilization is an art that has been practiced since prehistoric times. The first documentation of mobilization was made by Hippocrates (460 BC - 375 BC). He taught his students to apply a vertical manipulative thrust on a gibbus (prominent vertebra) and to give exercises afterward. Galen made reference to the manipulation of the spine for misalignment in a patient following trauma to the neck.[14]

For many centuries in England, bonesetters practiced manipulation as a family tradition. People consulted them to have their painful joints manipulated. Bonesetters still exist today in many European countries. In 1876, Sir James Paget (1814-1899), the renowned British surgeon, published his famous lecture, "Cases That Bonesetters Cure," in the British Medical Journal. Paget delineated the types of cases that were responsive to manipulative therapy. He exhorted his readers to "Learn them...imitate what is good and avoid what is bad in the practice of bonesetters." Paget's words fell on deaf ears. Orthodox medicine of the day found the rationale behind bonesetting untenable, an attitude probably justified in part even though patients who had visited bonesetters attested to their skill.[14]

Two major schools of thought of mobilization/ manipulation are osteopathy and chiropractic. Superficially, these two schools bear certain resemblances to each other with regard to the mechanistic approach to illness but beyond that, their scopes and philosophies are quite different.[14]

The history of osteopathy is intimately connected with Andrew Taylor Still (1828-1917). He studied medicine at the College of Physicians and Surgeons in Kansas City, Missouri. Still lost three of his sons in an epidemic of spinal meningitis, even though they had the best medical treatment available. Still became disillusioned with orthodox medicine as it was practiced during his day. A deeply religious man, the idea of osteopathy came to Still like a "revelation." He concluded that the human body possessed self-healing properties, that efficient functioning was dependent on unimpaired structure and that proper nerve and blood supply to the tissues was necessary for health maintenance. These concepts were contained in his "Rule of the Artery" which he proclaimed in 1874 and which became the basic concept of osteopathy. He founded the American School of Osteopathy in 1892 in Kirksville, Missouri.[14]

Today, osteopathic physicians (DO's) may be found in virtually every field of medicine and surgery as their backgrounds have expanded to encompass both osteopathic and allopathic knowledge.

Chiropractic began in Davenport, Iowa with Daniel David Palmer, a grocer. Palmer, having read some of Still's work, reported in 1895 that he "cured" the deafness of a janitor after he "adjusted" the latter's misaligned vertebra. Palmer's belief was that the spinal column was the controller of the human machinery and that all diseases could be traced to it. He formulated "The Law of the Spinal Nerve" as the basis for chiropractic. Palmer founded the first chiropractic school in Davenport in 1897. His adolescent son was its first graduate. Today there are 14 accredited chiropractic colleges in the United States recognized by the two major chiropractic professional associations, the American Chiropractic Association (ACA) and the International Chiropractic Association (ICA).

The basis of chiropractic philosophy is the theory of "subluxation." Chiropractors claim that subluxation in the spinal column interferes with nerve function and that this is the significant factor in disease causation. Manipulation of the appropriate area of the spine restores the natural alignment of the spine which, in turn, relieves the symptoms. Statements regarding the adjustment of the spine for disorders such as diabetes, various intestinal disorders, heart trouble and cancer are quite common in chiropractic literature.[14]

There is still no consensus as to the rationale behind spinal manipulations, but there exists a wealth of theories. Each school of thought has advanced its own rationale and has evolved manipulative techniques consistent with it.

The number of allopathic physicians (M.D.'s) who have recognized and used manipulative principles is growing, and several physicians have made remarkable contributions to its conceptualization.

James Mennell, M.D., who was once in charge of the Physical Medicine Department at St. Thomas' Hospital in London, published a book in 1952 entitled The Science and Art of Joint Manipulation. He pointed to the facet joints, postural strain and adhesions as causative factors in back pain. Later, his son John enunciated the concepts of "joint play" and "joint dysfunction."[14]

James Cyriax, M.D. was the orthopædic physician at St. Thomas' Hospital in London after James Mennell. More than any other physician, he has done a great deal to bring the usefulness of manipulation to the medical profession. His book, Textbook of Orthopædic Medicine, first published in 1954, is invaluable. Because of his ardent belief in the disc as a source of back pain problems, most of Cyriax' manipulative techniques are designed for the reduction of disc herniation. He claims that his rotatory maneuvers apply a torsional stress on the spine that exert a centripetal force that reduces the bulging disc material if the longitudinal ligaments are intact.[14]

The driving force behind a school of thought that has flourished in Scandinavia is Freddie Kaltenborn, who is a physiotherapist, a chiropractor and an osteopath. His philosophy is a synthesis of what he considers to be the best in chiropractic, osteopathy and physical medicine. He uses some of Cyriax's methods to evaluate the patient and mainly employs specific osteopathic and sometimes chiropractic techniques for treatment.[14] His refinement and development of treatment techniques is a vast contribution to understanding mobilization therapy.

In 1964 physical therapist Geoffery Maitland published his book, Vertebral Manipulation. He distinguishes between mobilization and manipulation and puts heavy emphasis on mobilization. His techniques are fairly similar to the "articulatory" techniques used by osteopaths. These involve oscillatory movements performed on a chosen joint in which the movement induced by the therapist is within the patient's available range of movement tolerance in order to release a fixed synovial joint. Because his techniques are of a gentle nature and are easier to learn, they have appealed to physical therapists and have gained much recognition, especially in Australia (where Maitland is a private practitioner in physiotherapy and a part-time instructor at the University of Adelaide) and in the United Kingdom. By using the word mobilization instead of manipulation, he has successfully eliminated the emotional aspects surrounding the subject, which has led to its better acceptance among members of the medical profession.[14]

RATIONALE/APPLICATION

Mobilization/manipulation techniques are passive movements applied to a joint (or soft tissue) in a specific manner to restore the full, free, painless range of motion of a joint. Such techniques must take into account the biomechanics of the joint in question as well as Fryette's Laws of Spinal Motion to be safe and effective (see Chapter 2, Basic Spinal Mechanics).

Indications for the use of mobilization techniques include joints that are painful, hypomobile or involve mechanical motion dysfunctions (subluxations and impingements). Gentle mobilization can also promote healing of injured tissues. Obviously, a muscle cannot be fully rehabilitated if the underlying joints are not free to move, and conversely, a muscle cannot move a joint that is not free to move. Thus, there are clear reasons to employ joint mobilization techniques.

The effects of mobilization/manipulation are both neurophysiologic and mechanical. The work of Wyke and others[3, 6, 16] in the area of joint mechanoreceptors explains why mobilization techniques can be effective in relieving pain, causing reflex inhibition of muscles and promoting relaxation (Fig 9-1). Mobilization techniques are mechanical because when they are

Type	Location	Receptor Appearance	Sensory Unit	Physiologic Function
I	Stratum fibrosum of capsule; ligaments Higher density in proximal joints	Laminated Ruffini-like corpuscle 300 μm wide 300–800 μm long	Myelinated parent axon and 2–6 corpuscles	Active at rest and during movement Low threshold for activation Slowly adapting
II	Junction of synovial and fibrosum of capsule; intra-articular and extra-articular fat pads Higher density in distal joints	Laminated, pacinian-like, conically shaped corpuscle 150–250 μm long 20–40 μm wide	Myelinated parent axon and 1–5 corpuscles	Active at onset and termination of movement Low threshold for activation Rapidly adapting
III	Collateral ligaments Not found in interspinous ligaments of cervical region	GTO-like corpuscle 800 μm long 100 μm wide	Myelinated parent axon and 1 corpuscle	Active at end of joint range High threshold for activation Slowly adapting
IV	Ligaments, capsule, and articular fat pads Absent in synovial tissue	Free nerve endings or lattice type endings	Thinly myelinated parent axon and terminal endings	Active only to extreme mechanical or chemical irritation High threshold for activation Slowly adapting

Figure 9-1. Characteristics of joint mechanoreceptors (reprinted with permission from Newton [13]).

employed into the range of restriction, they are moving into the area of plastic deformation of the soft tissue (collagen). An example of a stress-strain curve (hysteresis loop) appears in Figure 9-2. Simply stated, if a tissue is stretched only in its elastic range, no permanent structural change will occur. It is only when the tissue is stretched into the plastic range and beyond that permanent structural changes occur. Obviously, if stretched beyond the plastic range to the fatigue point, fracture will occur. For example, imagine bending the handle of a toothbrush back and forth rapidly. At first, there is much resistance, but as the bending continues, there is less resistance and the handle begins to bend further. Finally, it breaks. Judiciously applied, mobilization/manipulation techniques can stretch tissue and break adhesions effectively. Indiscriminately applied, they can tear tissue and cause sprains or strains of the joints.

One must have a basic appreciation of joint mechanics to effectively employ mobilization techniques. The reader should review Chapter 2 for a complete discussion of spinal biomechanics and a review of Fryette's Laws of Spinal Motion.

Joint play motions, first described by Mennell,[11] are involuntary, interarticular motions present in all

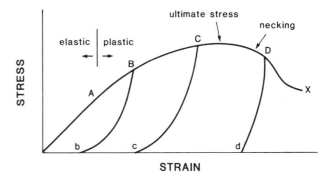

Figure 9-2. Stress-strain curve for collagen (hysteresis loop).

synovial joints. Joint play is necessary for painless, unrestricted, voluntary motion. Joint play movements occur by an external force (a therapist passively moving a joint) and include long axis distraction, tilts, glides and rotations. For example, distraction and P/A glide of the joints of the cervical spine would be joint play motions. They do not occur in voluntary active motions. However, the range of movement in these particular planes must exist (passively) in order for the full, unrestricted, voluntary motion to take place. Some refer to this concept as normal joint laxity or "slack."

Component motions are generally thought of as extra-articular movements that normally accompany active motions. They are not usually recognized, but are nonetheless necessary for full range of movement. Examples of component motions include spreading of the mortise of the ankle in dorsiflexion or the sliding of the radius along the ulna during elbow extension.[15]

Articular position of the joint as described by MacConaill and Basmajian[9] must be considered when performing joint mobilization. The close-packed position is at the extreme of one of the most habitual movements of the joint. It is the position in which the concave surface (smaller area) is in complete congruence with the convex surface (larger area). The capsule and ligaments are maximally taut and the two bones of the articular unit cannot be separated by traction across the joint surface. Joint mobilization should not be performed or attempted in the maximal close-packed position. If joint motion is to be avoided, this position can be useful during treatment. For example, the spinal segments above and below a segment to be mobilized may be "locked" into a close-packed position to isolate the mobilizing force to the desired level.

Any position that is not close-packed is considered loose-packed. The articular surfaces are not totally congruent and some parts of the capsule are lax. The maximum loose-packed position is the best position for early mobilization. In this position, the capsule is most relaxed. The bones of the articular unit can be drawn apart to the greatest extent by traction. This position is often described as the resting position of the joint. All examinations and the first treatment for restricted joint movement are performed from this position or from a position as close as possible to this. Subsequent treatments may be performed in positions nearer the close-packed position, but they are never performed in the maximum close-packed position. Generally speaking, rotation will cause a close-packed position. Likewise, extremes of all motions will tend to place the joint into more of a close-packed position, whereas mid-range of a joint movement will be closer to the loose-packed position. Full extension is the maximum close-packed position of the spine.[10]

The joint capsule is a richly innervated structure that is made up of two layers, the synovial lining on the inside and an external layer of dense, irregular collagen connective tissue. This outer layer of collagen fiber is somewhat thickened and immobile in joints that have a capsular pattern of hypomobility. This may be caused by increased collagen fiber that is laid down in response to injury or inflammation, or it may be caused by a binding together of the individual collagen fibers. These collagen fibers cannot be stretched like the yellow elastic fibers; rather, they must be mobilized in a more subtle manner and allowed to rearrange and loosen over a period of time. Articulating, stretching and traction techniques are more appropriate than manipulation to help rearrange and loosen the fibers.[7] If, on the other hand, joint hypomobility is due to impingement or subluxation where collagen changes have not yet occurred, manipulation may be more effective.[1,2]

Soft tissue massage, contract-relax techniques, passive stretching and active and passive range of motion exercises all increase the mobility of soft tissue in general. However, with the exception of certain contract-relax techniques, their effectiveness in mobilizing the joints is limited to stretching the contractile (muscle-tendon) tissue. Specific and general joint mobilization techniques are generally more effective in restoring mobility of the joints because they act specifically on the inert structures (capsule, ligament, cartilage and intervertebral disc). They can often be done with the joint in a comfortable mid-range position rather than at the often painful limit of range of motion.[16]

Contract-relax techniques can be effective in actually causing joint movement. If the joint is carefully positioned toward the direction of restriction, and the patient exerts a muscular effort, the muscular effort can cause the joint to move. These principles are inherent in some of the osteopathic "Muscle Energy Techniques" taught by some instructors and authors.[4,8,12] Muscle Energy Techniques can be very general or very specific to one joint, depending upon the degree of localization achieved by the specificity of the technique. In this chapter, both general contract-relax techniques and the more specific "Muscle Energy Techniques" will be discussed. The more advanced osteopathic evaluation scheme and Muscle Energy Techniques are beyond the scope of this text, and are discussed in depth in other works.[4,8,12] They are included in brief form in this chapter for the sake of completeness and to stimulate further interest in the reader.

Because of pain, mobilization cannot always be performed in the most restricting direction. In such a case, it is performed in directions other than, or possibly opposite to, the direction of restriction. Restoration of mobility in one direction will usually increase mobility in other directions as well. For example, a rotational mobilization is likely to increase range of motion in all other planes of motion. Therefore, if mobilization in one direction is particularly painful, beneficial results can often be obtained by initially mobilizing in less painful directions. Many times, the first mobilization treatment performed consists of gentle tractions applied to the joint structures with five to ten second holds. The purpose is to relieve the pain. Gradually, the mobilization may be increased.

Increasing joint mobility is one of the most frequent reasons joint mobilization is performed. As soft tissue injuries and inflammations heal, stiffness is inherent. Left alone, the joints may become hypomobile. The untreated hypomobile joint will soon begin to show signs of joint degeneration. To avoid this pathological chain of events, mobilization techniques and/or exercise must be used. The earlier they are started in the treatment regime, the more benefit obtained, provided they are not aggravating to any soft tissue pathology present.

Joint mobilization is not a panacea. It does, however, have a place in the armamentarium of the physical therapist. It has a place among the modalities aimed at reducing human suffering and increasing quality of life. It is unfortunate that practitioners of mobilization have made exaggerated claims and that some practitioners of orthodox medicine find it difficult to admit their own ignorance of the subject. Fortunately, joint mobilization is quickly becoming a more widely known and accepted treatment modality, and most practitioners of joint mobilization are improving their clinical decision-making skills to use it appropriately and skillfully.

Using a Three-dimensional Mobilization Table

A three-dimensional (3-D) mobilization table can enhance the effectiveness and ease of many of the techniques described in this chapter. The table shown in Figure 9-3 has many potential uses, including positional stretching, mobilization and traction, and many clinicians consider them indispensable in the treatment of spinal patients. The use of a 3-D table and a basic understanding of spinal biomechanics allows for endless options in joint mobilization. The therapist's only limitation is his or her imagination. The 3-D table allows the clinician to work on passive range of motion in all planes in an unweighted position. It can be used to position a patient to make accessory mobilization more specific to a physiologic motion. Finally, it can be used very effectively in combination with traction to find the position of most relief or maximize the centralization of lumbar herniated nucleus pulposus (HNP) symptoms.

JOINT MOBILIZATION METHODS

Joint mobilization is a form of passive movement done to restore joint play, component motion and/or range of motion. Most of the mobilization techniques shown in this text for the spine involve accessory motion techniques.

Joint mobilization includes the following:

Articulations are graded, oscillating movements done to restore joint play, component motion or range of motion to a hypomobile joint. They are graded as follows:

Grade 1 - Gentle movements of small amplitude done at the beginning of available range.

Grade 2 - Gentle movements of larger amplitude done into available mid-range of a joint.

Grade 3 - Moderate movements of large amplitude done through the available range of the joint and into the resistance.

Grade 4 - Oscillating movements of small amplitude done at the end of range and into the resistance.

Grade 5 - Thrusting movements done to the anatomical limit of the joint.

A progressive articulation is done in a progressive step-wise manner from the beginning of the range into the resistance.

A stretch articulation is done in a smooth manner from the beginning of the range into the resistance (Fig 9-4).

Grades 1 and 2 are primarily performed to maintain joint mobility, promote tissue healing and relieve pain. They are primarily neurophysiologic in effect. Grades 3 and 4 and progressive articulations are done to increase joint mobility. For example, Grades 1 and 2 are often indicated in the subacute stage of a joint sprain or inflammation to guard against joint hypomobility, to relieve pain, and promote healing, whereas Grade 3 and 4 and progressive and stretch articulations are indicated in more advanced stages of hypomobility or situations involving joint impingement or motion restrictions. Grade 5 mobilizations are thrust techniques used to gain full joint mobility, and are especially helpful when their purpose is to mobilize a subluxed or impinged joint.[10]

The rules of mobilization are as follows[11]:

1. The patient and therapist must be relaxed.

2. The procedure must be relatively pain free.

3. When possible, the therapist should stabilize one bone and move or mobilize the other.

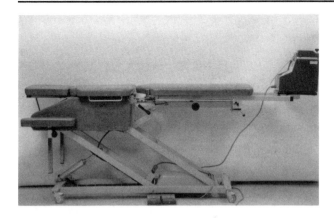

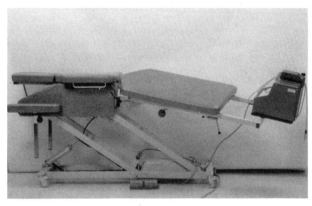

Figure 9-3. A three-dimensional mobilization table. The table has many uses, including positional stretching, mobilization and traction.

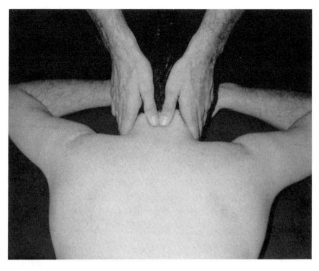

Figure 9-5. Central P/A mobilization for the cervical spine.

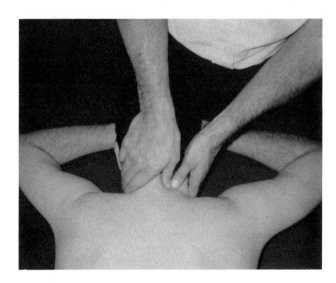

Figure 9-6. Unilateral P/A mobilization for the cervical, thoracic and lumbar spine.

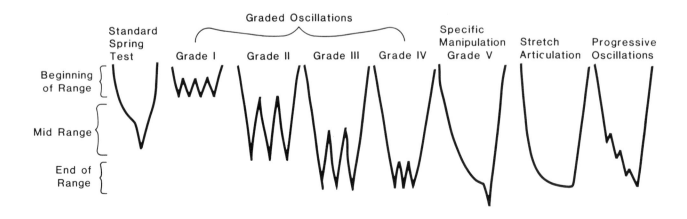

Figure 9-4. Grades of mobilization.

4. The first treatment must be done gently to get a chance to observe the patient's reaction.

5. The therapist should always compare and observe the vertebral levels above or below to gain knowledge of individual patient differences.

6. When possible, the therapist should examine one joint and one movement at a time.

7. The therapist should not examine for joint mobility if active joint inflammation or active traumatic injury is present.

8. Lever arms of force should be kept as short as possible.

Mobilization, like any other evaluation or treatment skill, cannot be learned or developed entirely by the reading of a textbook. There is no substitute for clinical practice and experience. It is reasonable to assume that the beginner will feel some insecurity and uncertainty when attempting these techniques for the first time. With perseverance, these techniques can be perfected. It is often beneficial to bring a spinal model into the treatment room to help both with patient education and to remind the therapist where his or her hand placement should be. Patients will appreciate the explanation and will not be aware the therapist is using the model as a guide!

The following techniques are the ones we have found to be the most helpful in the treatment of joint dysfunctions. The arrows indicate the directions of the mobilizing forces.

P/A Accessory Mobilizations - General

P/A accessory mobilizations are an extremely valuable tool for the physical therapist. One should not try to classify them as specific to any physiologic motion (flexion, extension, rotation or sidebending), but simply as accessory mobilization techniques designed to increase the general ability of a particular spinal segment to move. In fact, P/A accessory mobilizations are often considered palpatory techniques and are classified as part of the palpation examination by many authors and clinicians.[5] P/A accessory mobilizations can be performed to any area of the spine. One advantage to performing P/A accessory mobilizations is that they are segment specific and allow the therapist to detect changes in the joint feel during performance of the technique. To perform P/A accessory mobilizations, the patient lies prone in a position of spinal neutral. Either central or unilateral techniques can be employed.

For the cervical spine, a central technique is performed by placing the thumbs together as shown in Figure 9-5 and applying an anterior force on the spinous process of a vertebra. Unilateral P/A techniques are performed by using the same thumb contact, but applying the pressure lateral to the midline on the articular pillar (Fig 9-6). The thumb contact on the spinous process should be as broad as possible to avoid unnecessarily sharp contact pressure.

Central P/A's in the thoracic and lumbar spine are most effective and comfortable when the therapist uses the ulnar border of the hand. The hand is rolled in slightly toward the palm so that the contact point is on the hypothenar eminence rather than on the bony pisiform so that patient and therapist comfort is maximized (Fig 9-7). Unilateral P/A's in the thoracic and lumbar spine are done using the thumbs over the transverse processes. It should be noted that in the thoracic spine the transverse process is approximately a finger width lateral to the spinous process. This distance may be even greater in the lumbar spine. The transverse process may not actually be felt, especially in the lumbar spine where it is covered by lumbodorsal fascia and erector spinæ muscles. The inability to feel the transverse processes directly does not make this a poor technique. The therapist will be able to visualize and feel differences in P/A mobility through the soft tissue.

To get a pure P/A glide of an intervertebral joint with the patient lying prone, it is often necessary to angle the pressure cephalically, caudally, medially or laterally to take into consideration the curves of the spine.[5]

The basic P/A accessory mobilizations can be made more specific to a physiologic motion by changing the positioning of the patient manually or incorporating a three-dimensional mobilization table. The purpose is to take up the slack into the direction of the motion barrier with the P/A pressure applied in that position. For example, a P/A accessory mobilization for a lumbar segment becomes more specific for extension if the patient assumes the prone-on-elbows position or the therapist positions the mobilization table into extension.

Cervical Spine

Vertebral Artery Testing

Before attempting to test or mobilize the upper cervical spine, the therapist should perform the vertebral artery test. The vertebral artery test is a well-known screening procedure performed to ensure that the movements performed during cervical mobility testing or treatment will not compromise the circulation of the vertebral artery. Most clinicians are taught to perform the test during the initial examination. However, the integrity of the vertebral artery should be reassessed any time the therapist plans to perform testing or treatment that will increase the available range of motion of the cervical spine. A detailed description of the vertebral artery test is contained in Chapter 4, Evaluation of the Spine.

Cervical Spine Techniques

Twelve basic cervical mobilizations are presented in this text. The first five techniques discussed are similar to the segmental mobility tests described in Chapter 4. These five techniques are: forward bending, backward bending, rotation, sidebending and side gliding. For all of these techniques, the patient is positioned supine with his or her head extending over the end of the treatment table, resting on the therapist's hip (Fig 9-8). The therapist's hands are placed to cradle the patient's head and neck with the index fingers supporting the articular pillars superior to the segment to be mobilized (Fig 9-9). Graded passive movements and stretching techniques are most effective with these techniques.

Cervical Forward Bending

The forward bending mobilization is done by lifting the head and neck straight upward with both hands. The patient's cervical spine should be flexed to about 30°. To start, the therapist's knees should be somewhat flexed. The therapist then alternately extends and flexes the knees slightly to keep the patient's head in correct position as the mobilization force is applied (Fig 9-10). The mobilizing force is applied and directed through the index fingers, but maximal hand contact is maintained with the neck and head so they are carried along with the movement. Using the proximal interphalangeal joints (PIP's), the principle contact is made with the index fingers against the articular pillars of the neck. One should be careful not to use the fingertips with these techniques as this will cause discomfort.

Cervical Backward Bending

For cervical backward bending, the patient's neck is held in a neutral, mid-range position. Then, backward bending is done in similar fashion as forward bending except that the head and the portion of the neck superior to the point of contact of the index fingers is not carried along with the movement. Rather, as the mobilizing force is applied upward by the index fingers, the head and the portion of the neck superior to the force are allowed to fall into backward bending. Thus, a backward bending force is effected to the cervical

joints superior to the contact, especially to the segment immediately superior to the contact point (Fig 9-11). This technique can also be applied successfully to the first two or three segments of the thoracic spine.

Cervical Rotation

The cervical rotation mobilization is similar to the forward bending technique described above except that it is done to only one side at a time with the head and neck held in a neutral, mid-range position. For example, to do left rotation, the PIP contact of the right hand lifts upward onto the right articular pillar while the left hand supports the head and neck. As the upward mobilizing force is initiated against the right articular pillar, the therapist will immediately sense that left rotation is occurring. The therapist should then continue to apply the mobilizing force, following the arc of rotation that is naturally occurring. The head and neck are carried along with the movement (Fig 9-12).

Cervical Sidebending

The cervical sidebending mobilization uses the same positioning as the cervical techniques previously described. The neck is held in a neutral, mid-range position. The radio-palmar surface of the index finger near the metacarpophalangeal joint (MCP) is placed against the lateral aspect of the articular pillar. The mobilization force is applied in a medial and slightly inferior direction, causing the segment below the point of contact to sidebend to the same side as the mobilizing force. The opposite hand supports the head and neck (Fig 9-13).

Cervical Side Gliding

The cervical side gliding mobilization also uses the same basic position as the cervical techniques previously described. The mobilizing force is applied in a medial direction through the index finger as it contacts the lateral aspect of the articular pillar, causing movement to occur at the segment below the contact. The point of contact on the index finger is on the palmar surface of the MCP joint. The main difference between this technique and that of cervical sidebending is that in the side gliding technique, the patient's head is carried to the side with the movement. This is accomplished by a shift of the therapist's hips in the direction of the movement (Fig 9-14). In the sidebending technique, the head and neck actually tilt as sidebending occurs around the fulcrum created by the therapist's index finger.

Most therapists agree that cervical side gliding is an easy technique to learn and it is one that is usually comfortable for the patient. Side gliding is a technique

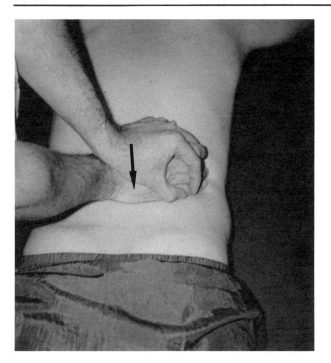

Figure 9-7. Central P/A mobilization for the lumbar spine. Using the ulnar border of the hand is more comfortable for the patient.

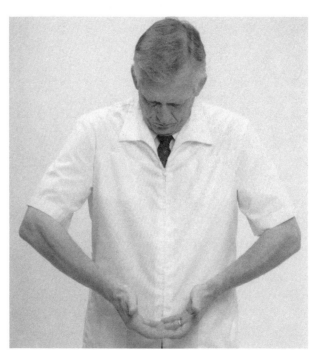

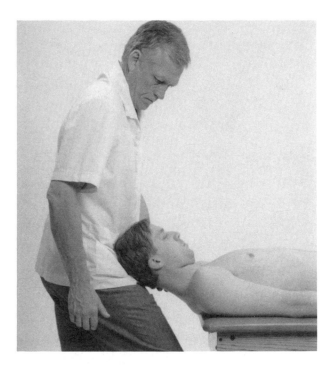

Figure 9-8. The patient's head rests against the therapist's anterior hip for cervical mobilization techniques.

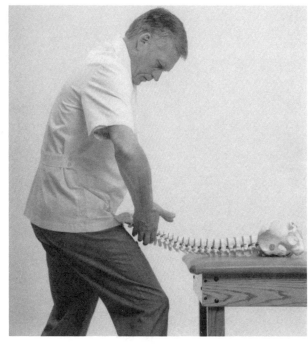

Figure 9-9. Position of the therapist's hands for cervical mobilization.

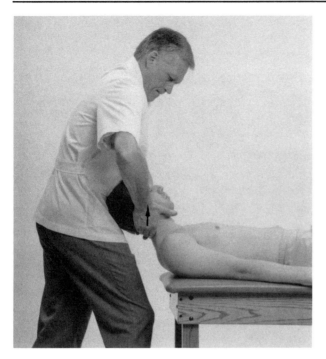

Figure 9-10. Cervical forward bending mobilization.

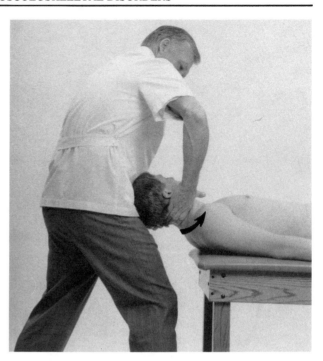

Figure 9-12. Cervical rotational mobilization.

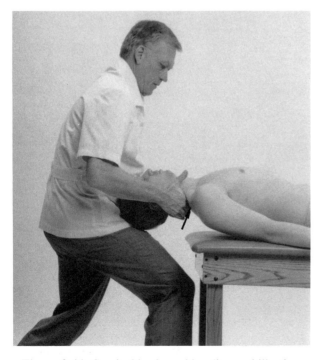

Figure 9-11. Cervical backward bending mobilization.

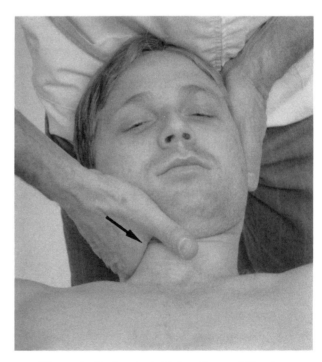

Figure 9-13. Cervical sidebending mobilization.

with which an inexperienced therapist can gain confidence. It is also a good technique to use if the patient is apprehensive or uncomfortable with the idea of having the head and neck moved passively by the therapist. This technique can be used to demonstrate to the patient that some movement can occur without discomfort.

Upper Cervical Rotation (C1-2)

When a rotational restriction of C1-2 is found, the passive mobility testing position can be used for treatment (see Chapter 4). Contract/relax or Muscle Energy Techniques (MET's) are the easiest methods of treatment. MET's are discussed in further depth near the end of this chapter.

Rotation is the major motion of C1-2. Approximately 40-45° of rotation to either side occurs at this joint. As discussed in Chapter 2, taking up range of motion (in any joint) in one plane decreases its ability to move in another plane. Therefore, by fully flexing the cervical spine, all of the joints below C1-2 are taken to end range in that plane, thus decreasing their ability to rotate.

The patient lies supine. Holding full flexion, the therapist rotates the patient's head toward the direction of restriction, taking up slack. The therapist places his or her thumbs along the patient's maxilla on either side. The patient is then asked to actively rotate in the opposite direction (Fig 9-15).

Patients often have a tendency to turn too hard. The righting reflex can be used to decrease this tendency. The patient is asked only to look with the eyes to one side or the other, gently activating suboccipital musculature. Motion is resisted by the therapist for a count of five. The patient relaxes and the head is turned further into the motion restriction or barrier. This can be repeated two or three times prior to rechecking active range of motion to determine the effect of treatment.

Manual Cervical Traction

The manual traction mobilization technique shown in Figure 9-16 may be done as a straight midline pull, or may be done in combination with passive range of motion in any plane. The radial border of the mobilizing hand makes contact with the base of the occiput, while the palmar surface supports the head. The thumb and middle finger grasp inferior to the occipital bone. The other hand cradles the chin to provide stabilization. The operator is cautioned not to apply much force through the chin. Passive range of motion of the neck may be done while traction is being applied. Movements should be carried out slowly and may be held for a few seconds as a stretching technique. Successful use of this technique will depend greatly on the therapist's ability to grip comfortably but very firmly at the base of the occiput. Manual cervical traction is helpful when used as a trial to determine the advisability of using mechanical cervical traction.

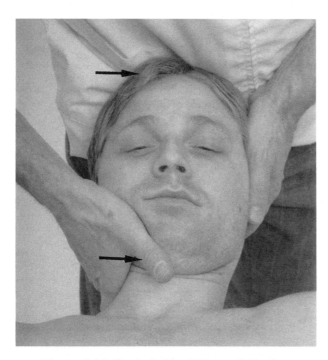

Figure 9-14. Cervical side gliding mobilization.

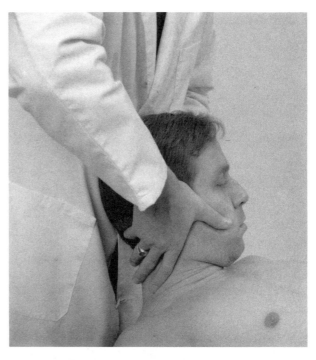

Figure 9-15. Upper cervical rotational mobilization. The cervical spine is fully flexed before upper cervical rotation is performed.

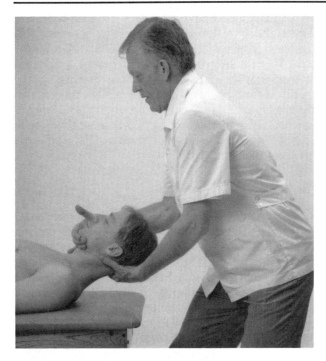

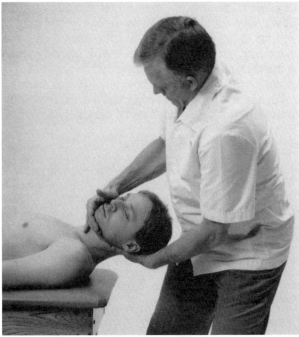

Figure 9-16. Manual cervical traction techniques. A) Traction with a straight pull; B) Traction with cervical rotation. Flexion, extension, axial extension (head back, chin in position), sidebending, or combinations of these motions can also be incorporated.

Manual Cervical Traction With a Towel

Many therapists have difficulty applying manual traction for any period of time, have a tendency to apply too much force through the mandible, or have hands too small to obtain a sufficient grip. Using a rolled towel can decrease these difficulties and make it easier to apply multidirectional mobilization along with the traction.

The example shown in Figure 9-17 is for treatment of a patient with limitation in extension, right sidebending and right rotation. The patient lies supine and the towel is placed perpendicular to the spine, below the occiput. The ends are brought together and twisted to the right. The therapist places his or her left hand distal to the towel with the thumb on the left side of the patient's neck and fingers on right side of neck, forming a "U" around the neck. The towel is used as a hand hold, or extension of the occiput.

The therapist's right hand grasps the towel from the right side, just above the forehead and perpendicular to the neck. Keeping the wrist locked in neutral, the therapist brings the elbow into the side, further twisting the towel to the right (Fig 9-18A). The towel should be held as if grasping a carton of milk rather than like shaking hands.

The therapist should be positioned so that the left arm is straight at the elbow. The right elbow is locked at the therapist's side, feet are a little more than shoulder width apart and the back is upright. Traction is applied by the therapist sitting down, not by pulling with the arms (Fig 9-18B).

Cervical flexion/extension can be added or subtracted by the therapist flexing or extending the knees. Sidebending can be added by shifting weight from one foot to the other. Rotation can be brought about by sidebending at the waist. When working on left rotation, the therapist switches hand positions so as not to be working across his or her body (right hand distal to towel around neck, towel twisted left, left elbow to the side).

Manual Cervical Traction With a Strap

A strap can also be used to obtains sufficient grip for manual cervical traction. A two inch web strap is positioned as shown in Figure 9-19. The strap crosses the therapist's shoulders and around the backs of his or her hands at the level of the middle and ring fingers. As the therapist leans back slightly, the strap tightens, ensuring a firm, yet comfortable, grip. The therapist can change the direction of pull by flexing or extending the knees or shifting weight in the same way as when using a towel for traction.

Inhibitive Cervical Manual Traction (Occipital Release)

Inhibitive manual traction is a mobilization technique that applies mild traction to the cervical

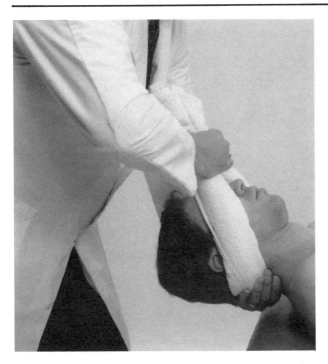

Figure 9-17. Manual cervical traction with a towel - starting position.

muscles and spine and incorporates a muscle relaxation technique through direct pressure on suboccipital muscle/tendon origins at the base of the skull. The therapist rests the back of his or her hands on the treatment table with the fingers extending upward. The patient's head is balanced on the therapist's

fingers, with the fingers contacting points just inferior to the inferior nuchal line. The balance is maintained with a slight amount of traction for up to several minutes (Fig 9-20). Often, a release or relaxation of the suboccipital muscles is felt after several seconds or minutes. This technique is often useful for relieving cervical headaches caused by tension of the suboccipital musculature.

Cervical Contract-Relax Techniques

In the cervical spine, hold-relax or contract-relax techniques are quite effective forms of mobilization. The cervical spine can be specifically positioned in a combination of the three planes of motion (flexion/extension, rotation and sidebending) to "lock" a specific segment prior to the patient exerting the muscular effort. If this is done, the techniques are more like the Muscle Energy Techniques described later in this chapter. The MET's are effective in mobilizing a specific joint. These have already been discussed in reference to the upper cervical spine.

Contract-relax or hold-relax techniques can also be more general, with the therapist positioning the patient's cervical spine toward the direction of restriction, without incorporating all three planes of motion to affect a specific segment. If the patient then exerts a muscular effort, the effect is more general to all of the soft tissues at multiple levels. Either single motions or a combination of motions can be effective. For example, if the patient lacks right rotation and

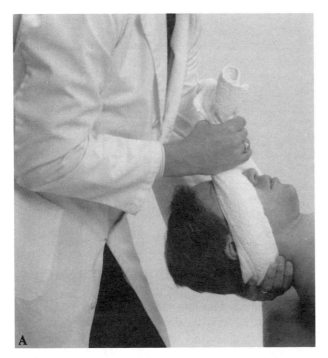

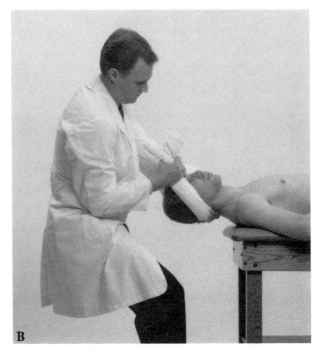

Figure 9-18. Manual cervical traction with a towel. A) The therapist brings his arm close to his side to twist the towel tight; B) Traction is applied by the therapist sitting down as shown.

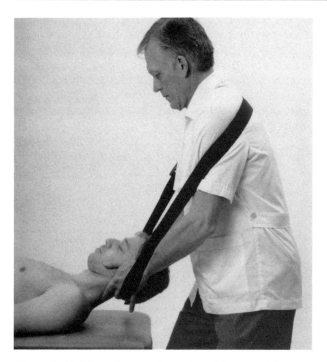

Figure 9-19. Manual cervical traction with a strap. The strap ensures the therapist retains a firm, yet comfortable grip.

extension, the patient's cervical spine can be positioned into right rotation and then extension as much as possible without recreating the symptoms. The patient then performs a gentle muscular contraction into left rotation (Fig 9-21). When the patient relaxes, the

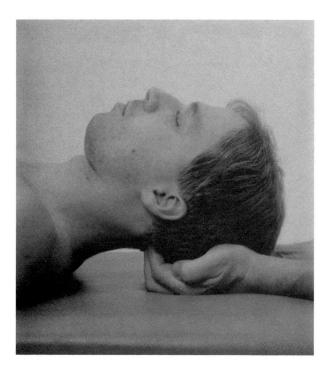

Figure 9-20. Inhibitive manual traction (occipital release).

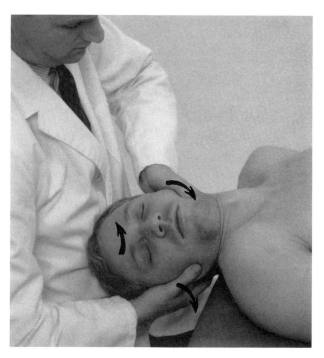

Figure 9-21. Cervical contract-relax technique. The patient shown lacks cervical right rotation and extension. The therapist positions the patient toward the motion barriers, then asks the patient to gently try to turn the head toward the left.

therapist repositions the cervical spine into more right rotation and extension as tolerated, and repeats the contraction two or three times.

Cervical Self-Mobilization Techniques

Self-mobilization of the cervical spine is done by having the patient grasp and stabilize the cervical spine as shown in Figure 9-22. The points of stabilization are the vertebrae below the segment to be mobilized. For example, if level C2-3 is to be mobilized, the patient stabilizes the C3 vertebra and does not allow movement to occur from that point inferiorly. Then, active forward and backward bending, rotation and/or sidebending are done. The greatest mobilizing force is concentrated at the level just superior to the stabilization. The patient may change the segment to be mobilized by moving the stabilization superiorly or inferiorly.

Upper Thoracic Spine and 1st Rib

Four upper thoracic mobilizations are presented in this text. One is an extension technique, two are rotational techniques and one is a sidebending technique. The techniques discussed for the 1st rib are similar to the 1st rib segmental mobility tests discussed in Chapter 4.

Upper Thoracic Extension-Sitting

An extension mobilization for the upper thoracic area can be done either by stabilizing the segment below that to be mobilized and moving the head and neck back over it or by holding the head steady and pushing the upper thoracic spine anteriorly under it.

The therapist forms a "V" with the thumb and forefinger, which is flexed at the PIP and DIP joints. The points of contact are the thumb and PIP of the forefinger on the transverse processes below the level to be mobilized. The spinous process is located in the notch of the "V." The patient is positioned at the edge of a chair and the therapist cradles the head with the chest and forearm. The therapist hugs the patient's head to the chest. The patient's nose should be in the bend of the elbow and the therapist's volar forearm cradles the opposite side of the head. The therapist's little finger cups around the patient's occiput (Fig 9-23A).

The patient's head should not be squeezed, but held gently. If the head is to be moved, this is accomplished by the therapist transferring weight, rather than pushing with the arm. The arm simply holds the patient's head to the chest.

In Figure 9-23B, the left hand stabilizes with enough force anteriorly to not allow any motion of the trunk posteriorly. The head and neck are moved back over the stabilizing hand by the therapist transferring weight from the right to left foot.

In Figure 9-23C, the head is held steady with the contact hand pushing in an anterior direction so that the trunk moves under the head and neck. Work on postural awareness can be added to this technique. The patient is asked to actively make a lumbar lordosis

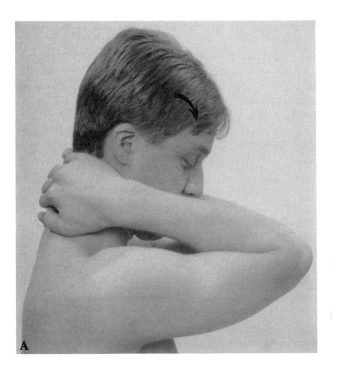

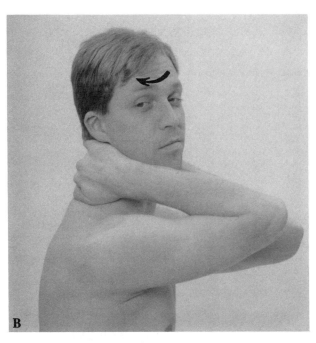

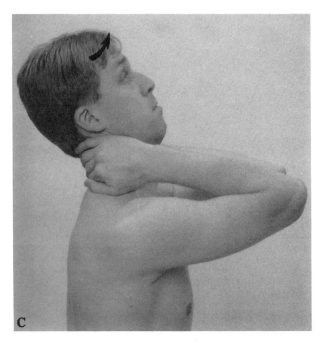

Figure 9-22. Cervical self-mobilization. A) Upper cervical flexion to stretch the suboccipital muscles; B) Upper cervical rotation; C) Mid-cervical extension.

while the head is held stationary. Thus, the patient gets an idea of the effect of improved sitting posture and actively helps the therapist so that less anterior force is required with the contact hand.

Slight distraction can be added to either technique, simply by the therapist standing up slightly or extending the knees.

Upper Thoracic Rotation-Prone

The rotational technique shown in Figure 9-24 may be done either with the patient prone with pillows under his or her chest or with the patient seated resting his or her head and arms forward on a treatment table. A 3-D mobilization table can be used instead of pillows under the chest. Lateral pressure in opposite directions is applied to the spinous processes at two adjacent levels. The inferior segment, or base, is the segment stabilized, with the mobilizing force applied to the spinous process of the superior segment. This spinous process is moved in the opposite direction of the rotational movement desired (the spinous process moving right imparts left rotation into the segment). Graded passive movements (articulations) and stretches can be used with this technique. Thumb contacts are effective when mild or moderate specific mobilization is desired. However, thumb contacts are sometimes uncomfortable if strong pressure is exerted because of the small contact area of the thumbs. Therefore, pisiform (mobilizing) and thenar eminence (stabilizing) contacts are more effective if vigorous mobilization is desired. For maximum effect the patient's head should be turned in the same direction as the desired mobilization.

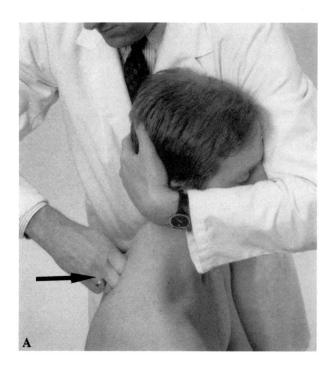

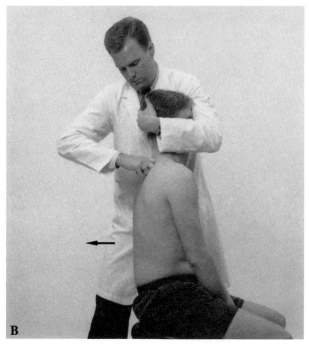

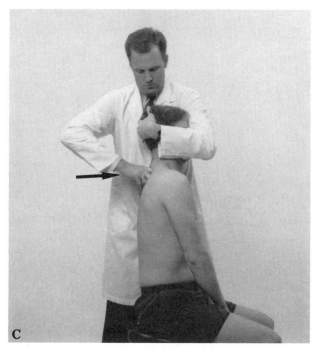

Figure 9-23. Upper thoracic extension technique. A) Starting position; B) The therapist pushes the head and neck posteriorly by transferring his weight from the left to right foot, while stabilizing firmly with the right hand; C) An alternate technique. The therapist stabilizes the head with the right arm while pushing the upper thoracic spine anteriorly with the left hand.

Upper Thoracic Rotation-Sitting

Figure 9-25 shows another upper thoracic rotational mobilization. When the head and neck are rotated, the spinous processes move in the direction opposite to the movement. For example, as the head and neck are rotated to the left, each spinous process

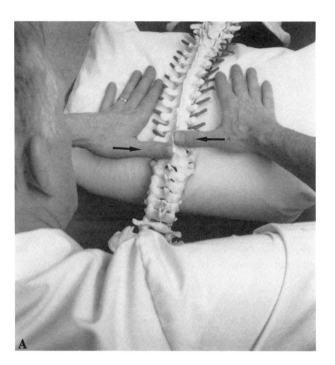

is observed to move to the right on its base. If a specific segment is manually blocked from moving, the rotational movement is prevented from occurring below that point and a greater rotational force can be directed to the segment above the point of stabilization. Such a technique is done with the patient sitting and with the therapist's hands positioned as shown in Figure 9-25. The thumb is held against the lateral aspect of the spinous process to stabilize while the opposite hand rotates the patient's head and neck to the opposite side to take up slack. The mobilizing force is then directed through the thumb. Graded passive movements and stretches can be used with this technique.

Upper Thoracic Sidebending-Sitting

The sidebending mobilization technique for the upper thoracic spine is similar to the rotational technique discussed above. With the patient seated, the therapist sidebends the head and neck while blocking movement of the spinous process at the selected level with his or her thumb (Fig 9-26). Normally the spinous processes move in the same direction as the movement being performed. The thumb prevents this movement from the point of stabilization inferiorly and directs an increased sidebending force to the segment above the point of stabilization. This technique should be done in three distinct steps as follows: 1) Stabilize with the thumb;

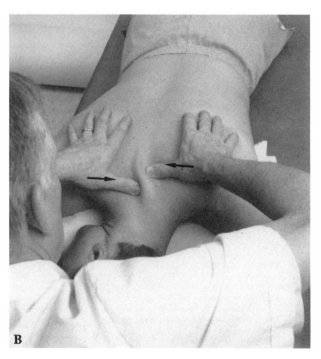
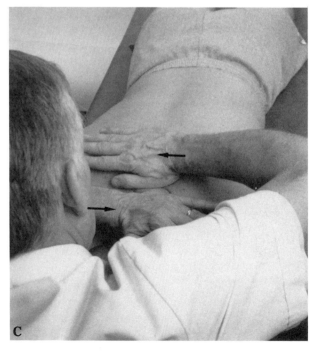

Figure 9-24. Upper thoracic right rotation technique. A) Contact positions for the thumbs; B) The inferior thumb stabilizes as the superior thumb directs a lateral force against the spinous process; C) A contact using the pisiform and thenar eminence is often more comfortable for the patient and therapist.

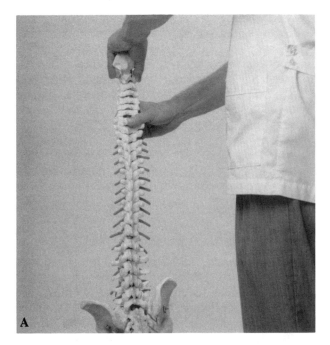
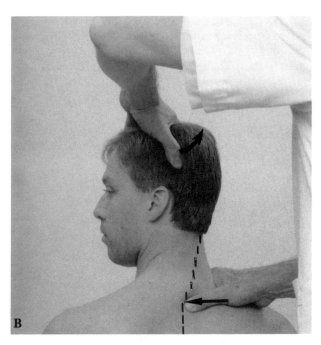

Figure 9-25. Upper thoracic left rotation technique. A) The thumb stabilizes laterally against the inferior spinous process; B) The patient's head is rotated to the left to take up slack, then the mobilization force is directed through the thumb.

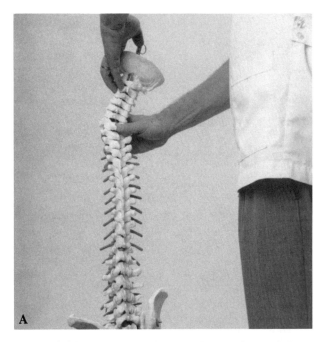
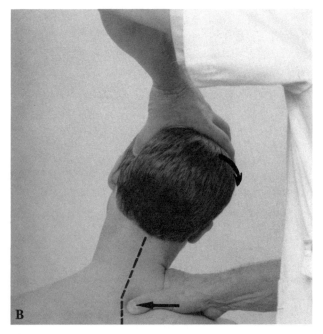

Figure 9-26. Upper thoracic right sidebending technique. A) The thumb stabilizes laterally against the inferior spinous process; B) The patient's head is sidebent right to take up slack, then the mobilization force is directed through the thumb.

2) Take up slack by passively sidebending the head and neck; and 3) Mobilize with the thumb. Graded passive movements and stretches can be used with this technique.

The two previous techniques can be modified by changing the hand hold on the patient's head to one in which the therapist cradles the patient's head in his or her arm and against the chest (Fig 9-27). This affords more head control and enables greater force to be applied. Sidebending in one direction with rotation in the opposite direction may be combined to increase the effectiveness of these techniques. An obvious disadvantage to this technique is that an uncomfortable stress may be applied to the cervical spine as the slack is taken up. If this occurs, the technique shown in Figure 9-25 or 9-26 should be substituted.

Caudal Glide of the 1st Rib-Prone

Caudal glide of the 1st rib is described here with the patient lying prone, although the techniques can also be done in sitting or supine. In prone, the therapist palpates the 1st rib by placing a thumb underneath (anterior to) the muscle belly of the upper trapezius right next to the cervical spine. A caudally-directed pressure is applied (Fig 9-28A). The first firm resistance felt caudally will be the 1st rib. The therapist then applies pressure onto the 1st rib. Either a prolonged stretch or the graded articulation mobilizations can be performed. The mobilization can be fine-tuned by changing the placement of the thumb slightly and applying the mobilization force in a slightly more anterior-caudal or posterior-caudal direction as desired.

A more general technique involves the therapist placing the web space of the hand over the upper trapezius with the thumb anterior and the fingers posterior. A caudal force can then be applied (Fig 9-28B).

With either of the above techniques, the patient's neck can be positioned in sidebending toward the side of mobilization to put the anterior and middle scalenes on slack, or away from the side of mobilization to put the scalenes on stretch. The therapist can also ask the patient to inhale deeply, as the therapist resists the pump handle motion of the 1st rib during inhalation. As the patient exhales, the therapist can follow the rib inferiorly to take up the slack. Either a prolonged stretch or oscillation can be performed or the deep breath can be repeated as desired.

Mid and Lower Thoracic Spine

Five techniques appropriate for the mid and lower thoracic spine are shown here. One is for forward bending, two are rotational techniques, one is for backward bending and one is a traction/backward bending technique.

Thoracic Forward Bending-Prone

The forward bending technique is shown in Figure 9-29. The patient's thoracic spine is flexed over a pillow or bolster, or a 3-D table is used. When anterior pressure is directed to the transverse processes of a thoracic vertebra, it causes that vertebra to forward bend on the vertebra inferior to it. Such a force may be imparted by the hypothenar eminence of one hand, through the fingertips placed over the transverse processes of a segment. The pisiform bones may also be used as contacts, and many clinicians prefer this technique (Fig 9-30 A&B). The transverse processes are located approximately one level higher than the spinous processes of their corresponding segments. The transverse processes can only be palpated indirectly so their approximate position must be determined in relation to the spinous processes. Thus, the transverse processes of a vertebra can be found at one level higher and approximately one inch lateral to the midline. Graded passive movements, stretches and thrusts may be used with these techniques.

Thoracic Rotation-Prone

The forward bending techniques just described can be modified to produce rotation by placing the fingertip contacts on the transverse processes at <u>adjacent</u> levels. The rotation produced is in the direction of the more inferiorly placed contact. This technique is shown in Figure 9-31. If a more forceful mobilization is required, this technique can be modified using pisiform contacts as shown in Figure 9-30 C&D.

Thoracic Rotation-Supine

The rotational technique shown in Figure 9-32 also uses contact with the transverse processes at two adjacent levels. In this technique, the therapist makes a fist and places it so that the thenar eminence makes transverse process contact on one side while the flat surfaces of the middle phalanges (knuckles) make transverse process contact at the opposite adjacent level. The spinous processes lie in the hollow created between the fingers and the thenar eminence. This contact is maintained as the therapist applies a mobilizing thrust through the patient's arms and chest as he or she rolls the patient over the fulcrum produced by the fisted hand. Rotation is in the direction of the thenar eminence. This technique can be modified to cause an extension mobilization by rotating the hand so that the thenar eminence and knuckle contacts are at the same vertebral level.

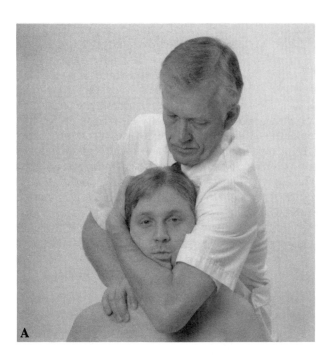

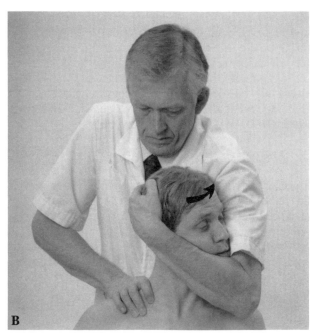

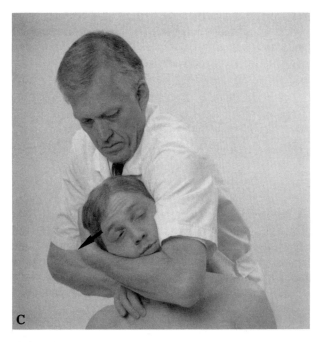

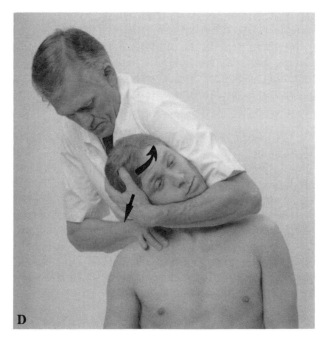

Figure 9-27. Upper thoracic rotation and sidebending techniques using an alternate stabilization method. A) The therapist's thumb still stabilizes, but by cradling the patient's head, the therapist has greater control over cervical movements; B) Rotation; C) Sidebending; D) Sidebending and rotation combined.

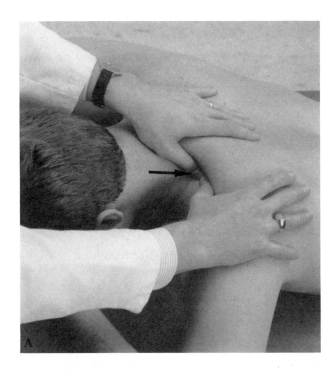
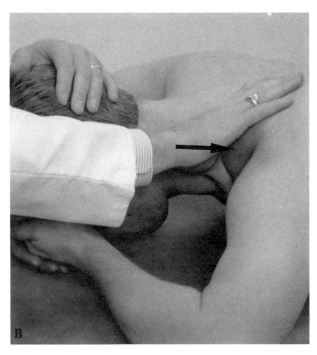

Figure 9-28. Caudal glide of the 1st rib in prone. A) The thumb is placed anterior to the upper trapezius muscle belly and a caudally-directed pressure is applied. The first firm resistance felt is the 1st rib; B) Alternate technique using the web space of the hand.

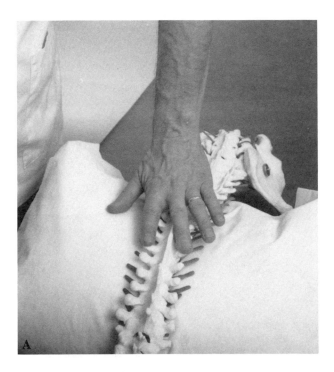
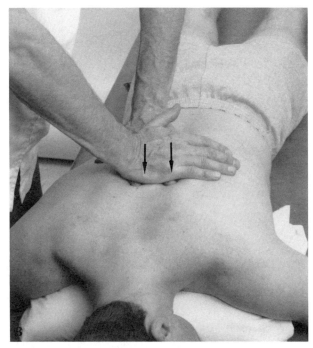

Figure 9-29. Thoracic forward bending mobilization. A) Finger and hand placement on the transverse processes; B) Anterior pressure directed by the opposite hand.

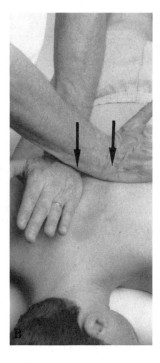

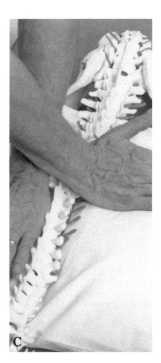

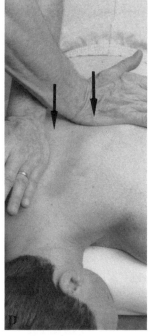

Figure 9-30. A&B) Thoracic forward bending mobilization using pisiform contacts; C&D)Left thoracic rotation mobilization using pisiform contacts. Note the rotation mobilization contacts are on adjacent transverse processes, while the forward bending mobilization contacts are on parallel transverse processes.

Thoracic Backward Bending

A backward bending mobilization force can be given by direct pressure on a spinous process with a pisiform contact as shown in Figure 9-33. For a more specific effect, the patient should be positioned in thoracic extension with pillows, a bolster or a 3-D table. The mobilization occurs at the segment inferior to the spinous process being contacted. Therefore, it is important to avoid contact with the segment below the pisiform contact so that it remains free to move. The therapist can ensure correct technique by making sure that the thumb of the contact hand is pointing toward the patient's head. That way, the segment below is free to move. Graded passive movements, stretches and thrusts can be used with this technique.

Thoracic Backward Bending/Traction

A traction-backward bending technique is shown in Figure 9-34. A rolled bath towel or pillow stabilizes the level above the segment to be mobilized. Depending upon the level being mobilized and the height of the therapist and the patient, it may be necessary for the therapist to stand on a stool or platform to obtain the correct position. The patient holds his or her arms crossed with the hands on opposite shoulders. The therapist reaches around the patient with both arms and grasps the patient's elbows and lifts upward and slightly backward. The amount of backward bending can be varied. The technique is often effective when

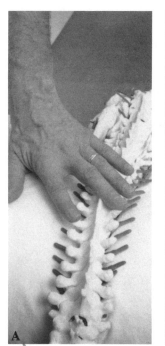

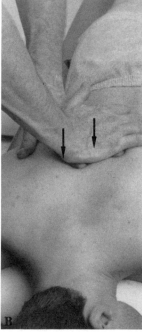

Figure 9-31. Thoracic left rotation mobilization. A) Finger placement on adjacent transverse processes; B) Anterior pressure directed by the opposite hand.

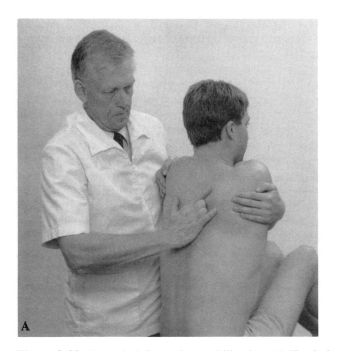

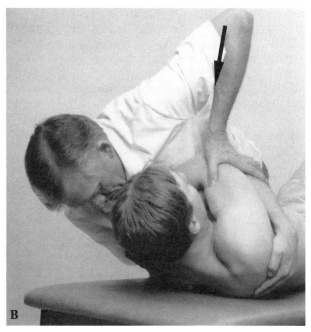

Figure 9-32. Thoracic left rotation mobilization. A) Hand placement on transverse processes; B) As the patient lies down over the fulcrum, the therapist directs a posterior thrust.

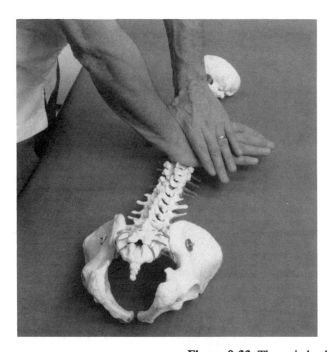

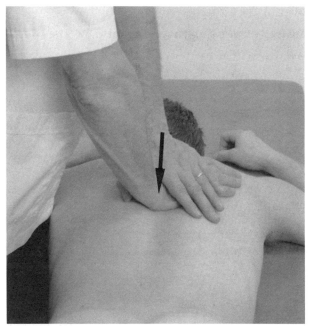

Figure 9-33. Thoracic backward bending mobilization.

done as a slow stretch and may involve a thrust at the end of the stretch. The thrust can be done by the therapist raising on his or her tiptoes then dropping suddenly onto the heels. The patient's weight is totally or partially supported by the therapist. This technique can also be done with the patient sitting on a stool. Mennell describes an alternate technique that involves the therapist standing back to back with the patient to effect the mobilization at the lumbar level. In this instance, the therapist's hip acts as a fulcrum as the patient is lifted into extension with traction.[11]

Ribs

P/A Glides-Prone

The rib mobilization shown in Figure 9-35 is done with the patient lying prone with pillows under the chest. The transverse processes are stabilized with the hypothenar eminence placed parallel to the spine on the opposite side of the rib to be mobilized. The therapist's forearms are crossed and the mobilization force is directed anteriorly and laterally through the hypothenar eminence that is contacting the posteromedial aspect of the rib. Graded passive movements, stretches or thrusts may be used with this technique. Working with the patient's breathing can also augment the mobilization. The therapist can resist rib movement during inhalation and/or can follow the rib anteriorly and perform an oscillation, a thrust or a prolonged stretch at end range during exhalation.

Lumbar Spine

Seven basic techniques for the lumbar spine are presented. Four are rotational techniques, one is an extension technique, one is a sidebending technique and one involves sidebending and may also incorporate rotation. The thoracic backward bending techniques shown in Figures 9-33 and 9-34 are also effective mobilization techniques for the lumbar spine.

Lumbar Backward Bending-Prone

Lumbar extension mobilizations are performed with the patient lying prone. A 3-D mobilization table, pillows or the "elbow prop" position can be used to pre-position the patient into varying degrees of extension, depending upon the amount of force desired. The therapist uses a pisiform contact to apply pressure in an anterior direction to the lumbar spinous process (Fig 9-36). The mobilization occurs at the segment inferior to the spinous process being contacted. Therefore, it is important to avoid contact with the segment below the pisiform contact so that it remains free to move. The therapist can ensure correct technique by making sure that the thumb of the contact hand is pointing toward the patient's head. Graded passive movements, stretches and thrusts can be used with this technique.

Lumbar Rotation-Prone

The rotational technique shown in Figure 9-37 is performed with the patient lying prone. The lateral aspect of the MCP joint of the thumb is used to stabilize the lateral aspect of the selected spinous process. The thenar eminence and heel of the hand also stabilize along the lateral aspect of the spinous processes superior to the MCP stabilization. The therapist's other hand grasps the anterior rim of the ilium of the side opposite the stabilization and lifts upward and medially to take up the slack. The mobilizing force is then given with the hand that is stabilizing against the lateral aspect of the spinous processes. This technique is specific to the L5-S1 segment if the L5 vertebra is being mobilized. Although this technique becomes less specific as the mobilization force moves superiorly, the greatest mobilizing force is always directed to the segment just inferior to the contact point of the MCP joint of the thumb. For example, if the third lumbar spinous process is contacted, the mobilization force is directed to the three segments between L3 and S1 with the L3-4 segment receiving the greatest force. Graded passive movements and stretches are effective with this technique. Thrusting is usually not used with this technique. This technique can also be effective in the lower and mid-thoracic spine. It is most effective when done in three distinct steps: 1) Stabilize against spinous processes; 2) Take up slack by rotating the pelvis; and 3) Mobilize with the hand that is stabilizing against the spinous processes.

A 3-D table enhances the effectiveness of this technique. For maximum effect, the therapist should use the table to rotate the spine in the opposite direction before stabilizing. This way the therapist is in better control and has greater range in which to take up slack. This technique can be combined with the sidebending technique shown in Figure 9-41. If the patient is in neutral flexion/extension, the rotation and sidebending should be in opposite directions. If the patient is positioned in flexion or extension, the rotation and sidebending should be in the same direction, following Fryette's Laws of Spinal Motion.

Lumbar Rotation-Prone

The rotational technique shown in Figure 9-38 is also done with the patient lying prone. The mobilizing force is directed on the transverse process with a pisiform/hypothenar eminence contact. The transverse

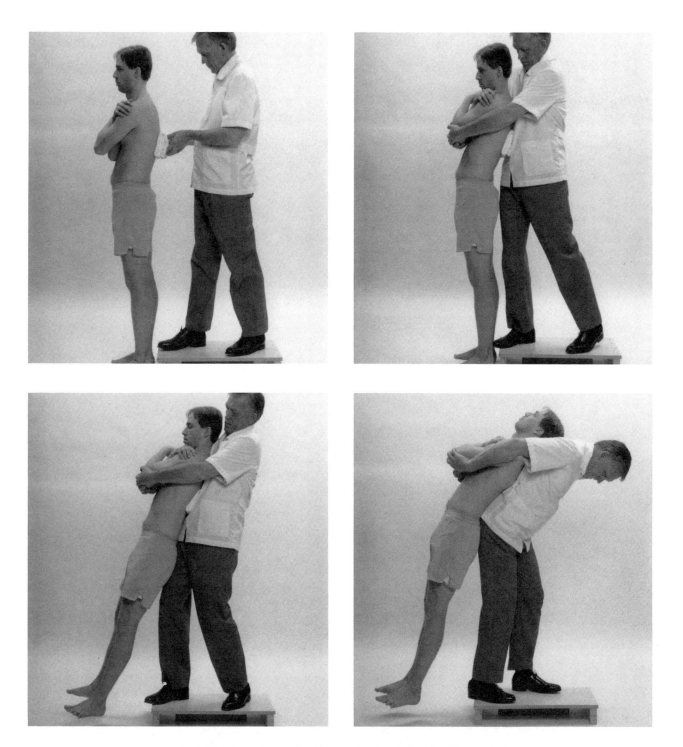

Figure 9-34. Thoracic and lumbar traction/backward bending technique.

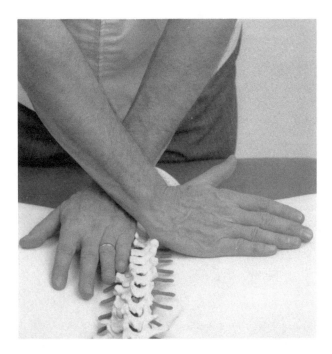
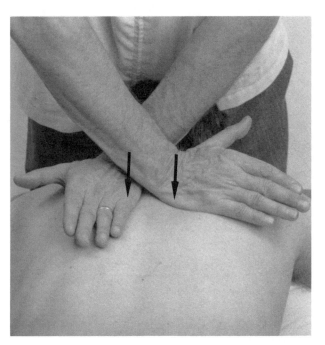

Figure 9-35. Rib mobilization.

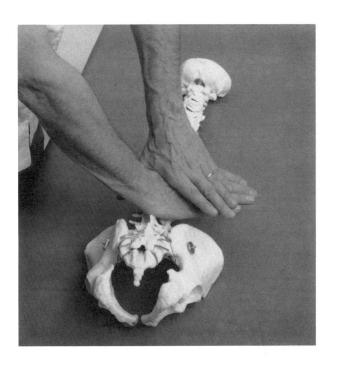
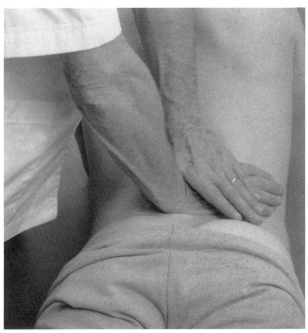

Figure 9-36. Lumbar backward bending mobilization.

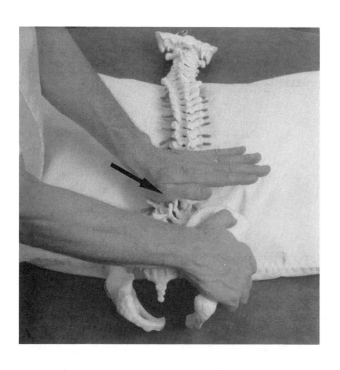
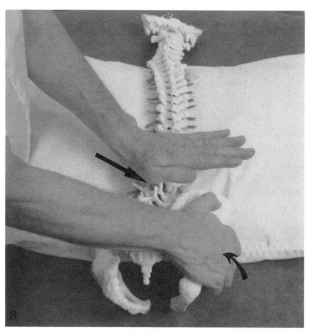
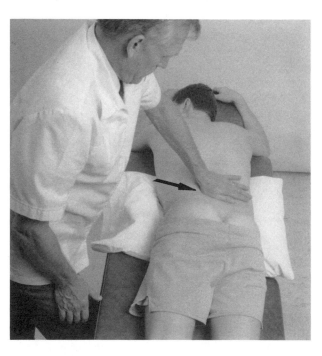
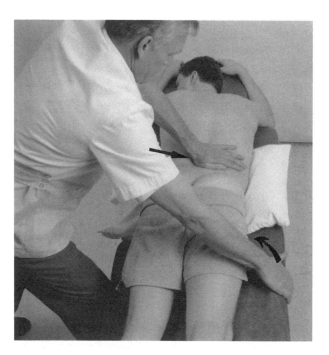

Figure 9-37. Lumbar left rotation mobilization. A) The left hand stabilizes against the spinous process; B) The right hand takes up slack by pulling the ilium posteriorly, then the mobilizing force is applied with the left hand; C) Alternate technique: the table is pre-positioned in right rotation; D) The therapist moves the table to take up the slack before mobilizing.

process of L1 is smaller and partially shielded by the 12th rib and the L5 transverse process is usually shielded by the iliac crest. Therefore, hand placements for L2, 3 and 4 are shown as only these transverse processes are prominent enough to be contacted by the hypothenar eminence. The transverse processes can only be palpated indirectly through soft tissue, therefore the contact is sometimes only approximate to the level desired. This technique is thus semi-specific to the level described and may be used when general hypomobility is present rather than hypomobility at one specific level. Each transverse process is contacted

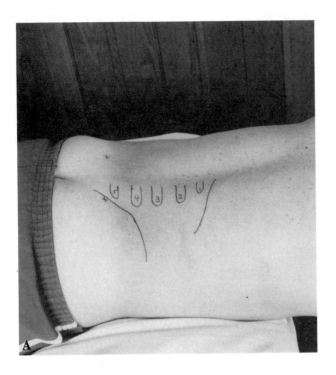

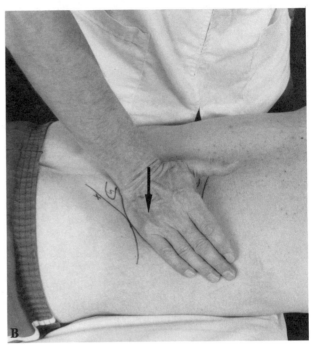

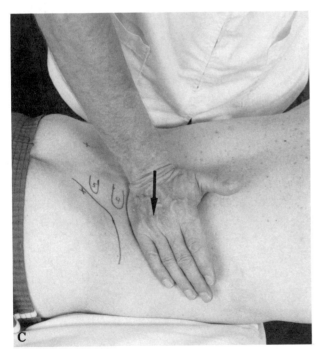

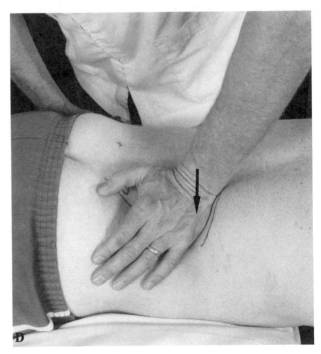

Figure 9-38. Lumbar left rotation mobilization. A pisiform contact is used to direct force anteriorly onto the transverse process. A) Approximate locations of the transverse processes; B) Contact on the L4 transverse process; C) Contact on the L3 transverse process; D) Contact on the L2 transverse process.

by placing the hypothenar eminence perpendicular to the spine. The L4 transverse process is slightly medial and superior to the posterior rim of the iliac crest. The L2 transverse process is found slightly inferior to the 12th rib. The L3 transverse process is midway between the L2 and L4 contacts. The pisiform contact should always be as close to the spinous process as possible with the mobilizing force directed posteroanteriorly. This causes the vertebra to rotate on its base. For example, when the L4 transverse process is the contact, the L4-5 segment receives most of the mobilization force. If the contact is on the left side, the direction of the mobilization is right rotation. Graded passive movements and stretches are effective with this technique and it is an especially useful technique when gentle, semi-specific mobilization is indicated.

Lumbar Rotation-Supine

The rotational technique shown in Figure 9-39 is a semi-specific technique that can be effective in the mid and lower thoracic spine and in the lumbar spine. It can also be used as an effective self-mobilization or home treatment technique. The patient lies supine with the knees and hips flexed as the pelvis is rotated. The degree of knee and hip flexion determines the general level of spinal mobilization. If the knees and hips are flexed completely to the chest, the mobilization is directed into the mid-thoracic spine. As the amount of flexion is decreased, the level of the mobilization moves lower into the thoracic and the lumbar spine. If

the patient's lower rib cage is stabilized, the mobilization becomes specific to the lumbar spine.

Graded passive movements and stretching techniques are most effective with this technique. Gentle hold-relax and contract-relax muscle stretches are also effective.

Lumbar Rotation-Supine "Lumbar Roll"

The rotational technique shown in Figure 9-40 is the classic "lumbar roll" mobilization that can be effective for articulation, stretch and manipulation. It is a specific technique in that it can be isolated to one segment and uses principles of ligamentous locking and facet apposition to gain specificity. The patient is positioned on the side opposite the desired direction of mobilization. The therapist faces the patient and places

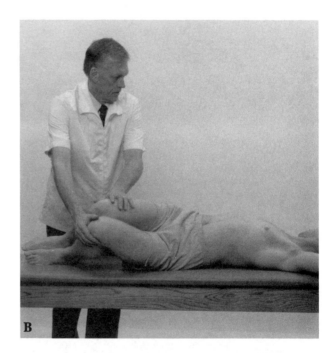

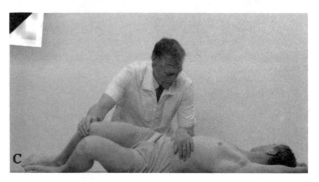

Figure 9-39. Rotation techniques. A) Mid and lower thoracic mobilization; B) Lumbar mobilization; C) Lumbar mobilization with added stabilization across the lower ribs.

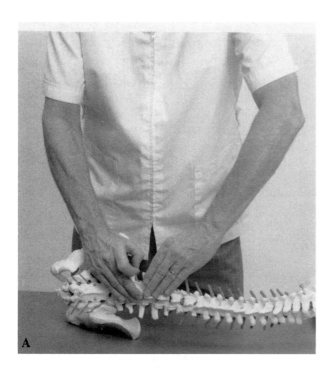

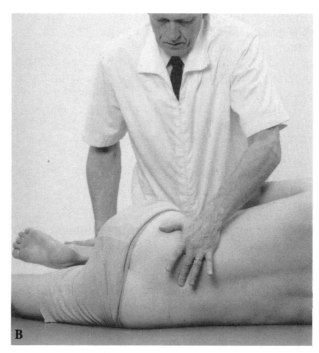

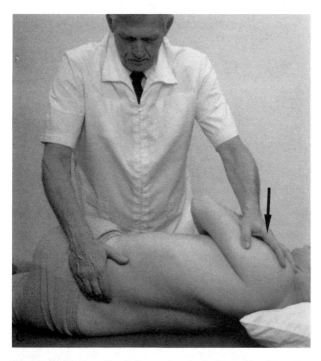

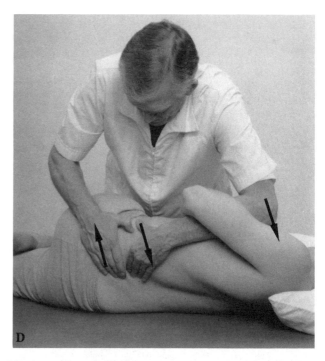

Figure 9-40. Lumbar left rotation technique - the "Lumbar Roll." A) Position of palpating hands. B) Flexion of the lumbar spine by flexing the patient's hip until the therapist feels the inferior segment move; C) Rotation of the patient's spine until the therapist feels the superior segment move; D) Force is imparted by rotating the lower segments toward and the upper segments away from the therapist.

the cephalad hand over the patient and palpates between spinous processes at the desired level for mobilization. With the caudal hand, the therapist gains a secure hold on the lower portion of the patient's top leg. He then imparts passive flexion to the lumbar spine by flexing the patient's hip and knee using his or her own hip as a balance point for the patient's knee. The therapist is actually shifting his or her pelvis to move the patient's lower body. With the palpating hand, the therapist feels for flexion to occur at the desired segment. When the therapist feels the inferior spinous process begin to move, he or she stops and lowers the leg to the table, "locking" the spine in flexion at that point. The therapist then imparts rotation down to the segment by rotating the trunk. This is done by pulling the patient's inferior arm toward the therapist and/or pressing the superior shoulder backward. Rotation is stopped when movement is palpated at the superior spinous process of the desired segment. In effect, this "locking" of the lower segments in flexion and upper segments in rotation causes the mobilizing force to be focused at the one desired level. The actual mobilization is accomplished by rotating the pelvis and lower segments in a direction toward the therapist and the shoulder and upper segments in a direction away from the therapist. Some of the mobilizing force is directed through the therapist's forearms to the patient's pelvis and shoulder, but it is important to concentrate as much force in the fingers as possible when doing this mobilization, to keep the lever arm as short as possible. The fingers are moved to the lateral aspects of the spinous processes to produce the rotational force. The fingers in contact with the inferior spinous process are on its lateral aspect closest to the table. The fingers in contact with the superior spinous process are on its lateral aspect on the top side. The therapist pulls the pelvis and inferior spinous process toward him- or herself and pushes the superior spinous process and shoulder away. The thumb may be used instead of the fingers for the superior contact.

Lumbar Sidebending-Prone

The sidebending technique shown in Figure 9-41 is done with the patient lying prone. As the hip is abducted, the lumbar spine sidebends. If a stabilizing force is placed against the lateral aspect of the spinous process, sidebending is prevented from that point superiorly. The lateral aspect of the MCP joint of the thumb is used to stabilize the lateral aspect of the selected spinous process in exactly the same way as the rotation technique shown in Figure 9-37. The technique is done in three steps: 1) The lateral aspect of the MCP joint, the thenar eminence and the heel of the hand are used to <u>stabilize</u> along the lateral aspect of the spinous processes; 2) The hip is abducted to <u>take up slack</u>; and 3) The therapist applies force against the

spinous processes to <u>mobilize</u>. This technique concentrates the greatest sidebending force at the segment just inferior to the point of contact of the MCP joint. If the patient is large or if vigorous mobilization is necessary, it may be necessary to use one therapist to stabilize and mobilize and an assistant to maintain abduction of the patient's leg. If both legs are carried along in the desired direction, more force can be imparted. This is accomplished easily with the use of a 3-D mobilization table.

For maximum effect using a 3-D table, the therapist should use the table to sidebend the spine in the opposite direction before stabilizing. This way the therapist is in better control and has greater range in which to take up slack. This technique can be combined with the rotation technique shown in Figure 9-37. To be effective, the patient must be positioned in flexion or extension and the rotation and sidebending must be in the same direction, following Fryette's Laws of Spinal Motion.

Lumbar Sidebending/Rotation - Sidelying Positional Stretch or Unilateral Traction

The sidelying positional stretch is a mobilization technique that involves sidebending and may also incorporate rotation (Fig 9-42). The patient is positioned on his or her side over a six to eight inch roll. The roll is positioned between the crest of the ilium and rib cage to achieve the maximum amount of sidebending at a specific area. As the spine bends over the roll, the facet joints are separated and the muscles and ligaments are stretched on the superior side. If the pelvis is allowed to roll forward and the shoulder backward, a rotational component is added and even more separation and stretching is achieved. Even more stretch can be obtained if the patient's top leg is allowed to hang over the edge of the treatment table.

Because this technique opens the neural foramen on the superior side, it can be thought of as a type of unilateral traction to the superior joints. Therefore, it can be used for nerve root impingement problems and for joint hypomobility and muscular tightness. When used for nerve root impingement, one must distinguish between an impingement arising from a disc protrusion with a lateral shift and an impingement caused by narrowing, thickening, osteophyte formation (lateral spinal stenosis) or a disc fragment in the intervertebral foramen. In the latter instance, the patient should be placed with the side of the impingement up. In the former instance, the treatment goal is to correct the lateral shift. This would be accomplished by placing the patient on the side of pathology. This technique to correct a lateral shift should be done only if centralization of the patient's symptoms occurs (see discussion of HNP in Chapter 5, <u>Treatment of the</u> <u>Spine by Diagnosis</u>). Positional stretches are usually done up to a maximum of ten minutes. They are also effective for home or self-treatment.

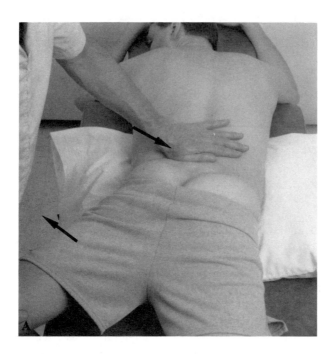

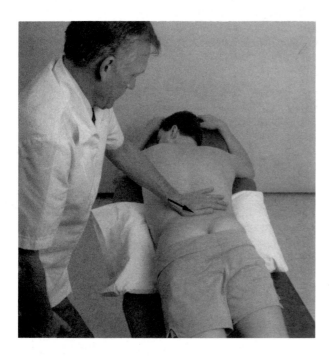 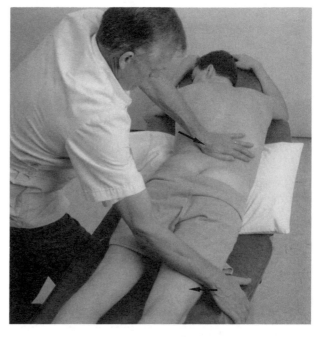

Figure 9-41. Lumbar left sidebending technique. A) The left hand stabilizes; the hip is abducted to take up slack before mobilization, then the mobilizing force is applied with the left hand; B) Alternate technique: the table is pre-positioned in right sidebending; C) The therapist moves the table back to the left to take up slack before mobilizing

Coccyx

If the coccyx is found to be positioned in extension, mobilization can be an effective form or treatment (Fig 9-43). The mobilization is performed with the patient prone over one or two pillows under the pelvis. The mobilization is done with the index finger inserted internally into the rectum and the thumb placed externally to grasp the coccyx. A-P glides and traction can both be effective.

Muscle Energy Techniques - An Osteopathic Treatment Approach

General Principles

Muscle Energy Techniques (MET) for joint mobilization are becoming quite popular among certain physical therapists who have advanced skills in mobilization. MET's have been developed primarily by osteopathic physicians, most notably Drs. Fred Mitchell Sr. and Jr. For sake of completeness, a brief description of the principles on which these techniques are based follows. As these techniques can be quite complicated without first-hand instruction, they are considered to be beyond the scope of this basic text

and are introduced to stimulate the reader into pursuing higher level skills.

The mobilization techniques discussed up to this point are primarily passive in nature; they require specific positioning of the patient and his or her relaxation. The forces imparted by the therapist may then be directed either into the restriction or away from it to gain joint mobility and/or stretch soft tissue. Thrust and oscillation techniques are passive in nature.

Muscle Energy Techniques, on the other hand, are active in nature. MET's may be likened to PNF contract-relax techniques except that they employ submaximal rather than maximal contractions. In fact, these techniques may be isotonic (where the counterforce is less than the force of the patient's muscular contraction, producing motion into or toward the motion barrier); isometric (where the counterforce meets the force of the patient's muscular contraction, producing no joint motion); and isokinetic (where the counterforce increases during contraction to meet changing contraction forces as the muscle shortens and its force increases[12]). Generally, MET's for joint mobilization are gentle, isometric contractions as opposed to maximal isometric contractions that tend to tighten and compress the joints. MET's employing hard maximal contractions are useful for loosening tight muscles and fascia, however. The safe and effective use of MET's depends upon a thorough understanding of the osteopathic evaluation schemes described by Mitchell, Moran and Pruzzo, by Phillip Greenman and by others.[4,8,12] The discussion included in this text is only a summary of the comprehensive explanations contained in their works, and is intended to be an introduction to some of the concepts we teach. The basic concepts for the employment of MET's may be summarized as follows:

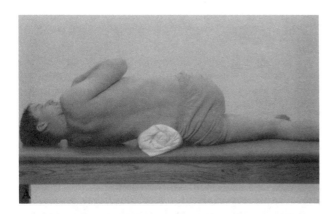
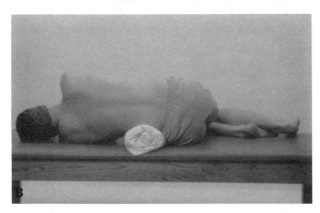

Figure 9-42. Positional stretch. A) Left sidebending; B) Left sidebending and right rotation.

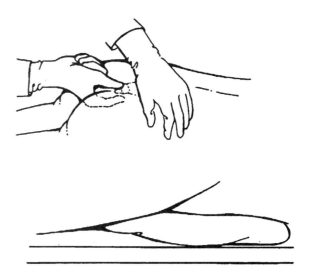

Figure 9-43. Position for coccyx mobilization.

After a positional and motion assessment of the spinal segments in question has been done, the patient is placed in a position corresponding to and facilitating the impartation of motion. The patient is then stabilized and the slack at the particular spinal segment is taken up in all three planes. The patient is then asked to perform a submaximal isometric contraction against a counterforce in a direction that will produce the desired effect. These techniques are particularly safe and gentle, especially in the upper cervical spine where risk of vertebral artery compromise is present with thrust and rotatory techniques.

Manual therapy techniques for the spine are usually taught to the beginner via assessment through the spinous processes because they are easily palpated. Problems sometimes arise using this method when one is trying to determine whether a joint dysfunction is on the left or right side. For example, palpating the T5 spinous process to be offset to the left of T6 determines only that the vertebral body may be rotated to the right. By palpating between the spinous processes, one might detect that two adjacent spinous processes are closer together than the spinous processes of two other adjacent segments. Does this mean that the superior element is backward bent or that the inferior element is forward bent? To clarify this problem, osteopaths indirectly palpate the transverse processes through fascial planes to determine the exact position of the facets as well as their ability to move in all three planes of motion. Thus, the lesion can be precisely defined and a treatment maneuver prescribed that exactly corresponds to the dysfunction. The basic principles governing the use of MET's are outlined as follows:

1. Motion Barriers - Normal joints all have physiological barriers to motion at opposite ends of their ranges of motion. These barriers are produced by the protective resiliency and elasticity of the soft tissues. Any other factor impeding the free motion of the joint between these range limits is considered to be pathological. In the normal spine, both in backward and forward bending, the facets at each segment should glide symmetrically in superior and inferior directions (open and close). This means that in flexion, the facets on each side should fully open and in extension the facets should fully close (Fig 9-44).

2. Positioning - Motion takes place in all three planes simultaneously. Positioning of patients for both active and passive techniques should account for motion in all planes. Fryette's Third Law of Spinal Motion applies here in that if motion is introduced into a segment in any plane, motion in the other planes is reduced. This means, for example, that if a spinal segment is positioned in extension, the available range for sidebending and rotation is reduced. If the segment is positioned in both extension and sidebending, the available range for rotation is even further reduced.[12]

3. Diagnosis and Treatment - Diagnosis and treatment by MET is based on the dysfunctional position of the segment and the motion restriction. The motion restriction is the opposite of the dysfunctional position. For example, a segment that is restricted in extension, right rotation and right sidebending (motion restriction) is said to be flexed, left rotated and left sidebent (dysfunctional position). Lesioned segments are named by their dysfunctional positions. A segment that is flexed, right rotated and right sidebent is called an FRS_R.

Two Lesions That Appear Similar But Are Very Different

Figure 9-45 shows two figures that appear to represent identical lumbar facet lesions. However, functionally and from an osteopathic treatment aspect, they are very dissimilar. In Figure 9-45A, the left facet will not close. This has been determined because during backward bending, the transverse process on the right becomes more prominent and during forward bending, the transverse processes become more equal. Positionally, the lesion is described as flexed, right sidebent, and right rotated (FRS_R). Its motion restriction will be in extension, left sidebending and left rotation.

Conceptually, by having the patient perform the motions of backward bending and forward bending in the above example and by palpating the change in position of the transverse processes, the following deductive thought process might occur: Since the left facet will not close, this means that the right facet is already in an extended (closed) position. Having the patient actively recruit extension of the entire spine will force the transverse process on the right to become more prominent (it will come from an extended position into more extension). In forward bending, the left facet is already in an open position. Since the right facet is free to move, the transverse processes tend to become more symmetrically placed. This does not

Vertebral Motion by Facet Function	
1. Forward Bending	Facets Open
2. Backward Bending	Facets Close
3. Sidebending Right	Right Facet Close
	Left Facet Opens
4. Sidebending Left	Right Facet Opens
	Left Facet Closes

Figure 9-44. Facet functioning during physiological motions.

mean that the left facet has moved into closure, only that the right facet has moved into opening.

In Figure 9-45B, the right facet will not open. In this example, a similar line of reasoning will apply. When the patient forward bends, the right transverse process becomes more prominent. When he or she backward bends, the transverse processes become more equal. Positionally, this lesion is described as extended, right sidebent, and right rotated (ERS_R). Its motion restriction will be in flexion, left sidebending and left rotation.

Since the position and motion restrictions of these two lesions are different, it stands to reason that they should be approached differently from a treatment aspect to restore motion. To illustrate this, the following brief descriptions of MET's for the two examples are given so that the reader may appreciate the differences:

Example Treatment For a Lumbar Segment That is Flexed, Right Rotated And Right Sidebent

Figure 9-45A - The left facet will not close. It is diagnosed by the posterior prominence of the right transverse process when the spine is in a hyperextended position. It is described as flexed, right rotated and right sidebent (FRS_R).

Lateral Recumbent Technique (Fig 9-46):

1. The patient is sidelying on a table on the side of the more posterior transverse process. The therapist stands at the side of the table facing the patient. The patient is close to the edge of the table.

2. The patient's head is supported by a pillow and the lower leg is straight with the upper leg flexed at the hip and knee.

3. The therapist's left hand palpates the interspinous space of the involved segment while the right hand reaches under the knee of the patient's uppermost leg to extend the patient's lower leg at the hip joint until the extension movement is localized to the lesioned segment (Fig 9-46A).

4. The therapist repositions his or her hands, placing the right hand in a position to palpate movement of the spine while the left hand introduces rotation down to the segment by moving the patient's upper shoulder backward toward the table surface. The patient is instructed to inhale, and as he or she exhales the rotation is produced, localizing movement to the segment (Fig 9-46B).

5. The patient is then instructed to grip the edge of the table behind him or her (Fig 9-46C).

6. The therapist repositions the hands again. The hand that rotated the shoulder palpates the segment. The opposite hand grasps the patient's uppermost leg at the ankle .

7. The therapist lifts up on the patient's upper leg to sidebend to the desired level, then presses down with his or her elbow on the patient's knee to rotate to that level. Finally, the therapist extends the upper leg to localize extension to the segment (Fig 9-46D).

8. The patient is instructed to pull the upper foot down toward the table. After a 5-10 second contraction, the patient relaxes.

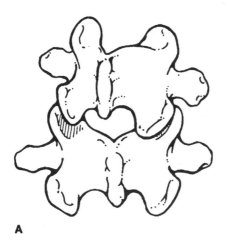
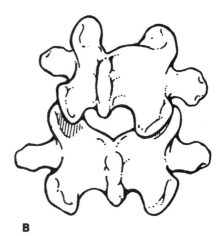

A   **B**

Figure 9-45. A) Lumbar facet lesion in which the left facet will not close; B) Lumbar facet lesion in which the right facet will not open. The two lesions appear identical but are very different from a treatment standpoint.

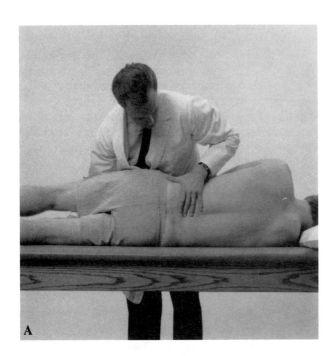

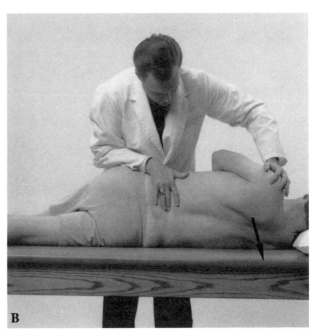

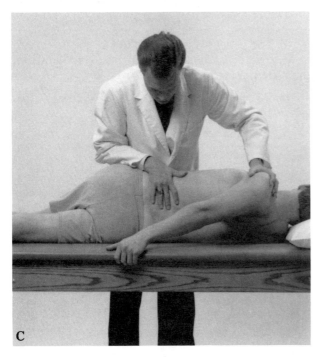

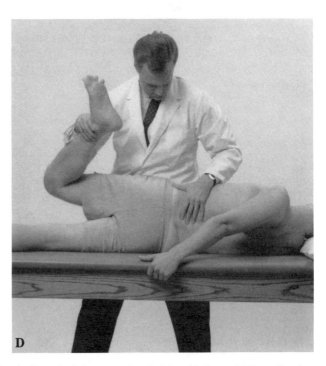

Figure 9-46. Lumbar muscle energy technique for segment that is flexed, right rotated and right sidebent. A) Localization of extension; B) Localization of left rotation; C) The patient grasps the table to stabilize his position; D) Final localization of sidebending, rotation and extension.

9. The therapist localizes movement to the segment again, then sidebends, rotates and extends again.

10. Steps 8 and 9 are repeated three times. The patient is retested and treatment is repeated if necessary.

Example Treatment for a Lumbar Segment That is Extended, Right Rotated and Right Sidebent

Figure 9-45B - The right facet will not open. It is diagnosed by the posterior prominence of the right transverse process when the spine is in a hyperflexed position. It is described as extended, right rotated and right sidebent (ERS_R).

Lateral Recumbent Technique (Fig 9-47):

l. The patient lies on his or her side, but with the chest toward the table surface. The patient lies with the prominent transverse process on the top side. In this example, the patient will be on his or her left side.

2. The therapist stands at the side of the table facing the patient. The therapist's left hand palpates the interspinous space below the vertebra to be treated, while the right hand flexes the hips so that flexion is localized to the involved segment (Fig 9-47A).

3. While supporting the knees against the body, the therapist lowers the patient's feet until sidebending to the left is localized to the segment (Fig 9-47B).

4. The patient is then asked to reach toward the floor until rotation to the left is localized to the segment (at times, this step can be omitted since rotation may be localized simultaneously with sidebending).

5. The therapist instructs the patient to lift his or her feet up toward the ceiling against unyielding resistance (isometric right sidebending hold/relax). The patient maintains the contraction for 5-10 seconds and then relaxes. The force required is approximately five pounds.

6. The segment is localized again by sidebending (dropping patient's feet further), flexing and rotating if needed.

7. Steps 5 and 6 are repeated three times.

8. The patient is retested and the treatment is repeated if necessary.

Summary of Muscle Energy Techniques

While a beginner may initially have difficulty performing the two techniques described, the purpose

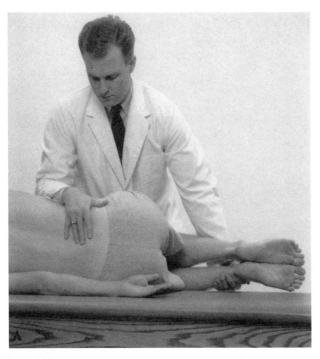
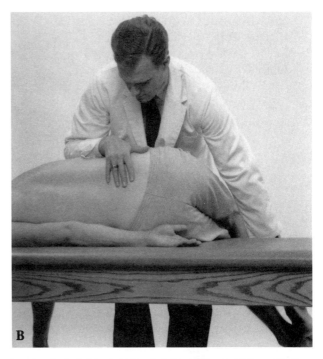

Figure 9-47. Lumbar muscle energy technique for segment that is extended, right rotated and right sidebent. A) Localization of flexion; B) Final localization of left rotation and sidebending.

of the above examples has been to show the nearly opposite approaches that are employed for two different types of dysfunctions. The unskilled practitioner may apply the same treatment to two very different joint dysfunctions just because they may appear similar. That is not necessarily bad. In many cases, a simple rotational mobilization or stretch successfully normalizes spinal movement. However, the clinician will find there are cases where a precise identification of the movement dysfunction as it occurs in all three planes and a specific muscle energy technique (as described in this chapter) are necessary to normalize segmental function.

The range of possibilities for MET's in application to the spine is almost unlimited. These techniques are gentle, safe and neurophysiologically based. As the physical therapist grows in his or her knowledge and skill in mobilization, MET's should become a part of his or her regular treatment regimen, balancing active versus passive and specific versus non-specific techniques.

REFERENCES

1. Burkart S: Personal Communications. Physical Therapy Department, University of West Virginia, Morgantown WV 1980.

2. Cyriax J: Diagnosis of Soft Tissue Lesions. Textbook of Orthopædic Medicine, Vol 1, 8th edition. Bailliere-Tindall, London 1982.

3. Freeman M and Wyke B: The Innervation of the Knee Joint: An Anatomical and Histological Study in the Cat. Joul Anat 101:505-532, 1967.

4. Greenman P: Principles of Manual Medicine. Williams and Wilkins, Baltimore MD 1989.

5. Groom D: Cervical Spine and Shoulders. The Saunders Group, Minneapolis MN 1992. Course Manual.

6. Halata Z: The Ultrastructure of the Sensory Nerve Endings in the Articular Capsule of the Knee Joint of the Domestic Cat (Ruffini Corpuscles and Pacinian Corpuscles). Joul Anat 124:717-729, 1977.

7. Kaltenborn F: Manual Therapy of the Extremity Joints. Olaf Norlis Bokhandel, Oslo 1976.

8. Lee D: Principles and Practice of Muscle Energy and Functional Techniques. In Modern Manual Therapy of the Vertebral Column. G Grieves, ed. Churchill Livingstone, London 1986.

9. MacConaill M and Basmajian J: Muscles and Movements. Williams and Wilkins, Baltimore MD 1969.

10. Maitland G: Vertebral Manipulation, 2nd edition. Butterworth, London 1968.

11. Mennell J: Back Pain. Little-Brown, Boston MA 1964.

12. Mitchell F, Moran P and Pruzzo N: An Evaluation and Treatment Manual of Osteopathic Muscle Energy Procedures. Mitchell, Moran and Pruzzo Associates, Valley Park MI 1979.

14. Nwuga V: Manipulation of the Spine. Williams and Wilkins, Baltimore MD 1976.

15. Paris S: The Spine. Atlanta Back Clinic. Atlanta GA 1975. Course Notes.

16. Polacek P: Receptors of the Joints: Their Structure, Variability and Classification. Acta Fac Med Univ Brunensis 23:1-107, 1966.

CHAPTER 10

SPINAL TRACTION

INTRODUCTION

This chapter presents and discusses the effects of spinal traction, the indications and contraindications for spinal traction, the types of spinal traction, and effective spinal traction techniques. The authors have included a summary of the literature on this subject and an introduction of new ideas. A portion of this chapter deals with the rationale of using spinal traction for the treatment of herniated nucleus pulposus (HNP) and other spinal nerve root syndromes. Detailed descriptions of proper positioning and considerable discussion of the forces necessary to achieve therapeutic results with spinal traction are included. The importance of using proper equipment for mechanical spinal traction is stressed. Spinal traction can be extremely effective treatment for certain musculoskeletal disorders, but the authors emphasize that there is a wide variety of traction technique available and the therapist must use his or her evaluative and clinical problem solving skills to decide upon the correct administration of traction techniques.

Reference to the use of tractive forces for the treatment of back problems can be found in antiquity. Certainly, Hippocrates and other early medical authors have described the use of traction in their writings. However, even into the first half of this century, the literature has been devoid of details of the techniques used, including the body type and weight of subjects, amounts of force used, duration of treatments, etc. Opinion varied as to indications, contraindications, weights and techniques.

Many physicians, therapists and patients recall the poor results of the continuous, or "bed" traction

that was common for many years. These poor results caused many physicians and therapists to become uninterested in using spinal traction. However, numerous authors claim traction is an effective and beneficial method of treatment when used appropriately and correctly. [8, 9, 18, 21-23, 25-28, 36, 42, 53, 54, 57, 60-63, 70] Other studies, however, have shown either poor results of treatment or that the positive effects of traction were of limited or marginal significance. [5, 37, 55, 67] Perhaps the conflicting results reported in the medical literature are due to the wide variety of techniques and types of traction used, many of which have not been subjected to truly randomized studies. Other studies that may be regarded as "scientific" because they have been controlled or blinded are nevertheless faulted because they essentially have compared "apples to oranges" and have drawn faulty conclusions.

For example, a frequently cited study by Pal, et. al., concluded that any benefit derived from continuous traction devices (bed traction) is due to the enforced immobilization rather than actual traction forces on the lumbar spine, since the traction forces applied in the study were not sufficient to overcome the frictional force between the bed and the lower half of the body. [55] In another study, Weber compared patients treated with traction to a control group who had simulated traction. The study showed that there was no significant difference between the two groups and concluded that traction is ineffective. [67] However, the traction force used in Weber's study was only one-third the patient's body weight, a force that is considered minimum and probably not even enough to overcome inertia and friction. Unfortunately, studies like these are often cited as proof that all forms of lumbar traction are worthless.

The word traction is a derivative of the Latin "tractico," which means a process of drawing or pulling. To achieve separation between two objects or surfaces, two opposing forces are required - traction and countertraction. Various authors have suggested the word "distraction" as being more descriptive. If the term "distraction" is used, the reference relates to the joint surfaces and suggests that these surfaces move perpendicular to one another. This is not always the case, as one can see in the spinal segment. As traction is applied, the movement produced at the segment is a combination of distraction and gliding.

EFFECTS OF SPINAL TRACTION

Correctly performed, spinal traction can cause many effects. Among these are distraction or separation of the vertebral bodies, a combination of distraction and gliding of the facet joints, tensing of the ligamentous structures of the spinal segment, widening of the intervertebral foramen, straightening of spinal curves and stretching of the spinal musculature.

The relative degree of flexion or extension of the spine during the traction treatment determines which of these effects are most pronounced. For example, greater separation of the intervertebral foramen is accomplished with the spine in a flexed position during the traction treatment, whereas greater separation of the disc space is achieved with the spine in a neutral position.

INDICATIONS FOR SPINAL TRACTION

Herniated Nucleus Pulposus with Disc Protrusion

Spinal traction is indicated for the treatment of herniated nucleus pulposus (HNP).[8,9,21-23,25-28,36,42-45,53,57] There is evidence that a disc protrusion can indeed be reduced and spinal nerve root compression symptoms relieved with the application of spinal traction. Mathews[45] used epidurography to study patients thought to have lumbar disc protrusion. He applied sustained traction forces of 120 lb for 20 minutes and showed that the protrusions were flattened and that the contrast material was drawn into the disc spaces. He also found recurrence of the bulging defects later (Fig 10-1). Gupta and Ramarao[21] also used epidurography to demonstrate reductions of lumbar disc protrusions in 11 of 14 patients treated with 60-80 lb of weight. The weight was applied for intermittent periods every three to four hours for 10-15 days. They also found definite clinical improvement in the patients in whom defects were reduced (Fig 10-2).

A recent study by Onel, et. al., is particularly convincing. This study used computed tomographic investigation to evaluate the effect of static horizontal traction on disc herniations. Changes occurring under the effect of a traction load of 45 kg (99 lb) were evaluated in 30 patients with lumbar disc herniation. The herniated disc material was retracted in 11 (78.5%) of the median, six (66.6%) of the posterolateral and four (57.1%) of the lateral herniations (Fig 10-3). The clinical improvement in the median and posterolateral herniations was far better than in the lateral herniations.[53]

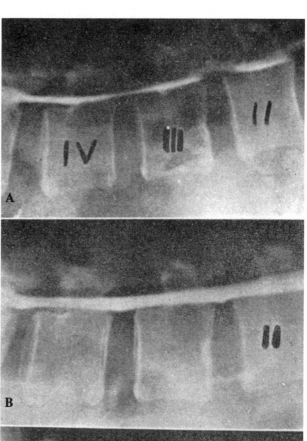

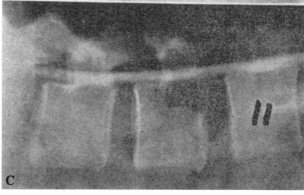

Figure 10-1. A) A disc protrusion before traction; B) The disc protrusion is being reduced with traction; C) The protrusion partially returns after traction is released (copied with permission from Mathews [44]).

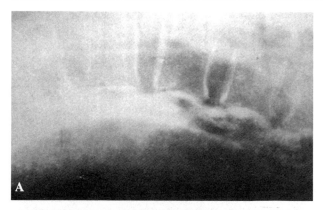

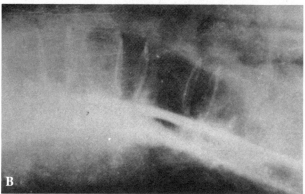

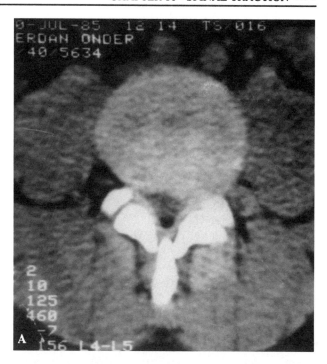

Figure 10-2. A disc protrusion being reduced by traction. A) Before traction; B) During traction (copied with permission from Gupta and Ramarao [21]).

Onel concluded that since the widening of discal space under the effect of traction causes a decrease in intradiscal pressure,[48] the negative intradiscal pressure "sucks back" the herniated nuclear material. Furthermore, the widening of the intravertebral disc space causes a stretching of the anterior and posterior longitudinal ligaments. Since the median and posterolateral herniations are located anterior to the posterior longitudinal ligament (PLL), the PLL may help to push the herniation back into place. Therefore, the effect of traction on HNP seems to be due partly to the suction effect of the negative intradiscal pressure and partly to the pushing effect of the PLL.[53]

The Onel study described two cases in which the traction increased both the amount of herniated nuclear material and the patient's symptoms. These two patients had fragmented discs, which were probably out of reach of the suction effect of the traction. One patient he described had a calcified disc, and no subjective or objective change was obtained with this patient.

Studies such as these show that traction can indeed separate lumbar vertebræ and lead to decreased pressure at the disc space with a resulting suction

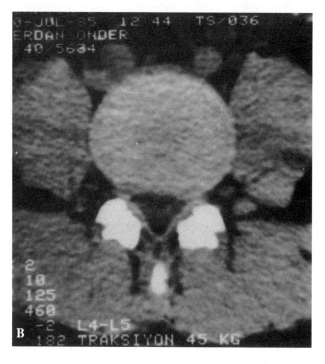

Figure 10-3. A disc protrusion being reduced by traction. A) Before traction - a left lateral HNP at L4-5, with invasion of the neural foramen by herniated nuclear material; B) During traction - regression of the herniated nuclear material from the discal space and neural foramen (copied with permission from Onel, et. al.[53]).

force. In addition, material can be drawn from the epidural space into the disc space. Similarly, it may be concluded that any anatomical correction produced is unstable. Thus, if patients are not carefully treated with a total management regimen, traction alone is likely to be unsuccessful. The patient must be carefully monitored as the traction treatment is administered. While the treatment may not be pain free, the patient must at least be able to relax to allow the treatment to be effective. The rules of centralization and peripheralization of the patient's symptoms (discussed in Chapter 5, Treatment of the Spine by Diagnosis) must be followed closely. Distinguishing between central symptoms and peripheral symptoms is extremely important and should govern all activities, including the application of spinal traction, spinal mobilization and exercises.

As with all conservative treatment approaches for HNP, patient education and a gradual, cautious return to activities are necessary if the traction is to be successful. Once the disc protrusion is reduced by spinal traction and spinal nerve root symptoms have been relieved, the rest of the principles discussed in Chapter 5 must be applied.

While the above discussion is directed to treatment of lumbar HNP and there is very little specific information in the medical literature about traction treatment for cervical HNP, the authors feel that much of what has been discussed is generally applicable to cervical HNP as well.

Degenerative Disc/Joint Disease

The argument is often raised that although traction can cause separation and widening of the intervertebral foramen and intervertebral disc space, the effect will only be temporary. It is true that the separation shown on x-rays will at least partially disappear soon after traction has been discontinued. If traction is applied to a patient with a narrowed intervertebral foramen or to one who has osteophyte or ligamentous encroachment, the disc space and intervertebral foramen are obviously not restored to their original size and structure.

Therefore, the relief experienced by these patients after the traction treatment must be explained from another basis. We already know that the pathology seen on x-ray or in CT scans does not necessarily correlate to the degree of symptoms present.[1,19,32,38-40,59,68,69] Many people have narrowing of the disc space and intervertebral foramen without signs and symptoms of spinal nerve root impingement. Previously asymptomatic patients in whom degenerative changes or osteophytes have been present for some time will have a sudden onset of symptoms related to a certain activity or position. A very fine line must exist between cases in which encroachment or irritation of the spinal nerve root occurs and does not occur. The traction treatment must somehow move,

separate or realign the segment in such a way as to relieve the impingement.

Goldish speculates that the degenerated disc may benefit from traction because lowering intradiscal pressure by traction may affect the nutritional state of the nucleus pulposus.[20]

Joint Hypomobility
(Soft Tissue Stiffness)

Traction may be regarded as a form of mobilization since it involves the passive movement of joints by mechanical or manual means. Any condition of joint hypomobility may respond favorably to traction. One argument against using traction for mobilization is that it is nonspecific and simultaneously affects several joints. However, when traction is applied to a series of spinal segments, each segment in that series receives an equal amount of traction. If the force applied is sufficient to mobilize the involved segment, it is irrelevant that other segments are also receiving the same amount of traction unless, of course, traction is contraindicated at those other segments. If this is the case, a more specific technique of joint mobilization should be selected.[56, 61]

Facet Impingement

When facet joints become restricted due to mechanical impingement, manual mobilization and manipulation techniques are often used to free the restrictions. Manual techniques that isolate the individual joints are often the preferred techniques. However, traction is another treatment option that can release an impinged facet joint. If the traction force across the joint is sufficient to release the restriction it will produce the desired results. Traction as a treatment for facet impingement is relatively ineffective in the thoracic area and it should not be used if traction is contraindicated at any segment that receives the traction force.

Muscle Spasm

Both traction and stretching exercises can relieve muscle spasm. Traction can also decompress or separate painful joint structures. If the pain is relieved by traction, muscle spasm will be relieved as a result of relaxation of nociceptive reflexes.[20]

CONTRAINDICATIONS FOR SPINAL TRACTION

Traction is contraindicated in structural disease secondary to tumor or infection, in patients with vascular compromise and in any condition for which movement is contraindicated.[70]

Relative contraindications include acute strains and sprains and inflammatory conditions that may be aggravated by traction. Vigorous traction applied to patients with spinal joint instability may cause further strain. Other relative contraindications may include pregnancy, osteoporosis, hiatal hernia and claustrophobia.

TYPES OF LUMBAR TRACTION

Bed Traction

Bilateral leg traction and pelvic belt traction are methods used for applying traction in bed. The traction rope is pulled over a pulley at the foot of the bed and free weights are attached. Bed traction is applied for as long as several hours at a time. This long duration requires that only small amounts of weight be used because the patient's skin cannot tolerate prolonged traction at high poundages. Thus, it is generally accepted that this form of traction cannot separate the vertebræ when applied to the lumbar spine.[28]

It is often said that bed traction's main purpose is to keep the patient immobilized in bed. However, even when bed traction is applied continuously, the force is not enough to prevent the trunk muscles from moving the spinal segments. The patient is not truly immobilized. Therefore, some authors argue that bed traction is not any better than bedrest alone.[20] The authors of this textbook have found no scientific evidence that supports any beneficial effect of bed traction. After all, it has not even been proven that patient compliance with bed rest is improved with the use of bed traction. Deyo's study shows that excessive bedrest can actually be harmful. With the information available, it becomes increasingly hard to justify the use of bed traction at all.

Mechanical Table Traction

Mechanical table traction differs from bed traction in that the traction is applied for shorter time periods on a treatment table. Since mechanical table traction is not continuous, much higher forces can be tolerated without risking skin breakdown. A pelvic belt is used to provide the traction force and a thoracic belt is used to provide counter traction to prevent the patient's entire body from slipping down the table.

The most simple form of mechanical table traction involves the use of free weights hanging from a pulley system at the foot of the table. In this sense, it is similar to the bed traction described earlier except that it uses shorter time periods and heavier weights. Mechanical

gear or winch systems have also been used. The most common method of mechanical table traction used today involves a traction machine that is specially made to produce a traction force.

Mechanical table traction can be sustained (static) or intermittent. Sustained traction is applied with a constant force for a few minutes. Intermittent traction uses a mechanical device that alternately applies and releases the traction force every few seconds.

Mechanical table traction is most effective if a split table is used to reduce friction. It is very important that a mechanical traction device maintains constant tension. In other words, any slack developed as the patient relaxes during the treatment must be automatically taken up and the desired amount of traction maintained. The effectiveness of mechanical table traction can also be enhanced by using a three dimensional (3-D) table which will be discussed later.

Manual Traction

To apply manual traction the therapist grasps the patient and manually applies a traction force. Manual traction is usually applied for a few seconds, but it also can be applied as a sudden, quick thrust. It allows the therapist to feel the patient's reaction.[10, 29, 56] It is sometimes more difficult for the patient to relax with manual traction than with mechanical traction because the exact amount of force that will be applied cannot be anticipated. A steady prolonged stretch is also more difficult to maintain since the therapist eventually fatigues.

Manual traction can be used as an easy clinical test to determine if mechanical table traction will be helpful. The therapist either pulls on the legs while the patient is supine or lifts the patient by the elbows while the patient is sitting with the arms crossed. Specific techniques are shown later in this chapter.

Positional Traction

The patient is placed in various positions using pillows, bolsters or sandbags to effect a longitudinal pull on the spinal structures. This form of traction usually incorporates lateral bending and only one side of the spinal segment is affected.[56] Positional traction is inexpensive and can be used at home.

Autotraction (Lumbar)

A special traction bench composed of two sections that can be individually angled and rotated is used with autotraction. Patients apply the traction by pulling with their own arms and can alter the direction of the traction as the treatment progresses. Treatment sessions can last one hour or longer and are supervised by a clinician .[33, 36, 51]

Gravity Lumbar Traction

With gravity lumbar traction, the lower border and circumference of the rib cage are grasped by a specially made vest secured to the top of the bed. The patient is then tilted on a circular bed or specially made table into a vertical or nearly vertical position. In this position the free weight of the legs and hips (about 40% of the body weight) exerts, by gravity, a traction force on the lumbar spine.[4, 20]

Two other types of gravity traction have become popular through commercialization efforts. One technique uses specialized boots that attach to the subject's ankles. The individual is then able to suspend him- or herself from a frame into a fully inverted position. The other technique involves a device in which the individual is supported on the anterior thighs and is able to hang inverted with the hips and knees flexed. Both techniques will achieve a traction force of approximately 50% of the total body weight on the lumbar spine.[52] A study by Kane showed significant separation of both the anterior and posterior margins of the lumbar vertebral bodies at all levels as well as increased dimension of the intervertebral foramina using the inversion boot method. These techniques have some risks which will be discussed later. Most of the gravity lumbar traction devices are portable and can be used for home treatment.

Cottrell 90/90 Traction

Cottrell traction involves positioning the patient with the knees and hips bent at 90° and the pelvis tilted posteriorly to decrease the lumbar lordosis. A rope attached to a pelvic belt is draped over the top of an A-Frame. The patient pulls on the rope to lift the pelvis off the floor. This produces additional posterior pelvic tilt and lumbar flexion. A study comparing the supine position to Cottrell traction measured greater posterior disc distraction than anterior disc compression with the use of Cottrell traction.[20] However, flexing the hips to 90° alone also produces posterior distraction. Therefore it is questionable whether the Cottrell 90/90 traction device actually provides significant traction or whether its main effect is simply to flex the lumbar spine. Whatever the case, Cottrell traction can be used to distract the posterior elements and therefore can be effective for the patient with foraminal (lateral) stenosis. We feel Cottrell traction should not be used to treat HNP, except possibly in the very early stages of acute HNP when flexion is the only position the patient can tolerate (Fig 10-4). Cottrell traction is portable and can be used for home treatment.

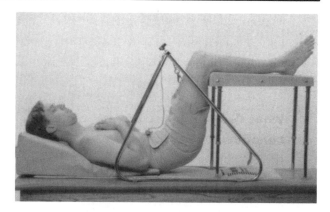

Figure 10-4. Cottrell traction.

E-Z Trac

The E-Z Trac™ consists of a portable frame and traction device capable of administering lumbar traction of up to 200 lb. It is hydraulic and can be preset to the desired poundage. It works best with the patient supine, but treatment can also be given in the prone position (Fig 10-5).

Lumba Trac™

The Lumba Trac™ consists of a rigid upholstered frame with a spring lever device capable of administering traction forces up to 150 lb (Fig 10-6). Like the E-Z Trac™, it is portable and does not require floor space when not in use. These devices are most useful for home treatment or in a small clinic where investing in a mechanical table traction set up may not be practical.

LUMBAR TRACTION TECHNIQUE

Many physicians and physical therapists routinely use cervical traction and appear reasonably satisfied with the beneficial results in patients with joint dysfunction, degenerative joint/disc disease and nerve root symptoms. Yet many do not use traction for treatment of similar conditions in the lumbar spine. We attribute this general attitude to inadequacies of equipment and lack of knowledge of effective traction techniques. With proper equipment and technique, the same satisfactory results that have been experienced with cervical traction can also be accomplished with lumbar traction.

Disappointment with bed traction caused many physicians and physical therapists to lose interest in any form of lumbar traction. Some patients are reluctant to have traction treatments, recalling the bed traction they received in years past. As previously mentioned, any benefit accredited to bed traction was probably

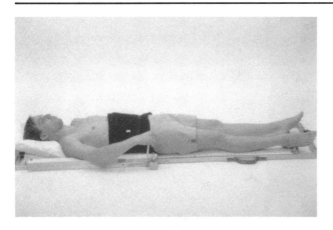

Figure 10-5. E-Z Trac™ traction.

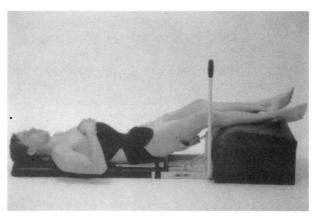

Figure 10-6. Lumba Tract™ traction.

the result of the rest and immobilization while the patient was undergoing treatment.

The coefficient of friction of the human body lying on a couch or mattress is 0.5. In other words, a force equal to one-half of the patient's body weight is required to move the body horizontally (Fig 10-7). It is necessary to move the lower one-half of the body horizontally before any force is effected to the lumbar spine (Fig 10-8). As one-half (0.5) of the body weight lies caudal to L3, a force equal to 0.5 X 0.5 = .25 or one-quarter of the body weight is all that can effectively cause a traction force if conventional bed traction techniques are applied.[28] Any force less than one-fourth of the patient's body weight will not be enough to overcome friction and any more than one-half will cause the patient to slide to the foot of the bed. Nowhere in the literature were these authors able to find any evidence that traction forces of one-fourth of the patient's body weight or less could effect any change in the structures of the lumbar spine.

The following points are essential to the administration of therapeutically effective lumbar traction:

1. The traction force must be great enough to effect a structural change (movement) at the spinal segment. Cyriax[9] reported a visible separation with sustained traction of 120 lb for 15 minutes. Other studies have reported measurable separation in the lumbar spine at forces ranging from 80 to 200 lb.[23, 34, 45] Judovich[28] advocated a force equal to one-half of the patient's body weight on a friction-free surface as a minimum to cause therapeutic effects in the lumbar spine. It is not necessary that the first treatment be administered at that weight, and it must be remembered that the minimum weight necessary to cause a measurable separation will not always be enough to produce satisfactory results. Conversely, clinical experience has shown that some patients have pain relief with forces of less than one-half the body

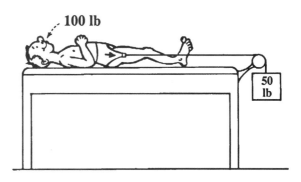

Figure 10-7. A pull of 50 pounds is necessary to slide a 100 pound person horizontally on a couch or mattress.

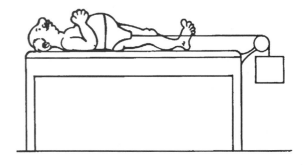

Figure 10-8. It is necessary to move the lower one-half of the body horizontally before any traction force is effected to the lumbar spine.

weight. It is important to assess the patient's reaction and results of the treatment after each visit. Adjustments can then be made until satisfactory results are achieved.

The weights required to cause damage to the vertebral structures have also been studied. Ranier found that a force of 400 lb was necessary to produce a rupture of the dorsolumbar spine (T11, T12) in a fresh cadaver.[14] Harris[23] indicated that enormous traction forces were necessary to cause damage to the lumbar spine with the breaking load possibly being as high as 880 lb.

2.   A split table is necessary to eliminate friction. As mentioned previously, it is the effective traction force on the spine that is important, and any friction involved must be considered. A split table on frictionless guides essentially eliminates this factor (Fig 10-9).[20]

All the slack in the harnesses must be taken up before the split table is released. It is a good idea to begin the treatment with progressively stronger pulls with the split table locked. After two or three progressions, the split table is released during a rest phase if intermittent traction is used. If using sustained (static) traction, the table is released with care being taken to avoid a sudden jerk. This may be accomplished by holding or blocking the movement of the table top as the mechanism is released, then gradually letting the table apart manually.

3.   Patients must be able to relax. The amount of force alone does not determine the effectiveness of the traction treatment. Patient comfort is of utmost importance. If the patient is unable to relax during treatment, the treatment will probably be ineffective. Cervical traction studies show that narrowing of the intervertebral spaces can actually occur during the traction treatment in patients who are unable to relax.[13] The treatment must not aggravate the condition and patients must feel secure and well supported. It may be beneficial to administer modality treatments before the application of traction. Such agents as ice, heat, ultrasound and massage are often effective.

4.   The use of a heavy duty, non-slip traction harness is essential.[60, 61] If patients do not feel secure, they will almost certainly remain tense during treatment. An effective, one-size-fits-all heavy duty lumbar traction harness is seen in Figure 10-10. This harness is lined with a vinyl material that causes it to adhere to the patient's skin, thus eliminating the slipping that is common with cotton lined belts. Both the pelvic and thoracic pads should be placed next to the patient's skin (Fig 10-11). If clothing is left under the harness, it will be more likely to allow slippage. Clothing can also take some of the traction force if it

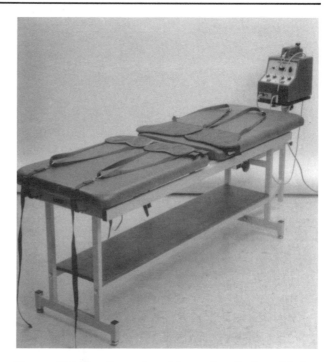

Figure 10-9. A split traction table, used to eliminate friction.

is bound tightly under both belts. Even something as simple as a strap around the patient's thighs will add support and help relaxation (Fig 10-12). The pelvic harness should be secured to the patient first. It is properly positioned when the top web belt crosses at approximately the umbilical line (Fig 10-13). The thoracic pads should be positioned so that they lie on the lateral-inferior chest wall. The thoracic pads are in proper position when both web belts are below the xiphoid process and are actually positioned and held on the inferior rim of the eighth, ninth and tenth ribs. The patient's arms should be placed through the thoracic harness when traction is given in the prone position. The anterior strap should always lie over the anterior aspect of the shoulder joint when the thoracic pads are in correct position. When properly positioned, the pelvic and thoracic belts will overlap slightly (Fig 10-14).

5.   The patient position (prone or supine) and the position of the pull straps of the pelvic belts (anterior or posterior) are used to determine the amount of flexion or extension of the patient's lumbar spine. There are four basic options for the position of the patient and pull straps: 1) Supine with a posterior pull; 2) Supine with an anterior pull; 3) Prone with a posterior pull; and 4) Prone with an anterior pull. The pelvic portion of the heavy duty traction harness described in this chapter should be prepared by threading the web belts one way for supine with a posterior pull and prone with an anterior pull (Fig 10-15A), and another way for supine with an anterior pull and prone with a posterior pull (Fig 10-15B).

CHAPTER 10 - SPINAL TRACTION **283**

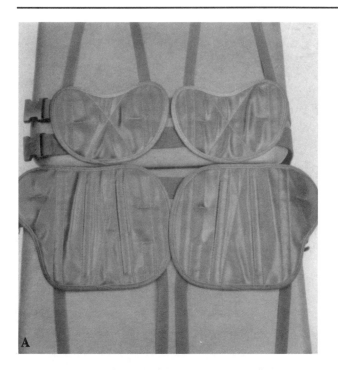

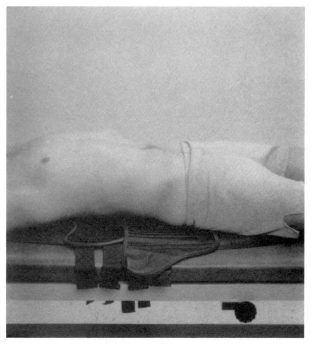

Figure 10-11. The traction harness should be placed next to the patient's skin to eliminate slippage.

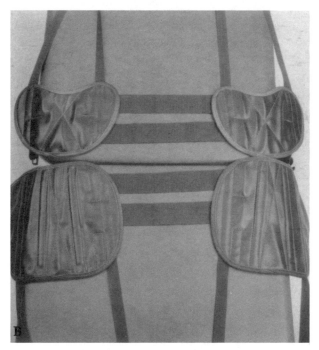

Figure 10-10. A heavy-duty lumbar traction harness. A) Adjusted for a small patient; B) Adjusted for a large patient.

The amount of flexion or extension desired will depend upon the disorder being treated and the comfort of the patient.[9, 60] In our experience, disc herniation is most effectively treated with the patient lying prone with a normal lordosis. However, this position is not always possible because the patient with acute HNP may not tolerate any position of normal lordosis. If this is the case the treatment must be given in flexion

initially with the goal of gradually working toward neutral lumbar lordosis.

Foraminal (lateral) stenosis is usually more effectively treated with the patient lying supine and the lumbar spine in a flexed (flattened) position. Joint hypomobility and degenerative disc/joint disease may be treated in either the prone or supine position.

The degree of flexion or extension in which the lumbar spine is positioned is determined by the goal(s) of the treatment. For example, if the treatment goal is to increase extension mobility, the patient should be positioned in as much extension as possible and the belts positioned for an anterior pull. In general, if the belts are positioned with an anterior pull the lumbar spine will be pulled more toward neutral or even into some extension. If the belts are positioned with a posterior pull, the lumbar spine will be pulled into flexion. Of course, the position of the legs and pillows or bolsters can be used to control the amount of flexion/extension also. However, patient comfort and the patient's ability to remain relaxed during the treatment are also important considerations when choosing the most beneficial position and no absolute rule applies. Variations of flexion, extension and lateral bending should be tried to find the most beneficial position for each patient.

There is often a postural component involved with disorders of the lumbar spine. Initially, traction

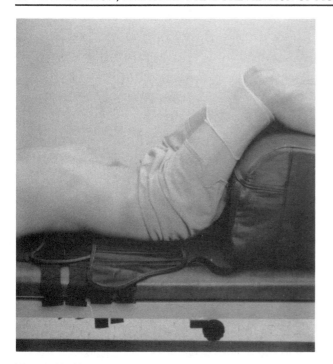

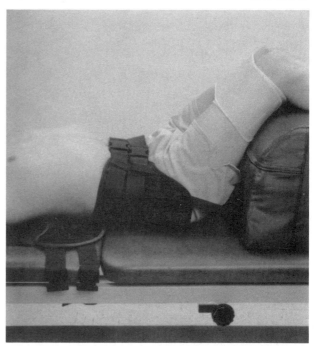

Figure 10-12. A strap placed around the patient's thighs will help the patient relax during supine lumbar traction.

treatments may have to be administered in positions that accommodate the patient's postural position. As progress is achieved, the treatment should be administered in positions that encourage the return to normal posture. For example, most patients with disc herniation will have a flattened lumbar lordosis and will be limited in spinal extension. One of the treatment goals will be to return this patient to normal posture. Although it may be impossible to place the patient in a position of normal lordosis initially, one will want to work in that direction as treatment progresses. Thus, it may be necessary to give the traction treatment in a position involving some flexion (supine with a posterior pull or prone with a posterior pull with the lumbar spine in flexion). Lumbar flexion is accomplished either with pillows or the use of a 3-D table as shown in Figure 10-16. However, as progress is noted and the patient is able to achieve a position of normal lordosis, the traction treatments should be given in a position that helps achieve the normal lordosis (prone or supine with an anterior pull).

Lumbar Traction in the Supine Position

When applying lumbar traction in the supine position, one should remember that it is not necessarily the position of the legs or the rope angle to the table that controls the amount of lumbar flexion/extension. The position of the legs controls hip flexion and has only a slight effect on lumbar lordosis. Likewise, the

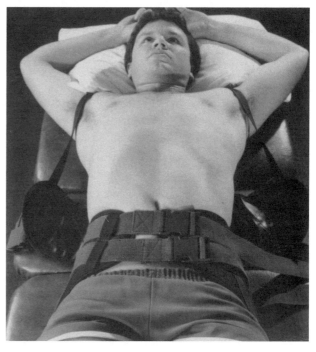

Figure 10-13. The pelvic harness is properly positioned when the top web belt is above the iliac crests and the web belt's top edge crosses at the umbilical line.

rope angle to the table does not always effectively control the amount of spinal flexion/extension. The choice of pelvic harness is probably most important because it determines the amount of spinal flexion achieved. If the pelvic harness pulls from the sides only, it is difficult to control the degree of lumbar lordosis. This is the reason a pelvic harness that pulls

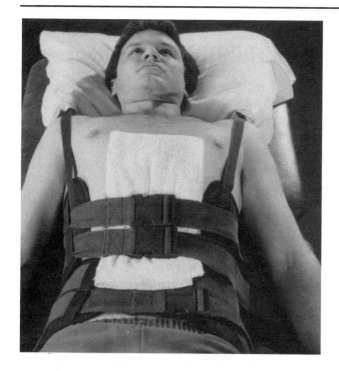

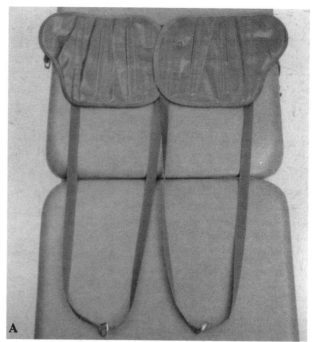

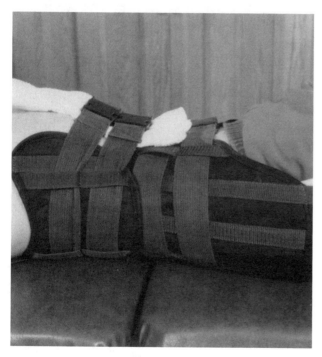

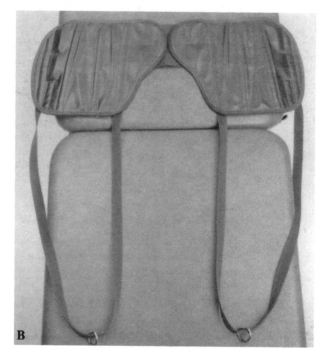

Figure 10-14. When properly positioned, the pelvic and thoracic pads will overlap slightly.

from the anterior or posterior is essential. The knees and hips can be flexed moderately for comfort, with a bolster or pillows under the lower legs. If flexion is desired a *posterior pull* should be used (Fig 10-17). An *anterior pull* will produce a normal to slight extension curve in the lumbar spine (Fig 10-18). The rope angle to the table should remain relatively in line. This is especially true if heavier poundages are used.

Figure 10-15. The web belts must be threaded into the pelvic harness correctly. This will vary depending upon the type of traction desired. A) Proper threading for supine with a posterior pull or prone with an anterior pull; B) Proper threading for supine with an anterior pull or prone with a posterior pull.

It should be noted that certain commercial traction tables are not recommended for heavy poundages unless a straight or 0° rope angle to the table is maintained.

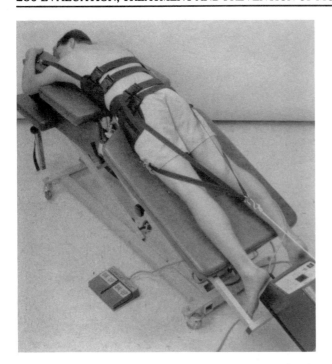

Figure 10-16. Prone lumbar traction with the spine in flexion. The 3-D table is flexed and the pelvic harness is threaded so that it imparts a posterior pull.

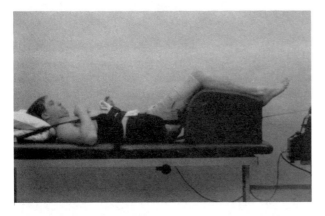

Figure 10-17. Supine lumbar traction with a posterior pull.

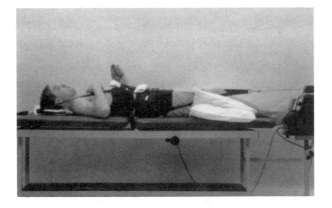

Figure 10-18. Supine lumbar traction with an anterior pull.

Lumbar Traction in the Prone Position

When using prone traction, the amount of lumbar flexion can be controlled with a 3-D table or pillows under the pelvis and, as mentioned above, by using the correct pelvic harness. If one desires to apply lumbar traction with the spine in a normal amount of lordosis or in extension, the prone position is probably best. The harness should be positioned with an *anterior pull*. The patient lies flat on the table and the rope angle to the table is varied to control the exact amount of lordosis (Fig 10-19).

For patients who cannot tolerate a neutral or extended position, prone traction can be especially effective. Pillows or a 3-D table are used to accommodate the patient's preference for a flexed posture. A *posterior pull* is used (Fig 10-20). Since this type of patient often has significant pain and or muscle guarding, the prone position is excellent for applying modality treatments and the traction can follow without moving the patient. Another advantage of prone traction is that the therapist can palpate the interspinous spaces to ascertain the amount of movement that is taking place during the treatment.

6. The traction mode (sustained or intermittent) selected will depend on the disorder being treated and the comfort of the patient. HNP-protrusion is usually treated more effectively with sustained traction or with longer hold-rest periods (60 second hold, 20 second rest) of intermittent traction. Joint dysfunction and degenerative disc disease usually respond to shorter hold-rest periods of intermittent traction. Some mechanical traction devices administer sustained traction relatively ineffective due to their inability to take up slack during the treatment. To be effective it is essential that a mechanical traction device continue to take up slack as the patient relaxes.[62]

7. The length of treatment is another important factor to consider. When disc protrusion is treated with spinal traction, the treatment time should be short. As the disc space is widened the intradiscal pressure is decreased.[48] It seems that this decrease in pressure will only be maintained for a short time, as osmotic forces will soon equalize pressure to that of the surrounding tissue. If equalization does occur, the suction effective on the protrusion would be lost. Theoretically, an increase in intradiscal pressure with respect to the surrounding tissue might result when the traction is released. Consequently, the patient may experience a sharp increase in pain after treatment. The author has not observed this adverse reaction in intermittent treatments of less than ten minutes and sustained treatments of less than eight minutes. Often, the first treatment is only three to five minutes long.

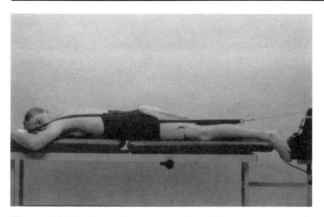

Figure 10-19. Prone lumbar traction with an anterior pull.

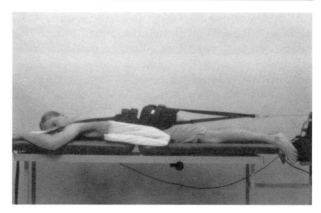

Figure 10-20. Prone lumbar traction with a posterior pull.

8. The use of progressive and regressive modes of traction can also be a treatment consideration. Certain mechanical traction devices can gradually increase the traction force at the beginning of the treatment and to gradually step down the force at the end of the treatment. Progressive-regressive application of traction is actually like a "warm up, cool down" period known to all trainers, therapists and physicians. The gradual application and removal of traction forces made possible with the progressive-regressive traction modes may enhance the potential effectiveness of traction in certain patients.[58]

Manual Traction

Paris uses manual lumbar traction for treatment of HNP. These techniques are sometimes used with a sudden thrust and can be directed unilaterally.[56] Kaltenborn also describes various manual traction techniques that can be used for spinal mobilization.[29] Manual traction can be helpful in testing the patient's tolerance to traction or to find the most comfortable direction in which to administer the treatment (Fig 10-21). The therapist either pulls on the legs as shown or lifts the patient by the elbows while the patient is sitting with the arms crossed. Manual lumbar traction is of questionable value in most cases because of the physical difficulty met when applying and sustaining forces great enough to be effective.

Positional Traction

Positional traction is applied by placing the patient in a side lying position over a rolled pillow or blanket. The roll should be approximately six to eight inches in diameter and should be placed at the level of the spine where the traction or separation is to occur. The effect is a unilateral stretch of the soft tissue structures, gapping of the facet joints and opening of the neural foramen on the side opposite to the roll. The technique can involve only sidebending or can also incorporate rotation (Fig 10-22). This technique may also be used

(sidebending only) to correct a lateral scoliosis sometimes seen in patients who have herniated lumbar discs.

Gravity Lumbar Traction

Gravity lumbar traction with the patient in an upright position has been claimed to be effective in the treatment of disc protrusion. The amount of force that can be applied is limited to approximately 40% of body weight.[4] A moderate amount of physical effort is also required from patients. Chest pain caused by the thoracic vest is sometimes a limiting factor. This form of traction is recommended only for medically screened, well-motivated patients whose body size and shape allows this form of treatment.[54] The program usually consists of one hour of traction twice daily.

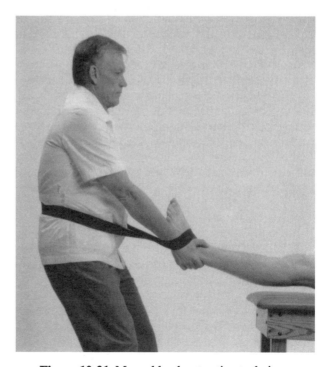

Figure 10-21. Manual lumbar traction technique.

This treatment time is not consistent with the previously mentioned theory that an initial suction force on the disc caused by the vertebral bodies separating is soon lost due to osmosis of body fluids into the disc.

Gravity traction with the individual inverted has been shown to separate the intervertebral disc and foraminal spaces and may therefore be an effective method of administering lumbar traction in certain cases.[30] There are some risks associated with gravity traction, however. Recent investigation has shown the inverted position can produce marked changes in heart rate and blood pressure in young adults. There is also evidence of increased ocular pressure and the potential for retinal damage.[35] Inversion traction may be dangerous for hypertensive individuals and those with cardiac anomalies or cerebral vascular disease. In any case, blood pressure, heart rate and patient comfort should be monitored closely during inversion and the patient should be acclimated to the inversion position on a gradual basis.[30]

Other disadvantages of gravity traction include difficulty controlling direction (flexion, extension and lateral bending) and force.

It is our opinion inversion devices can improve joint mobility and general flexibility effectively, but they do not offer the control of direction and, in some cases, the amount of force necessary when treating patients with HNP or degenerative disc/joint disease.

Unilateral Lumbar Traction

In some cases, lumbar traction involving a pull at a lateral angle to the midline of the body has been demonstrated to be more comfortable and more efficacious for unilateral disorders (including protective scoliosis) than is bilateral lumbar traction.[2, 3, 23, 51, 63] Although the technique seems sound, very little unilateral lumbar traction has been used clinically because of problems with patient positioning and with availability and adaptability of equipment. Lumbar traction involving a pull at a lateral angle to the midline of the body involves two problems: First, most commercially available traction equipment does not adapt to this technique. Second, when using equipment that does adapt to a lateral pull, the patient's body simply slides to the side of the table and aligns itself with the traction force and the pull on the lumbar spine remains straight (Fig 10-23). When attempts are made to stabilize the spine to prevent this realignment, the exact area of lateral bending is difficult, if not impossible, to control. For instance, when attempts are made to stabilize the patient with a belt across the torso, most sidebending occurs at the segment just inferior to the belt and the exact segment can only be determined by x-ray.

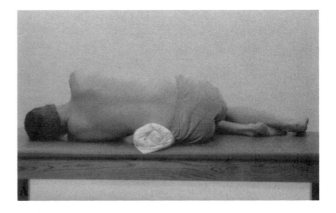

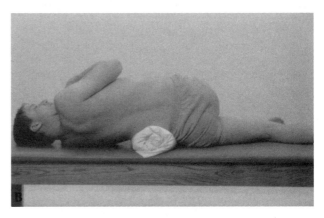

Figure 10-22. Positional traction. A) Left sidebending; B) Left sidebending and right rotation.

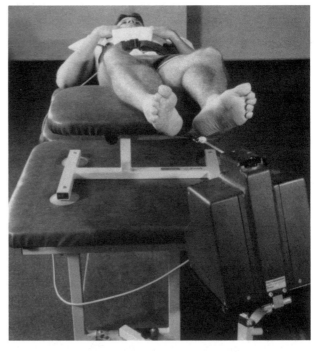

Figure 10-23. Ineffective unilateral lumbar traction. When using a unilateral traction technique that involves a lateral pull, the patient's body slides to the side of the table and aligns itself with the traction force.

The unilateral lumbar traction technique we prefer uses the conventional heavy duty traction harness described earlier. By hooking only one side of the harness to the traction source, or by varying the length of the harness straps between sides, effective unilateral lumbar traction can be administered. With this method, the lateral bending and separation of the vertebræ is uniform throughout the lumbar spine. The technique can be applied in either the prone or the supine position (Fig 10-24).

We have investigated the effects of unilateral traction to determine if vertebral separation occurs, where it occurs and whether a lumbar scoliosis occurs when the unilateral pull is applied. The information obtained is based on comparison of x-ray findings in one 200 lb man with no apparent lumbar disorder. This investigation was done with the subject in the supine position with a 100 lb pull from the right side only (Fig 10-24A). Measurements were taken from the lateral aspect of the inferior edge of the T12

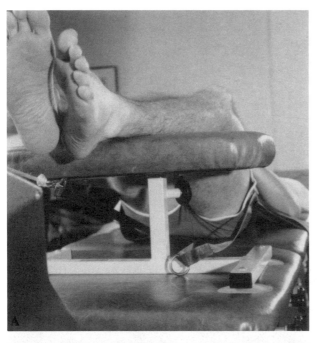
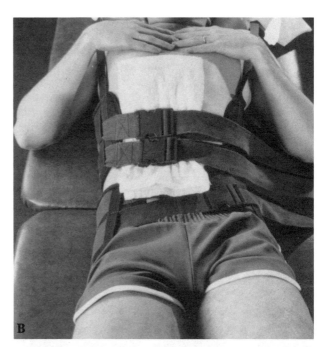
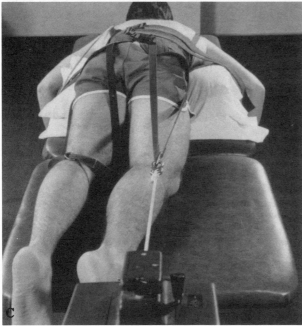
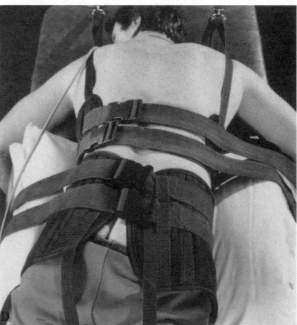

Figure 10-24. Effective unilateral lumbar traction. A&B) Supine traction with only the right pelvic belt hooked to the traction force; C&D) Prone traction with only the right pelvic belt hooked to the traction force.

vertebral body to the superior surface of the sacrum at a point adjacent to the lateral aspect of the L5 vertebral body. The unilateral traction produced a separation of 10 mm on the side of the pull and a separation of 2 mm on the side opposite the pull. Lumbar lateral bending of 12° was also observed with the curve being convex on the side of the pull. The separation and curve occurred uniformly throughout the lumbar part of the spine (Fig 10-25). These findings were then compared to supine sidebending at the same degree without the traction force, which showed a separation of 7 mm on the convex side and a narrowing of 11 mm on the concave side (Fig 10-26). Investigation of a patient with a lumbar disorder has revealed similar findings (see section on Unilateral Facet Joint Hypomobility).

The general indications and contraindications for applying conventional lumbar traction are also applicable to unilateral traction techniques. Complete and thorough evaluation and assessment are necessary before a patient receives lumbar traction. Part of that assessment should involve consideration of the factors that favor the unilateral or the bilateral techniques.

Whenever there are general indications for lumbar traction, a unilateral pull may be considered, especially if the disorder is unilateral. Often, the determining factor is the patient's comfort and his or her ability to relax with the treatment. A trial of manual traction can be done to ascertain if the patient is a suitable candidate for traction. The manual traction should be given at various degrees of flexion, extension and lateral bending to find the most comfortable and beneficial patient positioning.[63] When the disorder is unilateral, the most comfortable position will often be one that does involve some lateral bending of the spine along with traction. It is wise to take advantage of this more comfortable position in these cases.[63]

Three specific instances when unilateral traction may be preferred to the conventional bilateral technique are for unilateral facet joint hypomobility or facet impingement, protective lumbar scoliosis and lumbar scoliosis caused by unilateral lumbar muscle spasm.[63]

Unilateral Technique for Unilateral Facet Joint Hypomobility /Impingement

Conventional lumbar traction has been suggested as a mobilization technique for hypomobility or impingement .[60, 63] When the pathology involves the facet joints on one side only, a unilateral technique should be considered. The following is a case study of unilateral facet joint hypomobility or impingement involving the use of unilateral lumbar traction.[63]

The patient was a 17 year old, 155 lb athlete/student. The patient reported the onset of symptoms had occurred three months previously, after a compression type fall with the spine extended. The pain was only minor at first but had stiffened his spine. He had not sought medical help. When seen three months after injury, his chief complaint was that it

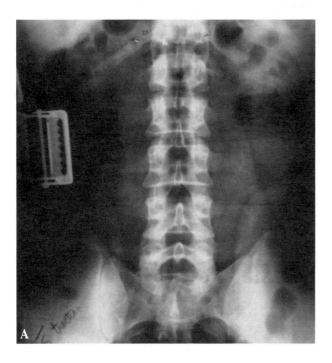
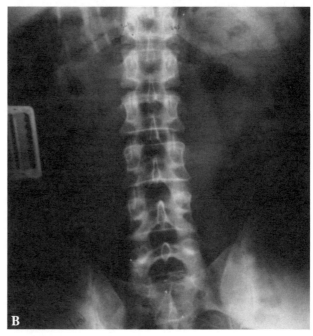

Figure 10-25. Effects of supine unilateral lumbar traction (A/P view). A) No traction force; B) A traction force of 100 pounds pulling from the right side only. Total vertebral separation from T12 to sacrum was 10 mm on the right and 2 mm on the left.

hurt in the area just lateral to the L5-S1 interspace on the right when he ran. He was otherwise doing the full activities of daily living for a 17 year old athlete/ student.

The x-ray revealed apparent narrowing of the right facet joint (Fig 10-27A). Mobility tests revealed hypomobility at the L5-S1 level with the greatest restriction in right rotation and left sidebending. Other clinical signs and symptoms supported the presence of facet joint hypomobility at that level. There were no positive neurological findings.

The patient was given continuous ultrasound for six minutes at 20 watts, followed by intermittent unilateral lumbar traction with a right sided pull of 100 lb for 10 minutes. An x-ray was taken while the traction was being applied, and it showed visible separation (mobilization) of the right L5-S1 facet (Fig 10-27B). The patient was nearly symptom free after two treatments, and received a total of four treatments. He returned to full activities of daily living, including varsity cross-country running, and remained symptom free for several months following the study.

Unilateral Technique for Protective Scoliosis

If a patient has an HNP and the protrusion is encroaching upon a spinal nerve root, lateral bending of the spine often offers relief. This is referred to as a "protective scoliosis." Many musculoskeletal problems involve lateral bending of the spine, and the protective scoliosis is only one of several possibilities. Most patients with protective scoliosis lean away from the side of the symptoms. However, when the disorder involves an HNP with a protrusion medial to the nerve root, the patient may bend toward the side of the symptoms. If the herniation is lateral to the nerve root (most common), the patient will bend away from the painful side (Fig 5-23). In all cases, the patient assumes the position that offers symptomatic relief.[15, 66]

When the patient with a protective scoliosis is placed in conventional bilateral traction, the scoliosis straightens as soon as the traction is applied, which may result in increased pain. The traction does not appear to be beneficial. On the other hand, if the scoliosis can be maintained while the traction is applied, the treatment may be given without increasing the patient's discomfort. Such a technique enhances the chances of achieving the desired results of the treatment.

A protective scoliosis differs from the condition McKenzie describes as a lateral shift.[46] With a protective scoliosis, the patient places himself in the most comfortable position. A lateral shift is a mechanical phenomenon that occurs when the nuclear gel moves laterally. It is difficult to distinguish between these conditions clinically unless manual correction is

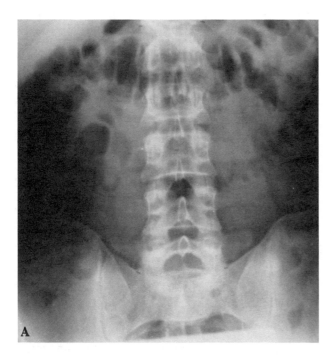
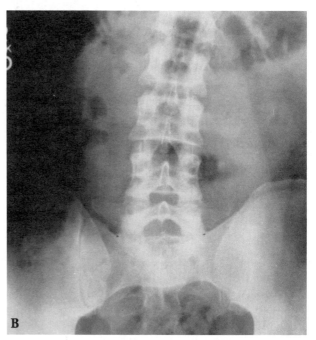

Figure 10-26. Effects of supine left sidebending (A/P view). A) No sidebending; B) Left sidebending. Total vertebral separation from T12 to the sacrum was 7 mm on the right, with an 11 mm narrowing occurring on the left.

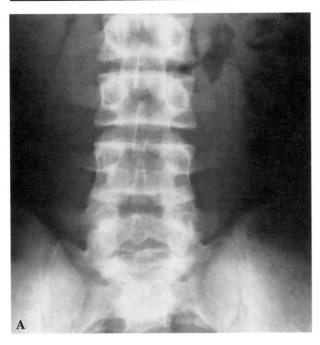 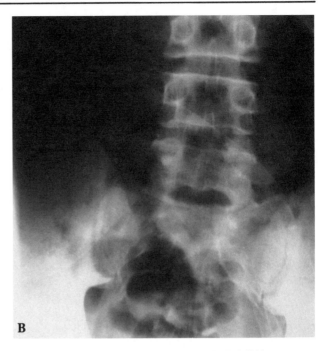

Figure 10-27. A) P/A x-ray showing a narrowed right facet joint and a position change of right rotation at the L5-S1 interspace; B) Intervertebral separation occurring with a 100 pound traction force from the right (reprinted with permission from Saunders [63]).

attempted. When manual correction causes increased peripheral symptoms, one may be dealing with a protective scoliosis and lumbar traction will be more effective if the scoliosis is not disturbed.

To maintain the protective scoliosis for the patient who leans away from the side of the symptoms, the pull should be from the same side as the symptoms. For the patient who leans toward the affected side, the traction pull should be from the side opposite that of the symptoms (Fig 10-28). Therefore, in either case the pull is from the convex side of the lumbar curve.

Unilateral Technique for Lumbar Scoliosis Caused by Muscle Spasm

Unilateral lumbar traction can also effectively in reduce a lumbar scoliosis caused by unilateral paravertebral muscle spasm in the lumbar area. To do this the unilateral pull should be from the concave side of the scoliosis[63] (Fig 10-29).

Three Dimensional Lumbar Traction

Postural changes accompany many of the spinal disorders treated by physical therapists. It is sometimes difficult to determine if the abnormal posture is the result of the pathological disorder, or if the postural change is the cause of the disorder. However, regardless of this relationship, return to normal posture is always one of the treatment goals. For example, the patient

with HNP-protrusion is often seen with a flattened lumbar spine and a lateral scoliosis. One of the goals of treatment should be to return this patient to normal posture. However, this is not always possible in the initial course of treatment. Attempts to straighten the lateral scoliosis or restore the lordosis often cause an increase in the peripheral signs and symptoms and a general worsening of the condition. When this is the case, traction is often the treatment of choice if it can be administered so the patient's flexed and laterally shifted posture is not disturbed. As previously discussed, the initial treatment is often given in the prone position with pillows under the lumbar spine to maintain flexion. The harness strap from the convex side of the scoliosis is hooked to the traction source.

Thus the traction treatment is given without disturbing the patient's postural position. On subsequent treatments, the amount of flexion and the amount of unilateral pull is lessened as the patient is gradually worked back into a normal postural position.

A 3-D table offers an advantage because the table can be positioned initially to accommodate to the patient's abnormal posture. As the traction force is being administered, the table can be adjusted gradually to return the patient toward the normal posture. Thus, the 3-D traction table offers considerable advantage, especially in the ease and convenience of administering treatment (Fig 10-30). The 3-D table shown is the same as the 3-D mobilization table depicted in Chapter 9, Mobilization Techniques. Therefore, the 3-D table

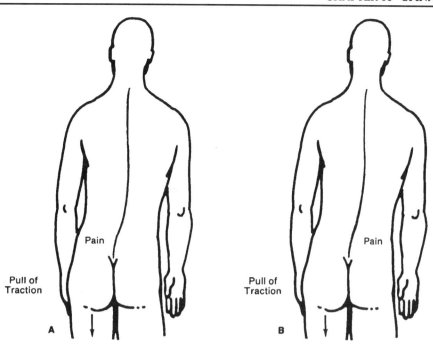

Figure 10-28. A) A patient with a protective scoliosis away from the side of the symptoms; B) A patient with a protective scoliosis toward the side of the symptoms. In both cases, the unilateral pull should be from the convex side of the curve, so that the scoliosis is maintained (adapted from Saunders [63]).

has a variety of uses and the clinician treating spinal patients would be well advised to consider obtaining at least one for use in the clinic. The variety of clinical applications allowed by a 3-D table are limited only by the clinician's imagination.

Home Lumbar Traction

Several types of traction described earlier (90/90, gravity, E-Z Trac™ and Lumba Trac™) can be used for home treatment. Home traction devices are most useful when used as an adjunct treatment for those patients who have had successful treatment with traction in the clinic and those who do not require a high degree of control and specificity of treatment technique. Those patients who require a high degree of control of poundage and positioning are better treated with the mechanical traction systems found in the clinic, at least initially.

TYPES OF CERVICAL TRACTION

Cervical Traction System using a Head Halter

Conventional cervical traction methods use head halters that fit under the chin anteriorly and on the occipital bone posteriorly. During a cervical traction treatment using one of the standard head halters, force is transmitted through the chin strap to the teeth and the temporomandibular joints become weight bearing

structures. A common problem from administering cervical traction is aggravation of the temporomandibular joints because of the force applied at the chin. The exact amount of force on the chin

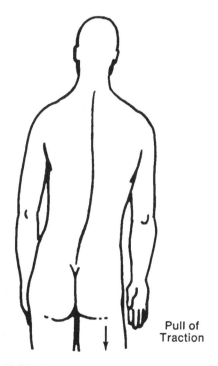

Figure 10-29. A patient with a unilateral muscle spasm causing a lumbar scoliosis. To stretch this condition, the unilateral pull should be from the concave side of the scoliosis (adapted from Saunders [63]).

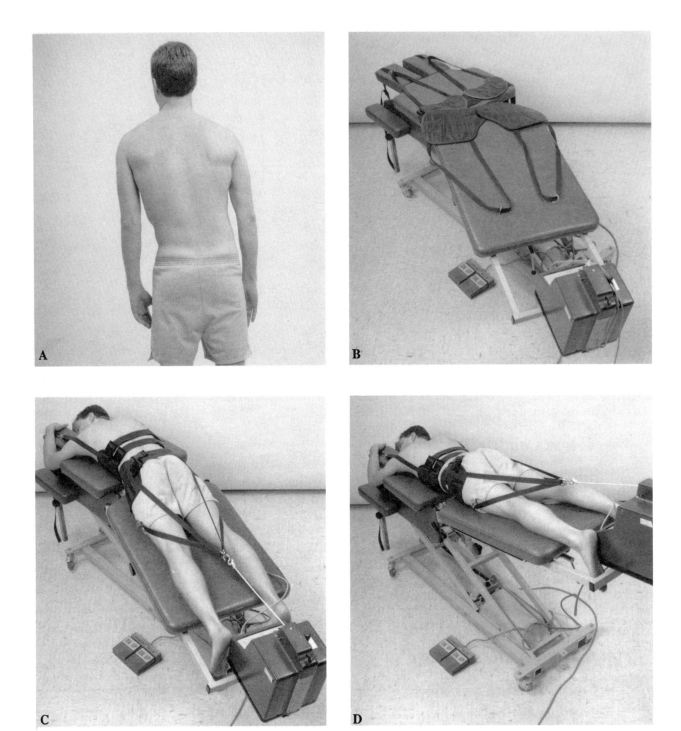

Figure 10-30. Three-dimensional lumbar traction techniques. A, B and C) The table is initially positioned in flexion and left sidebending to accommodate the patient's flattened lumbar lordosis and left lateral shift; D) After a few minutes of traction, the table is positioned in neutral and a bit of right sidebending (mild over-correction). Finally, the table can be extended for even more over-correction. The treatment progression may take place in one treatment or over several sessions, depending upon patient response.

depends upon the design and adjustment of the head halter, the direction (flexion or extension) of the traction force and the amount of the traction force. Some head halters are better than others (Fig 10-31). Nevertheless, even when the utmost care is taken to minimize the force on the chin, there often exists enough force to cause an undesirable effect on the temporomandibular joints.[16]

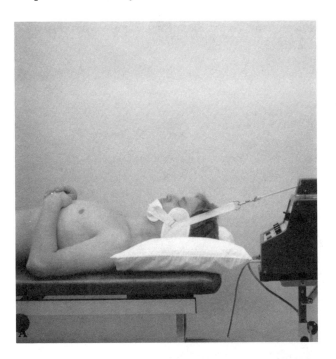

Crisp,[7] and Shore, Frankel and Hoppenfeld,[65] have drawn attention to the fact that during treatment some of the patients experience considerable discomfort in the temporomandibular joints. This is particularly true if an abnormal dental occlusion exists such as the absence of posterior teeth. In some cases, the discomfort is so great that the treatment has to be discontinued. With advancing age, the tissues become more susceptible to disruption and joint trauma which, in some cases, may be irreversible.[65] Franks suggests that cervical traction should be carried out with caution. He reports that, in the older patient particularly, excessive pressure on the jaw can lead to intracapsular bleeding and hematoma in the temporomandibular joint.[17]

The Saunders' Cervical Traction Device™

The cervical traction device shown in Figure 10-32 does not contact the chin or place any force on the temporomandibular joints. The device consists of a shaft that connects to the traction source of a commercial traction table at one end as the other end rests near the head of the traction table. Mounted on this shaft is a friction-free carriage that holds an adjustable V-shaped device. The V-shaped device fits against the back of the patient's neck just below the occipital bone. There is also a small head rest on the

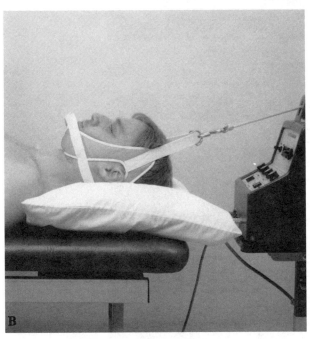

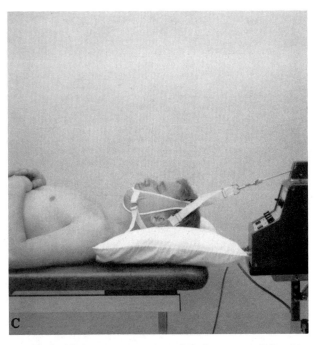

Figure 10-31. Three conventional cervical traction halters. A) Least desirable because more anterior placement of the chin pad causes potential for excess pressure on chin; B) Acceptable because of better force dispersion along the length of the mandible; C) Most desirable because of better force dispersion and its adjustability for use in the clinic (can use it for unilateral traction). For home use, "B" is most desirable because it is less expensive and less confusing for the patient to use.

carriage and a strap that fits over the patient's forehead to hold the patient's head in position as treatment is applied. Treatment is applied with the patient lying supine. This device allows complete control of head and neck positions both in flexion and in extension.

The Saunders Cervical Traction Device™ meets all the general requirements for applying cervical traction. It can be used in the optimal range of head and neck positions with any amount of force and duration (intermittent or sustained). The most favorable patient position (supine) is used and the chin and temporomandibular joints are not encroached upon.

Manual Cervical Traction

Cyriax advocates manual cervical traction and estimates that he exerts forces as high as 200 lb.[9] He often incorporates passive range of motion with the manual traction (Fig 10-33). Inhibitive manual traction is a technique used by Paris that has a beneficial relaxing effect as well as a tractive force[56] (Fig 10-34). Manual traction and inhibitive manual traction are described in greater detail in Chapter 9, <u>Mobilization Techniques</u>.

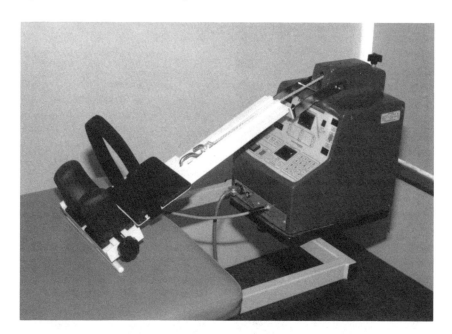

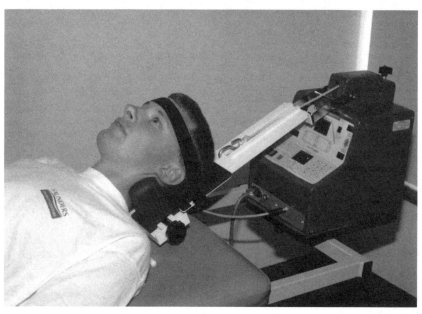

Figure 10-32. The Saunders' Cervical Traction Device. This device does not contact the mandible at all, thus eliminating the main problem associated with conventional cervical traction halters.

Unilateral Cervical Traction

Unilateral cervical traction can be incorporated if the therapist wants to direct a stronger force to one side of the cervical spine, or to maintain a protective scoliosis (see discussion under "Unilateral Lumbar Traction"). When using unilateral cervical traction, a stabilization strap must be used over the patient's chest. Otherwise, the patient will align himself with the angle of the rope and the unilateral effect will be lost (Fig 10-35). A unilateral effect may also be achieved by shortening only one of the two straps that attach the head halter to the traction source. Unilateral traction is achieved with the Saunders' Cervical Traction Device™ and the Saunders Cervical Hometrac™ by aligning the patient's body (trunk) at an angle to the direction of pull of the device (Fig. 10-35).

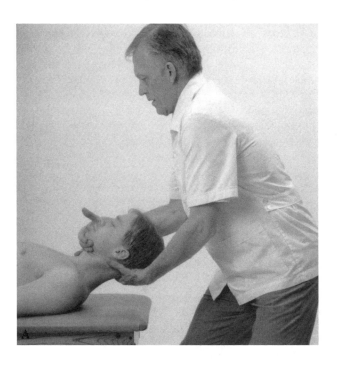

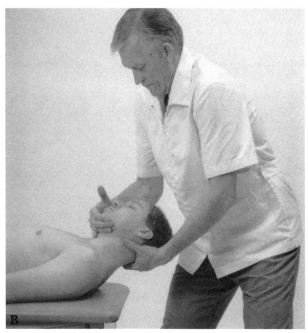

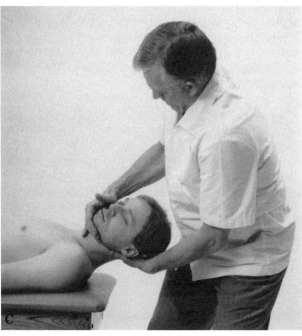

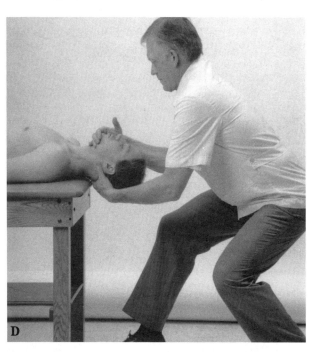

Figure 10-33. Manual cervical traction techniques. A) Traction with a straight pull; B) Traction with cervical sidebending; C) Traction with cervical rotation; D) Traction with cervical extension.

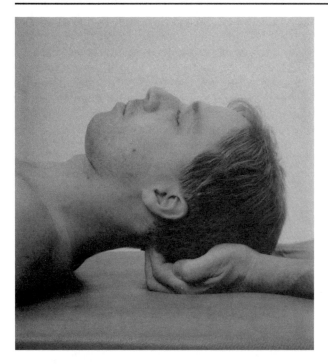

Figure 10-34. Inhibitive manual traction (occipital release).

Home Cervical Traction

Home cervical traction can be administered with either the head halter method, the Saunders Cervical Hometrac™ (Fig. 10-36), or the Saunders' Cervical Traction Device™. Since supine cervical traction has been shown to be much more effective than sitting, the commonly used over-the-door head halter method of home cervical traction is not recommended. If a head halter with rope, pulley and hanging weights is to be used, a system that allows the patient to lie in a supine position is preferred (Fig 10-37). The head halter system does require some physical agility to apply to one's self and some patients may require help using it at home. It also can apply excessive pressure to the TMJ, as mentioned earlier. The C-Trac™ device shown in Figure 10-38 can be used with a head halter or the Saunders' Cervical Traction Device™. The Saunders Cervical Hometrac™ and the C-Trac™ can be used in the clinic as well as at home.

CERVICAL TRACTION TECHNIQUE

Many of the considerations for lumbar traction technique are equally appropriate for cervical traction. In addition, the following points are essential:

1. The first question that should be resolved concerning cervical traction technique is seated versus supine positioning. Although both positions are commonly used, research reveals that the supine position is superior.[6, 13, 22] It is also of interest that some researchers have found compression or narrowing of the joint space with application of cervical traction. This narrowing is often attributed to muscle guarding and to the patient's inability to relax during traction. These findings are most common when patients are seated.[13]

2. Colachis and Strohm have demonstrated a relationship between separation of the vertebral bodies and the angle of pull. They studied angles of pull at 6°, 20°, 24° and found that as the angle was increased, the posterior separation of the cervical vertebræ also increased.[6] One must not forget, however, that the space available for the spinal nerve in the intervertebral foramen decreases with flexion beyond the neutral or straight position of the spine.[41] Therefore, if opening of the intervertebral foramen or mobilization of the posterior cervical structures is the desired effect, the most advantageous position for cervical traction is flexion of the cervical spine to 25-30°. This position effectively straightens the normal lordosis but does not go beyond that point. However, if greater separation is desired at the intervertebral disc space or if one is using traction to mobilize to improve cervical extension and/or axial extension (the head back, chin in posture), any amount of flexion would render the treatment less effective.

3. The angle of the rope to the table is not the only factor influencing the amount of flexion or extension administered. In fact, it is probably less important than the choice of head halters or cervical traction devices. If a poorly adjusted or constructed head halter is used, a different degree of flexion may be effected even if the angle of the rope to the table is within the recommended limits.[63] Many head halters are available. The most satisfactory seem to be those that position the head and upper cervical spine in a neutral or flexed position, enabling the pull to be exerted more at the occiput than at the chin (Figs 10-31 and 10-32). This is more comfortable for the patient and also exerts a force directly in line with the cervical spine. It is our experience that most patients are more restricted in cervical flexion in the upper cervical area and they lack extension mobility in the lower cervical/upper thoracic region. For these patients, a head halter/traction device that flexes the head and upper cervical spine and at the same time pulls from a relatively straight angle (to extend the lower cervical/upper thoracic) is ideal.

4. Judovich[27] found that 25-45 lb forces were necessary to demonstrate a measurable change in the posterior cervical spine structures. Jackson[26] confirmed this finding. In another comprehensive work, Colachis and Strohm[6] demonstrated that a tractive force of 30 lb produces separation of the cervical spine. A search of the literature disclosed no evidence of separation

occurring at lesser forces in the mid and lower cervical spine. Weights of 25-40 lb, therefore, appear necessary to produce vertebral separation. Daugherty and Erhard[11] demonstrated separation of the atlanto/occipital and atlanto/axial joints with 10 lb of traction. Therefore, it appears that less force is necessary when treatment is directed to the upper cervical area.

5. Research has been done concerning the forces necessary to cause damage to the cervical structures. Using fresh cadavers, Ranier[14] found that a tractive force of 120 lb was necessary to cause a disc rupture at the C5-C6 level.

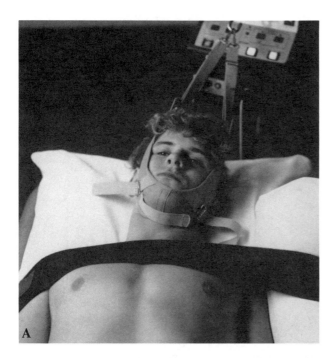

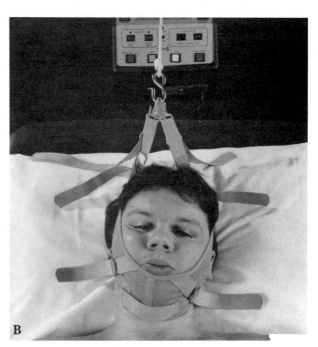

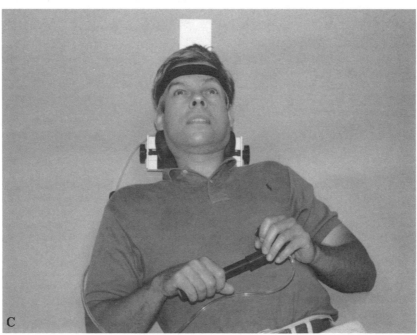

Figure 10-35. Unilateral cervical traction - right sided pull. A) Note the rolled pillow and strap to prevent the patient's body from sliding; B) The right side halter strap is shorter than the left; C) Unilateral cervical traction may be achieved with the Saunders Cervical Traction Device™ and the Saunders Cervical Hometrac™ by aligning the patient's body (trunk) at an angle to the direction of pull of the device.

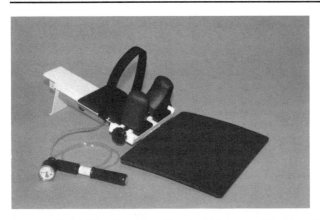

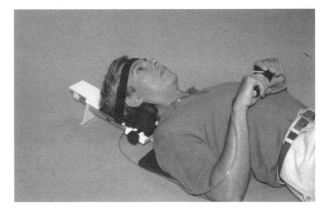

Figure 10-36. The Saunders Cervical Hometrac™ offers the same benefits as the Saunders Cervical Tracton Device™ in a portable model that can be used by the patient at home. Cervical traction forces of up to 50 lb may be achieved to provide either intermittent or sustained traction.

6. When receiving traction treatments, the patient must feel secure and be able to relax. The force of the traction must not cause so much pain that the patient cannot relax. The use of modalities before the traction treatment may help. Patient comfort should be considered when choosing between intermittent or sustained (static) cervical traction since either can be effective. For herniated discs, sustained traction or intermittent traction with a longer hold period (60 second hold, 10 second rest) is usually preferred.

7. Treatment time should be relatively short (five to ten minutes) when treating HNP. Times can be increased slightly for other conditions. Patient comfort should always be of primary consideration when determining duration of the treatment.

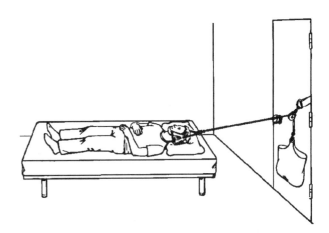

Figure 10-37. Supine home cervical traction device.

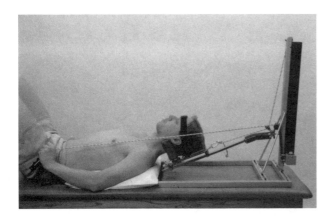

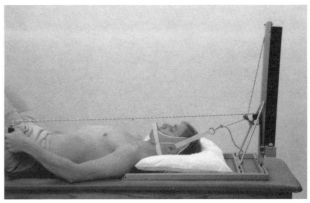

Figure 10-38. C-Trac™ cervical traction.

REFERENCES

1. Bigos S and Battie M: Acute Care to Prevent Back Disability: Ten Years of Progress. Clin Orthop and Rel Res 221:121-130, Aug 1987.

2. Brodin H, et al: Manipulation av Ryggraden. Scandinavicen University Books, 1966.

3. Brodin H: Manueli Medicine ooh Manipulation. Lakartidningen 63:1037-1038, 1966.

4. Burton C: Low Back Pain, 2nd Edition. Lippincott, Philadelphia PA 1980.

5. Christy B: Discussion on the Treatment of Backache by Traction. Proc R Soc Med 48:811, 1955.

6. Colachis S and Strohm M: Cervical Traction. Arch Phys Med 46:815, 1965.

7. Crisp E: Disc Lesions. Livingstone, Edinburgh 1960.

8. Crisp E: Discussion on the Treatment of Backache by Traction. Proc R Soc Med 48:805, 1955.

9. Cyriax J: The Treatment of Lumbar Disk Lesions. Brit Med Joul 2:14-34, 1950.

10. Cyriax J:Treatment by Manipulation. Massage and Injection. Textbook of Orthopaedic Medicine, Vol 2, 10th edition. Bailliere-Tindall, London 1980.

11. Daugherty R and Erhard R: Segmentalized Cervical Traction. Proceedings, International Federation of Orthopaedic Manipulative Therapists. B Kent, ed. pp. 189-195. Vail CO 1977.

12. De Lacerda F: Effect of Angle of Traction Pull on Upper Trapezius Muscle Activity. J Orth Spts Phy Ther 1: 205-209, 1980.

13. Deets D, Hands K and Hopp S: Cervical Traction: A Comparison of Sitting and Supine Positions. Phys Ther 57:255, 1977.

14. DeSeze S and Levernieux J: Les Tractions Vertebrales. Sem Hop Paris 27:2075, 1951.

15. Finneson B: Low Back Pain. JB Lippincott, Philadelphia PA 1973.

16. Frankel V, Shore N and Hoppenfeld S: Stress Distribution in Cervical Traction Prevention of Temporomandibular Joint Pain Syndrome. Clin Orth 32:114-115, 1964.

17. Franks A: Temporomandibular Joint Dysfunction Associated with Cervical Traction. Ann Phys Med 8:38-40, 1967.

18. Frazer E: The Use of Traction in Backache. Med J Aust 2:694, 1954.

19. Gall E: Lumbar Spine X-rays - What Can They Reveal? Occ Health and Safety 48:32-35, 1979.

20. Goldish G: Lumbar Traction. In Interdisciplinary Rehabilitation of Low Back Pain. CD Tollison and M Kriegel, eds. Williams and Wilkins, Baltimore MD 1989.

21. Gupta R and Ramarao S: Epidurography in Reduction of Lumbar Disc Prolapse by Traction. Arch Phys Med Rehabil 59:322-327, 1978.

22. Harris P: Cervical Traction: Review of Literature and Treatment Guidelines. Phys Ther 57:910, 1977.

23. Harris R: Massage, Manipulation and Traction. E. Licht, New Haven CT 1960.

24. Hickling J: Spinal Traction Technique. Physiotherapy 58:58, 1972.

25. Hood L and Chrisman D: Intermittent Pelvic Traction in the Treatment of the Ruptured Intervertebral Disc. J Am Phys Ther Assoc 48:21-30, 1968.

26. Jackson B: The Cervical Syndrome. Charles C Thomas, Springfield MO 1958.

27. Judovich B: Herniated Cervical Disc. Am J Surg 84:649, 1952.

28. Judovich B: Lumbar Traction Therapy. JAMA 159:549, 1955.

29. Kaltenborn F: Proceedings of the International Federation of Orthopaedic Manipulative Therapists. B Kent, ed. Vail CO 1977

30. Kane M: Effects of Gravity Facilitated Traction on Intervertebral Dimensions of the Lumbar Spine. Master's Thesis, U.S. Army-Baylor University Program in Physical Therapy, Academy of Health Sciences, Fort Sam Houston TX 1983.

31. Kapandji I: Spine. Vol 3 of The Physiology of the Joints, 2nd edition. Churchill-Livingstone, London-New York 1974.

32. Kraft G and Levinthal D: Facet Synovial Impingement. Surg Gynecol and Obstet 93:439-443, 1951.

33. Larsson V, et al: Auto-Traction for Treatment of Lumbago-Sciatica. Acta Orthop Scand 51:791, 1980.

34. Lawson G and Godfrey C: A Report on Studies of Spinal Traction. Med Serv J Can 12:762, 1958.

35. LeMarr J, Golding L and Crehan K: Cardiorespiratory Responses to Inversion. Phys Sportsmed 11:51-57, 1983.

36. Lind G: Auto-Traction: Treatment of Low Back Pain and Sciatica. Thesis, University of Linkoping, 1974.

37. Lindstrom A and Zachrisson, M: Physical Therapy on Low Back Pain and Sciatica: An Attempt at Evaluation. Scand J Rehabil Med 2:37, 1970.

38. Magora A and Schwartz A: Relation Between Low Back Pain and X-ray Changes IV: Lysis and Olisthesis. Scand J Rehabil Med 12:47-52, 1980.

39. Magora A and Schwartz A: Relation Between the Low Back Pain and X-ray Findings II: Transitional Vertebra (Mainly Sacralization). Scand J Rehabil Med 10:135-145, 1978.

40. Magora A and Schwartz A: Relation Between the Low Back Pain Syndrome and X-ray Findings I: Degenerative Findings. Scand J Rehabil Med 8:115-126, 1976.

41. Maslow G and Rothman R: The Facet Joints, Another Look. Bul NY Acac Med 51:1294-1311, 1975.

42. Masturzo A: Vertebral Traction for Sciatica. Rheumatism 11:62, 1955.

43. Mathews J and Heckling H: Lumbar Traction: A Double Blind Controlled Study for Sciatica. Rheumatol Rehabil 14:222, 1975.

44. Mathews J: Dynamic Discography; A Study of Lumbar Traction. Ann Phy Med 9:275-279, 1968.

45. Mathews J: The Effects of Spinal Traction. Physiotherapy 58:64-66, 1972.

46. McKenzie R: The Lumbar Spine. Spinal Publications, Waikanae New Zealand 1981.

47. Morris J, Lucas D and Bresler M: Role of the Trunk in Stability of the Spine. J Bone and Joint Surg 43A:327-351, 1961.

48. Nachemson A and Elfstom G: Intravital Dynamic Pressure Measurements in the Lumbar Discs. Scand J Rehabil Med (Suppl 1): 1, 1970.

49. Nachemson A and Morris J: In Vivo Measurements of Intradiscal Pressure. J Bone Joint Surg 46A: 1077-1092, 1964.

50. Nachemson A: The Lumbar Spine, An Orthopædic Challenge. Spine 1:50-71, 1976.

51. Natchev E: A Manual on Auto-Traction Treatment for Low Back Pain. Folksam Stockholm Sweden 1984.

52. Nosse L: Inverted Spinal Traction. Arch Phys Med Rehabil 59:367, 1978.

53. Onel D, et al: Computed Tomographic Investigation of the Effect of Traction on Lumbar Disc Herniations. Spine 14(1):82-90, 1989.

54. Oudenhoven T: Gravitational Lumbar Traction. Arch Phys Med 59:510, 1978.

55. Pal B, et al: A Controlled Trial of Continuous Lumbar Traction in Back Pain and Sciatica. Br J Rheumatol 25:181-183, 1986.

56. Paris S: The Spine. Atlanta Back Clinic. Atlanta GA 1976. Course Notes.

57. Parson W and Cummings J: Mechanical Traction in the Lumbar Disc Syndrome. Can Med Assoc Joul 77:7-11, 1957.

58. Petulla L: Clinical Observations With Respect to Progressive-Regressive Traction (Unpublished Article). Los Gatos, California 1983.

59. Quebec Task Force Study: Scientific Approach to the Assessment and Management of Activity Related Spinal Disorders. Spine 12:7S, 1987.

60. Saunders H: Lumbar Traction. J Orthop Sports Phys Ther 1:36, 1979.

61. Saunders H: Spinal Traction: A Continuing Education Module for Physical Therapists. University of Kansas, Independent Study, Division of Continuing Education, 1979.

62. Saunders H: The Use of Spinal Traction in the Treatment of Neck and Back Conditions. Clin Orthop and Rel Res 179: 31-38, Oct 1983.

63. Saunders H: Unilateral Lumbar Traction. Phys Ther 61:221-225, Feb 1981.

64. Shah J: Shift of Nuclear Material With Flexion and Extension of the Spine. In The Lumbar Spine and Low Back Pain. M Jayson, ed. Pitman Medical, London 1980.

65. Shore N, Frankel V and Hoppenfeld S: Cervical Traction and Temporomandibular Joint Dysfunction. Joul Am Dental Assoc 68(1):4-6, 1964.

66. Waitz E: The Lateral Bending Sign. Spine 6:388-397, 1981.

67. Weber H: Traction Therapy in Sciatica Due to Disc Prolapse. J Oslo City Hosp 23(10): 167-176, 1973.

68. Weisel S et al: A Study of Computer-Assisted Tomography - The Incidence of Positive CAT Scans in an Asymptomatic Group of Patients. Spine 9(6):549-551, 1984.

69. Witt I, et al: A Comparative Analysis of X-ray Findings of the Lumbar Spine in Patients With and Without Lumbar Pain. Spine 9:298-299, 1984.

70. Yates D: Indications and Contraindications for Spinal Traction. Physiotherapy 58:55, 1972.

CHAPTER 11

SPINAL ORTHOSES

INTRODUCTION

Many health care practitioners believe spinal supports and braces can be used effectively in treatment and prevention of musculoskeletal disorders.

Ninety-nine percent of 3,410 orthopædic surgeons surveyed in the United States reported prescribing spinal orthoses.[17] While there is no hard scientific evidence of the clinical effectiveness of lumbosacral supports and braces as a group, retrospective studies have documented acceptance by patients and improvement of symptoms in 30-80% of cases.[1, 11, 15]

Medical and industrial health and safety literature is filled with the pros and cons of using spinal supports and braces. Certain facts about the effects of spinal supports and braces have been known for many years while certain other effects remain unclear. We have not made many recent discoveries about the effects of spinal supports but we have seen a renewed interest in their use. The lower lumbar region is of particular interest because most back disorders occur in one or both of the lower two segments. This renewed interest seems to focus on prevention as well as treatment, and is especially evident in business and industry.

There seems to be an increased awareness and evidence of back injuries in sports. This also has created interest in use of lumbosacral supports and has led to development of new back supports, ideas and designs.

Perhaps another reason for the renewed interest in back supports and braces has to do with the recent changes in attitudes toward the treatment of musculoskeletal disorders. Most experts now agree that almost all back disorders can be treated most effectively by early intervention with exercise and patient education. We no longer tell patients to rest, take it easy, and wait until they are completely free of pain before starting exercises and activities. Many practitioners recognize that placing a support on patients often helps them return to full function sooner and avoid the well-documented harmful effects of prolonged immobilization and inactivity.[8, 10]

Physical therapists play an important role in determining the need for and selection and fitting of spinal braces and supports. This chapter will:

1. Discuss the effects of spinal braces and supports commonly used for the treatment of musculoskeletal disorders

2. Review the indications for spinal bracing

3. Review the types of spinal braces and supports

4. Discuss fitting procedures

5. Discuss total management of the patient using a spinal brace or support

Spinal orthoses can be grouped into three major categories: *corrective, supportive and immobilizing.* Corrective braces are used in the treatment of disorders such as idiopathic scoliosis and kyphosis and will not be considered here. This chapter will instead direct attention to the spinal braces and supports providing support and/or immobilization for conditions commonly seen by the physical therapist. The types of spinal orthoses discussed are lumbosacral corsets; chairback braces; Williams braces; sacroiliac belts; dorsal-lumbar corsets; Taylor™ braces; Knight-Taylor™ braces; hyperextension braces; the Saunders S'port All™ and Work S'Port™ back supports; soft cervical collars; hard cervical collars; Philadelphia collars; and two and four poster cervical braces.

EFFECTS OF SPINAL SUPPORTS AND BRACES

A review of the literature reveals the following effects of various spinal supports and braces:

1. Immobilization of the sacroiliac joints

2. Immobilization of the intervertebral joints

3. Increased motion of intervertebral joints adjacent to those that are immobilized

4. Transfer of part of the vertical load from the spine to other structures

5. Increase in intra-abdominal pressure (lumbar supports)

6. Decrease in intradiscal pressure

7. Decrease of venous return from the lower extremities (lumbar supports)

8. Control of lordosis or kyphosis

9. An awareness of correct posture

10. A placebo (psychological) effect for the user

11. Decrease of abdominal and/or spinal muscular activity

12. Increase of spinal muscular activity

Cervical Spine

There have been relatively few quantitative evaluations of the effects of cervical orthoses. Colachis and associates found that the soft collar did little to limit cervical motion and that the more rigid plastic collars were only somewhat more effective.[4] Johnson and associates found that, in general, increasing the length and rigidity of a cervical orthosis improved its ability to restrict motion.[9] However, lateral bending and rotation throughout the cervical spine and flexion-extension at the upper levels were not well controlled by any of the conventional orthoses.

The goals of cervical bracing vary according to the patient's problem. Certain cervical muscle and joint injuries may only require gentle support to remind the patient to restrict neck motion or to maintain proper posture. A flexible collar should satisfy these goals. A more rigid orthosis may be necessary to actually limit cervical motion. No orthosis, including the halo with skeletal fixation, restricts all motion.

Another function of cervical collars and braces is to transfer the weight of the head to the shoulders, thus unloading the cervical spine. Although no scientific study supports such an effect, clinical experience indicates that collars and braces that lift under the mandible and occiput do accomplish this task.

Thoracolumbosacral Spine

Back supports and braces have been used for the treatment and prevention of problems in the thoracolumbosacral spine for years. Proponents have cited the following reasons for their use:

1. Physically Restrict Motion or Movement. The ability of spinal braces to immobilize thoracolumbosacral rotation, flexion and extension has been studied extensively. Norton and Brown showed that lumbar flexion-extension was reduced but not eliminated by many of the braces that they studied. In many cases, however, they found increased motion toward the upper and lower margins of the braces they tested. Braces such as the chairback provided immobilization in the upper lumbar and lower thoracic spine, but considerable increase of lower lumbar movement resulted.[16]

According to Wasserman and McNamee, adequate fixation of the pelvis is essential to achieve restriction of motion in the lower lumbar region. However, they did find a 50% reduction in rotation at regions in the center of the garments they tested.[22]

For a back brace to physically restrict movement in the lumbosacral area effectively, it would have to be rigid and attach so it would immobilize the pelvis and the lumbar spine. Attempts to secure rigid back braces to the pelvis to immobilize the lumbosacral joint have generally proven impractical or uncomfortable. Thus, it appears that bracing can restrict movements in the thoracolumbar area effectively. However, in the lumbosacral area, physical restriction of movement may not be possible.

2. Serve as a Reminder to Avoid Undesirable Movements. If a back support or brace effectively limits movement in the lower lumbar spine, it is probably because it serves as a reminder that certain

movements, such as forward bending and twisting, are to be restricted. Many individuals report that their back supports help them remember to use good body mechanics. Thus, a properly fitted back support may help individuals avoid certain movements if they are properly educated and motivated about the support's purpose and function.

3   Help Individuals Achieve Proper Posture. One of the greatest benefits of a properly fitted back support may be the proprioceptive feedback it provides. Wearing a back support increases awareness of the position of the pelvis and lumbar spine. This constant awareness of body position makes it easier for the wearer to avoid undesirable postures.

4.   Increase Intra-Abdominal Pressure Which Decreases the Weight Bearing Load on the Spine. According to Morris, Lucas and Bresler, the action of the trunk muscles converts the abdominal and thoracic cavities into nearly rigid-walled cylinders.[12] Both cylinders are capable of transmitting part of the forces generated in loading the trunk and thereby of relieving the load on the spine itself. Generalized contraction of the trunk muscles, including the intercostals, the abdominals and the diaphragm, occurs when lifting weights of 100-200 pounds. The relatively simple mechanism of an upward push on the diaphragm by increased intra-abdominal pressure reduces the force on the spine. They found that an inflatable corset raised the standing and sitting intra-abdominal pressure by 25% but did not change the maximum pressure that was produced during heavy lifting. However, the activity of the abdominal muscles was markedly decreased when the inflatable corset was worn. They concluded that either the contracted muscles of the abdominal wall or the external pressure of the corset could act to contain the abdominal contents in a compressed state capable of transmitting the weight bearing force.

Nachemson and Morris studied the effect of an inflatable lumbar corset on intradiscal pressure. In all cases studied, there was a considerable (15-28%) decrease in the total load on the disc studied.[14]

In another study, Nachemson, Schultz and Andersson found that wearing a lumbar brace significantly unloads the spine in some situations, but has no effect in others. Lumbar spine compression was reduced by about one-third in a task involving trunk flexion.[15]

The implication is that a support may effectively unload the spine during certain activities but that an individual can create the same unloading effect through the contraction of the abdominal muscles that naturally occurs during heavy lifting activities. Thus, the greatest benefit of the support may be derived from the relatively constant unloading of the spine during normal activities. However, the unloading effect on the spine is not necessarily an added protection at all times during all activities.

Since almost all back disorders are the result of cumulative injury that results from even subtle activities like sitting or standing stooped for long periods of time, one would conclude that this relatively constant unloading is of great benefit. Even when individuals are active, such as when playing racquetball or basketball, they will not be contracting the abdominal muscles constantly. Therefore, it makes sense that a back support can help the abdominal muscles provide support.

5.   Stabilize the Pelvis and Lower Spine. By increasing intra-abdominal pressure, a back support effectively acts like the stays and support rings of a barrel. If the support rings are tightened and/or strengthened, the barrel is stabilized. When one tightens or contracts the abdominal, trunk and pelvic muscles, the spine is stabilized. A properly fit lumbar support, capable of increasing intra-abdominal pressure, acts in the same way.

In Summary

1.   Back supports have not been shown to physically immobilize the lower lumbar spine effectively.

2.   Back supports may provide proprioceptive feedback to remind individuals to use proper body mechanics and posture.

3.   There is evidence to support the concept that a properly fit back support will increase intra-abdominal pressure which, in turn, decreases vertical loading on the spine.

4.   The circumferential pressure of a back support provides a stabilizing effect on the pelvis and spine. While this stabilizing effect cannot be measured, clinical experience tells us that this is often the word that patients use to describe the effect of a back support.

There are critics of back supports. Some believe that the use of back supports, at least over long periods of time, will create dependency and weaken the abdominal muscles.[19] At least one study shows that with a back support the abdominal muscles are in a more relaxed state.[12] However, studies done to measure the effect of back supports on back and abdominal muscle strength show there is no weakening effect.[13, 20, 21]

Proponents argue that a properly fit back support may actually have a strengthening effect in some cases. If a support decreases pain and helps patients achieve proper posture and avoid potentially harmful movements, they may recover faster and become active sooner. The activity will actually strengthen the muscles instead of weakening them.[6, 10, 14]

The inability of back supports to stay in proper position has long been a criticism of lumbosacral supports and braces in general. If the back support rides up above the iliac crests, the lumbosacral area (where most back problems occur) may not be supported sufficiently. While the problem of a support or brace riding up may not be significant when an individual is relatively inactive, it often becomes a problem during recovery as the patient becomes more physically active. It is also a problem if a back support is to be used effectively as a preventive method in an active individual. A recent innovation involving attachment of a back support to a pair of elastic athletic shorts effectively solves this problem. This concept will be discussed in greater detail later in the section discussing the different types of lumbosacral supports and braces.

Sacroiliac Joints

Sacroiliac belts or supports serve to immobilize the sacroiliac joints by circumferential pressure around the pelvis. Most sacroiliac supports have a sacral pad that presses against the posterior sacrum to add further immobilization and proprioceptive input. The only effect of a sacroiliac support is immobilization and proprioceptive input, which can lessen symptoms.

INDICATIONS FOR SPINAL BRACING

In general, any patient with a musculoskeletal disorder who might benefit from immobilization, unloading of compressing forces on the spine and/or postural correction may be a suitable candidate for a spinal support or brace.

Perry found that opinion among orthopædic surgeons was divided concerning indications for braces, but that the majority of orthopædists did prescribe a support for treatment of post-operative fusions, spondylolisthesis and pseudoarthrosis.[17] The chairback brace was the most commonly prescribed device for these conditions. Interestingly, less than 25% of the orthopædists surveyed prescribed supports

for acute strain, post-operative discs, disc syndromes and chronic situations, with the lumbosacral corset being the device most often prescribed by this group.

Pain, Muscle Guarding and Spasm

The unloading/stabilizing and proprioceptive effects that a back support offers may alleviate pain effectively which, in turn, will reduce muscle guarding and spasm.

Acute Sprains and Strains

It seems reasonable that acute sprains and strains need protection from undesirable movements and activities and that proper posture must be achieved for normal healing to take place. At the same time we know that some activity is desirable to maintain strength and fitness and that the healing process is actually stimulated by careful movement and activity. The unloading/stabilizing effect the back support provides may also relieve the patient's pain. This, along with the proprioceptive feedback that helps the patient achieve proper posture and body mechanics, may allow safe movement and activity sooner than would be possible without the support. Since healing time with soft tissue injuries is relatively short, the use of supports with acute sprains and strains should be of short duration. Usually, a week or so is sufficient; certainly six to eight weeks is the longest treatment time, even in the most severe cases.

Post-Surgical Fusion, Laminectomy and Discectomy

Most orthopædic surgeons prescribe a support such as a lumbosacral corset or chairback brace for lumbar fusions and laminectomies, and a cervical support such as a soft collar, Philadelphia collar or four poster brace for cervical fusions and laminectomies. It is less common to use them following discectomies. The goal with such supports is to immobilize the area, thus relieving pain, and to remind the patient to restrict movement while allowing early ambulation and activities. Such supports are normally used for short periods of a few days to a few weeks.

Congenital or Traumatic Joint Instability

Congenital defects and severe injuries resulting in spinal joint instability may be a source of constant aggravation for the patient who attempts to lead an active life. In such cases, a back support or brace may let the patient participate in a vocation or in activities that otherwise would result in chronic pain and discomfort. Patients should be advised to use such support only when they need the protection. It is also wise for these patients to exercise regularly to maintain adequate strength of the spinal and abdominal muscles. One should also remember that it is not always possible to cause an immobilizing effect when the patient is doing full, normal activities. This is especially true in the lower lumbar and upper cervical spine. Again, the beneficial effect of the support is probably due to the unloading/stabilizing effect and the reminder to use good posture and body mechanics, and not to an actual restriction of movement.

If a spondylolisthesis is unstable, it can be a constant source of aggravation. Spondylolisthesis is frequently associated with hyperlordosis of the lumbar spine. In a hyperlordotic state, the shear forces between the two segments that are slipping apart are greatly magnified. Reduction of the hyperlordosis can reduce the shear forces. These cases can often be managed effectively with a support that lifts the abdomen upward and posteriorly. This moves the center of gravity posteriorly and reduces hyperlordosis.

Preteen children who participate in sports that require excessive lumbar lordosis (i.e., gymnastics) and teenagers who participate in contact sports are more frequently found to have spondylolysis.[6, 7] Such patients can be treated with a brace that maintains the spine in lumbar flexion during the healing phase, or provides pain relief.

Herniated Nucleus Pulposus-Protrusion

Herniated nucleus pulposus-protrusion is characterized by a bulging defect caused as the nuclear gel pushes against the outer rings of the annulus. Treatment is directed toward reducing those factors that increase the compression load on the disc. Spinal supports have been shown to reduce the intradiscal pressure in the lumbar disc by 25-35% in both the sitting and standing positions. Rotation and forward bending also increase intradiscal pressure and spinal bracing can help restrict these movements. Furthermore, a spinal support can remind the patient to avoid these movements and to maintain correct posture (lumbar lordosis) during recovery.

Cervical supports may also unload the disc by transferring the weight of the head onto the shoulders, but scientific research is unable to substantiate such claims. Such supports are sometimes help maintain the proper head and neck posture required during recovery of herniated disc syndrome.

Postural Backache (Lumbar Hyperlordosis)

Postural backache caused by weak abdominal muscles and excessive lumbar lordosis is probably most effectively treated with postural correction and abdominal strengthening exercises. Extreme cases may require a lumbosacral support, chairback brace or a Williams brace. When a support or brace is prescribed, it should be accompanied by an exercise program.

Fractures

Various types of fractures of the spine are often treated with braces or supports. In any case requiring immobilization and/or unloading of the spine, bracing may be considered. It must be remembered that conventional lumbar and cervical orthoses do not completely immobilize the spine. Even the halo with a plastic body vest does not totally restrict cervical movement. In general, the upper cervical and lower lumbar spine are the most difficult to immobilize and fractures in these areas will be the most difficult to support with bracing. It is common to use bracing for support of fracture after some healing has taken place and restricted movement is allowed. The fact that the brace reminds patients to restrict movement and maintain correct posture is often beneficial.

Compression fractures occurring in the upper lumbar and lower and mid-thoracic spine are often treated with braces. The goal of a bracing program for compression fractures is to keep the injured part of the spine in extension and to prevent flexion, thus keeping the vertebral body space as wide as possible and allow the vertebral body to heal with as much height as possible. The Jewett™ and Cash™ hyperextension braces are probably the most commonly used braces for treatment of compression fractures. Their sole function is to prevent flexion of the upper lumbar, lower and mid-thoracic spine and to remind the patient to maintain an extended posture.

While the hyperextension braces treat compression fractures effectively, it has been our experience that some patients (especially geriatric) cannot tolerate their rigid natures. In such cases, a Taylor™ brace or dorsal-lumbar corset may be a reasonable alternative. They offer less rigid support, but at least they offer some support and serve as reminders to the patient to avoid flexion. An added benefit of either of these supports is that they decrease the vertical weight bearing force on the spine by increasing the intra-abdominal pressure. The hyperextension braces do not provide this effect.

Since the majority of compression fractures occur in geriatric females and are associated with severe osteoporosis, these supports may be used as a part of a preventive program, too. Active extension exercises should be performed concurrently to enhance muscle strengthening, improved posture and prevent the trunk musculature deconditioning that is apt to occur when a sedentary person uses a back support. If the patient is instructed to avoid slumping into the brace and to maintain correct posture while in the brace, the patient may actually strengthen the postural muscles. For example, the shoulder straps of a Taylor™ or dorsal-lumbar corset should act as reminders to the patient to hold herself in correct posture. Their function is not to pull the shoulders back and hold the patient straighter. Likewise, the lordotic curve in a chairback brace is a reminder for the patient to stand and sit while actively maintaining the lordosis. This concept of "active bracing" is what the Milwaukee brace uses in the treatment of scoliosis. Patient education and compliance are the keys to appropriate use of bracing to prevent compression fractures.

Degenerative Joint/Disc Disease

Degenerative joint and/or disc disease is usually associated with soft tissue hypomobility (stiffness). Treatment for hypomobility of the spine should be directed toward mobilizing the restricted joints and tight muscles. In some cases, however, any mobilizing activity may tend to aggravate rather than relieve the pain and discomfort. The patient will report that any attempt to increase activities is accompanied by another flare up. In such cases, a support may at least allow the patient to participate in activities that would otherwise be too aggravating. On the other hand, degenerative joint/disc disease is sometimes associated with spinal segment hypermobility (instability). Spinal segment instabilities often respond favorably to treatment with a spinal support.

Prevention

Walsh and Schwartz reported substantially less lost time from work due to back injury after employees attended back school and wore a back support.[21] There was a statistically significant difference compared to control groups having either back school only or no intervention at all. Numerous businesses have reported considerable reductions in workers' compensation costs after implementation of back injury prevention programs that involved the use of back supports and lifting belts. While these reports are not comparative scientific studies, they do attract our attention and do merit consideration. We found 12 unpublished reports of businesses who claimed to have reduced workers' compensation with programs that, at least in part, used industrial back supports:

- Support Belts Can Bolster Prevention Programs. In Back Pain Monitor™ Edited by Debra Golden 9(4): 49-64, 1991 (Reports on three unpublished observations)

- Ergodyne Corporation, St. Paul, MN (Seven unpublished observations)

- Payless Cashways Lumber Company, Kansas City, MO (Unpublished observation)

- Home Depot, Atlanta, GA (Unpublished observation)

Perhaps, if we consider the nature of back disorders, the focus on prevention will become clearer. There is considerable evidence that almost all back disorders result from cumulative injuries and that many lifestyle and vocational factors contribute to an eventual problem.[2, 3, 5, 18] The back disorder may be developing long before the first episode of pain and the "back injury" is just that - an episode of pain usually caused by a relatively minor aggravation or injury. The episode usually goes away in a few days or weeks but then tends to recur intermittently. In other words, the back "problem" may be in existence but currently asymptomatic. Our treatment should, therefore, focus on preventing the next episode.

Injury prevention by external protection is common in sports medicine. Pads, helmets and supportive taping are routinely used in many sports. The use of a back support for the industrial athlete should be considered in the same way.

TYPES OF SPINAL ORTHOSES

The common types of commercially available lumbosacral supports and braces fall within five general categories:

Cervical

Soft (Foam) Collars (Fig 11-1)

Soft collars have very little, if any, immobilization effect. They do serve as a reminder to limit head and neck motion, especially flexion. They do not provide forces to position the head in certain postures. However, if they are properly positioned under the mandible and occipital line, they partially unload the cervical spine by supporting a portion of the weight of the head. They are sized according to neck circumference and height. Exact measurements will depend upon the desired head and neck position and expected function.

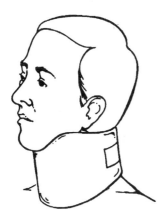

Figure 11-1. Soft cervical collar.

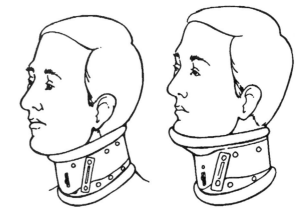

Figure 11-2. Hard cervical collars.

Hard (Plastic) Collars (Fig 11-2)

Hard collars serve basically the same function as soft collars, but do so with greater immobilizing and supporting effect. Most collars are adjustable. A chin support (plastic cup) may be added to the hard collar for additional support. These braces are also sized according to neck circumference and height.

Philadelphia Collar (Fig 11-3)

The Philadelphia collar is a molded plastic, semi-rigid orthosis designed to provide support effects similar to the other cervical supports described in this chapter. It is sized in small, medium and large. The Philadelphia collar is lightweight and may be more comfortable than other cervical orthoses. This collar may also serve as a foundation for cervical casting. This support is significantly more effective than the soft collar and is almost as effective as the more rigid four poster cervical brace in controlling flexion-extension between the occiput and third cervical vertebræ. It is less effective than other rigid braces at the middle and lower cervical levels.

Two and Four Poster Braces (Fig 11-4)

The two or four poster brace applies forces under the chin and occiput to restrict flexion and extension of the head and cervical spine. These orthoses include an anterior section consisting of a sternal plate, one or two uprights and a chin support, and a posterior section consisting of a thoracic plate, one or two

uprights and an occipital support. The two sections are connected by flexible straps between the chin and occipital supports and by over-the-shoulder straps between the thoracic and sternal plates. The uprights are adjustable for height and position of the chin and occipital supports. They are made of aluminum with

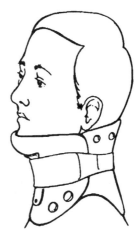

Figure 11-3. Philadelphia collar.

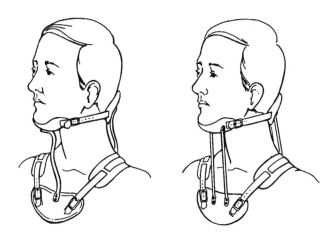

Figure 11-4. Two and four poster cervical braces.

leather or plastic padding of the parts that touch the body. A thoracic extension may be added to provide increased support and rotatory control. However, this may impart undesired thoracic movement to the cervical spine. The advantage of this support is that fine adjustments can be made and that it is more rigid than the soft or hard collars. This orthosis effectively restricts flexion in the mid-cervical spine. It is only partially effective in restricting lateral bending and upper cervical flexion-extension. This brace is sized small, medium and large.

Thoracolumbosacral

Dorsal-lumbar Corset (Fig 11-5)

The dorsal-lumbar corset is sized according to hip measurement and is available in several lengths and developments. Development is the difference between waist size and hip size. In other words, a size 36" (hip size) with a 6" development will have a 30" waist. The typical women's lumbosacral corset will have a 6-8" development, whereas a man's corset will have a 1-2" development. The dorsal-lumbar corset provides immobilization and support to the lower and mid-thoracic spine. The shoulder loops remind the patient to stand and sit up straight. They are not effective in holding the patient straighter and, if they fit too tightly, they will irritate the underarms.

The dorsal-lumbar corset is used for treatment of compression fractures and osteoporosis for patients who do not require or who cannot tolerate the more rigid support of a Taylor or hyperextension brace. Dorsal-lumbar corsets are also used for other conditions of the lower and mid-thoracic spine, such as sprains, strains and degenerative joint/disc disease.

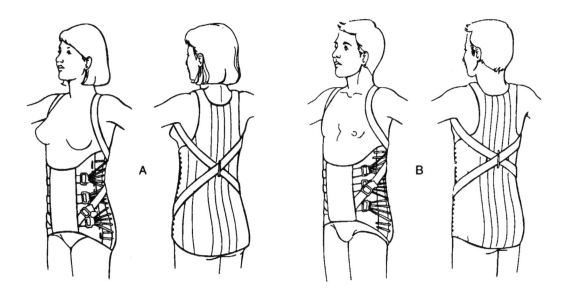

Figure 11-5. Dorsal-lumbar corset: A) Women's and B) Men's.

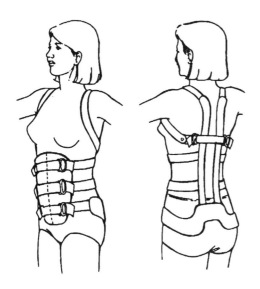

Figure 11-6. Taylor brace.

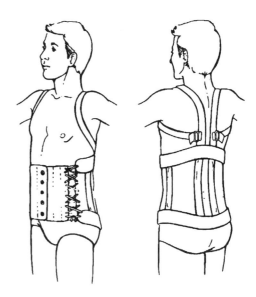

Figure 11-7. Knight-Taylor brace.

Semi-Rigid Dorsal-lumbar Braces (Taylor™ and Knight-Taylor™) (Fig 11-6 and 11-7)

The Taylor™ brace is similar to the chairback brace, except that the posterior uprights extend into the mid-thoracic region and there are straps that loop around the shoulders. The thoracic band may be absent. The Knight-Taylor™ brace is similar to the Taylor™ with the addition of lateral uprights and a full corset-like front. It is somewhat more rigid and restricts lateral bending better than the Taylor™. They are sized similar to the dorsal-lumbar corset and serve the same function, except that they provide a more rigid immobilization effect.

Hyperextension Brace (Fig 11-8)

The hyperextension braces (Jewett and Cash) provide a three-point fixation system consisting of posteriorly directed forces from the sternal and suprapubic pads and an anteriorly directed force from the thoracolumbar pad. This fixation system causes hyperextension and restricts flexion in the thoracolumbar spine. Control of flexion is achieved by the pads only; the frame should not contact the patient. With the patient seated in the prescribed posture and the orthosis properly adjusted and aligned, the sternal pad will have its superior border 1/2 inch inferior to the sternal notch and the suprapubic pad will have its inferior border 1/2 inch superior to the

symphysis pubis. Hyperextension braces are normally sized by height, hip circumference and chest circumference.

Lumbosacral

The Lumbosacral Corset (Fig 11-9)

Lumbosacral corsets are usually sized according to hip measurement and have a taller back than front. Most manufacturers feature styles with several different heights and developments. Most lumbosacral corsets have removable metal stays that fit in pockets along the length of the spine (Fig 11-9). The women's garment is usually made to cover more of the buttock area. This should be considered when fitting the garment as the stays should be bent to contour to the convex curve of the buttocks as well as concave (lordotic) curve in the lumbar spine. Doing this will help keep the corset from riding up during activity. For this reason, lumbosacral corsets are sometimes more effective for women than men. The lumbosacral corset is similar to the dorsal-lumbar corset with less height in the back and without the straps that loop around the shoulders. The most common lumbosacral corsets are made of a Dacron™ or cotton material, have a snap or zipper front, have 4-6" of size adjustment in the side panels and are washable. Some are made of elastic material and have front closures.

When fitting a woman's lumbosacral corset, it is important to choose a garment that does not crowd the

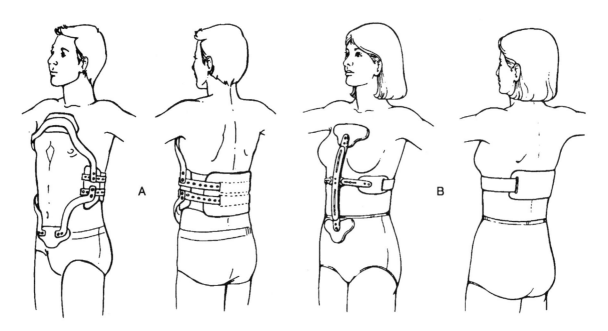

Figure 11-8. Hyperextension braces: A) Jewett and B) Cash.

breasts in front when the patient is sitting. The corset should come down onto the buttocks as far as possible if the lower lumbar spine is to be supported. The bottom front of the corset should just touch the angle of the hip when the patient is sitting. The front is always closed from the bottom up. The corset should be put on the patient and adjusted to the proper size and position before the metal stays are shaped and put into place. If possible, the stays should be shaped to the patient's normal standing lordosis. It is difficult to alter or physically control the lumbar lordosis with this type of support, but the corset can serve as a reminder of correct posture and the patient can alter his or her lordosis actively.

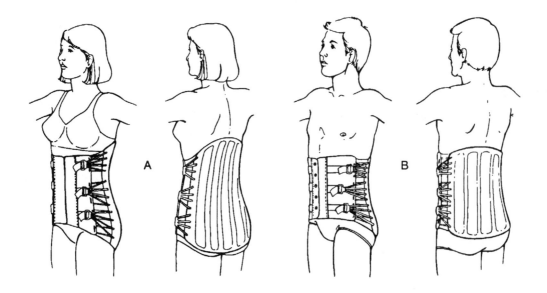

Figure 11-9. Lumbosacral corset: A) Women's and B) Men's.

The lumbosacral corset is a flexible support and restricts movement relatively ineffectively, especially lower lumbar movement, yet it can be effective as a reminder to the patient to avoid movement and to maintain correct posture. It effectively increases intra-abdominal pressure, thus reducing intradiscal pressure (vertical loading).

If the patient is in acute discomfort, the corset should be donned and doffed while lying down. If the condition is severe, the support is worn at all times when the patient is out of bed. In other cases, the patient may only wear the support while doing activities that might cause aggravation. The support is seldom worn while lying down and resting. While the lumbosacral corset is effective when the patient is relatively inactive, it becomes uncomfortable and tends to ride up as the patient becomes more active.

The Semi-Rigid Lumbosacral Braces (Chairback, Knight™ and Williams)

The chairback brace consists of two posterior uprights, pelvic and thoracic bands and a pie pan abdominal support anteriorly (Fig 11-10). The Knight™ spinal brace is similar to the chairback with the addition of lateral uprights and a full corset-like front. (Fig 11-11) It is somewhat more rigid than the chairback. These braces effectively restrict movement in the thoracolumbar region but are not necessarily effective in restricting mobility in the lumbosacral area. Studies actually show increased movement occurs in the lumbosacral area with the semi-rigid lumbosacral brace during moderate to vigorous activity.[16] Unless the goal is to physically restrict movement in the upper lumbar and lower thoracic area, the semi-rigid brace has no more to offer than a lumbosacral corset. They are usually not as comfortable, are more expensive and have the potential to actually increase mobility at the lumbosacral spine. Therefore, they would rarely be the correct choice for support of the lumbosacral spine.

These semi-rigid braces are fitted according to hip size and length from the mid-sacral to the lower thoracic spine. They are made of metal covered with leather or vinyl. They are somewhat cooler to wear than the lumbosacral corset.

The Williams brace (Fig 11-12) provides a three-point pressure system consisting of a posteriorly directed force from the pelvic adjustment strap and anteriorly directed forces from the pelvic and thoracic bands. This pressure system tends to limit lumbar extension and reduce lordosis. The brace also tends to limit lateral bending. The brace is made of metal covered with leather and has a corset front. This brace must fit relatively tightly to be effective. This can become a problem because patients often cannot tolerate the brace for very long. It is difficult to keep in place when the patient is active and especially when sitting.

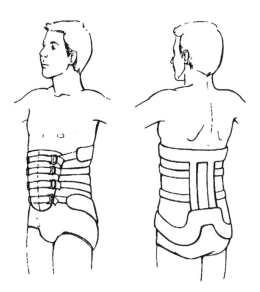

Figure 11-10. Chairback brace.

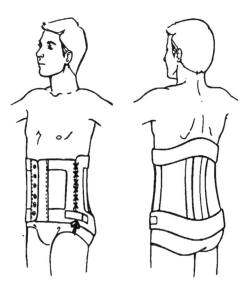

Figure 11-11. Knight brace.

The Lumbar Support or Belt (Fig 11-13)

Many types of lumbar supports or belts are available. Leather weight lifting belts and motorcycle belts have been popular for many years; now variations are becoming popular in industry. Most are made of fabric and elastic with Velcro™ or buckle closures. Many have flexible metal or plastic stays or a plastic panel in the back to provide some additional stabilization. Some feature adjustable side pull straps and some even have an air bladder that can be pumped up to make the garment fit tighter and conform to the shape of the body better. They are fitted by waist size.

Since it is nearly impossible to keep these types of supports or belts down over the iliac crests, especially when the wearer is active, it is questionable if any support or stabilization is afforded to the lumbosacral area. Perhaps their benefit is derived because they serve as a reminder to the wearer to practice proper posture and good body mechanics. Some studies show that lumbosacral supports increase intra-abdominal pressure, however, these studies were done using a corset with a wider front panel than many of the supports and belts described in this section.[1,4] Whether the narrower supports and belts that ride up above the pelvis and fail to cover the entire abdominal area have this effect has not been studied.

Lumbosacral Supports Designed to Stay in Place Saunders S'port All™ Back Support (Fig 11-14)

The difficulty of supporting the lower lumbar spine with a back support or brace has been discussed. Part of the difficulty lies in keeping the back support in its proper position. Stabilizing the pelvis and lower spine is vital because over 90% of back injuries occur in the lower two segments of the spine and some "back problems" actually occur in the pelvis. If the back support rides up above the iliac crests, the back support is not supporting either the pelvis or the lower two segments of the spine, which are positioned below the top of the iliac crests (Fig 11-15A).

Attempts to keep back supports and braces from riding up have included ideas such as groin straps, garter belts and crotch inserts. All have proven to be impractical and/or uncomfortable and irritating. A back support attached to elastic athletic shorts provides a satisfactory way to comfortably keep a back support in place. Because it is combined with an elastic athletic short, the back support stays in place to stabilize the hips and pelvis as well as the back (Fig 11-15B).

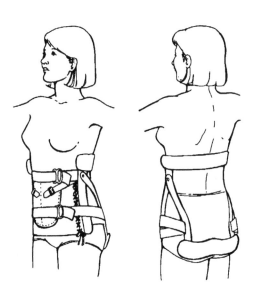

Figure 11-12. William's brace.

The one piece back support/athletic short is comfortable, non-restrictive and will not slip out of place even with vigorous movement. It is constructed of paneled elastic that conforms to body shape and features two separate tapered side pulls with adjustable straps designed to distribute support throughout the lumbar region. The attached elastic athletic short is

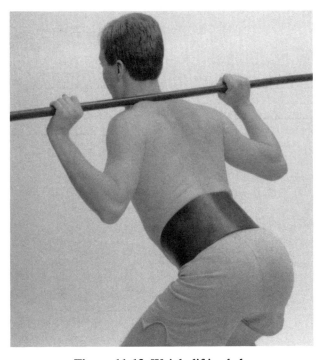

Figure 11-13. Weight lifting belt.

designed to offer graduated support for the quadricep, hamstring, groin, pelvis and abdominal areas. This garment is fitted by waist size.

Saunders Work S'port™ Back Support (Fig 11-16)

The Saunders Work S'port™ Back Support applies the same principle as the S'port All™ to a more traditional looking back support. The Work S'port™ combines a back support with an adjustable belt that can be looped through any pair of pants.

The elastic support attaches firmly to the belt underneath so that the Work S'port™ remains anchored over the lumbosacral area where support is needed most. Like the S'port All™, the Work S'port™ has detachable side pull straps that allow easy adjustment from light to strong support depending on the activity at hand.

The Work S'port™ is especially suited to individuals who need only intermittent support or jobs in which back supports need to be shared over shifts. It is also preferred by those who need a back support but do not want an undergarment.

Sacroiliac Joints

Sacroiliac Support Belt (Fig 11-17 and 11-18)

The sacroiliac belt partially stabilizes the sacroiliac joints and symphysis pubis by providing circumferential support around the pelvis. It is fitted by hip size. It must fit relatively tight to accomplish any degree of immobilization and must fit low around the pelvis to be effective. It is used post-partum, post-traumatic injury and for hypermobility of the sacroiliac joints. Various sacroiliac supports and belts are available commercially, ranging from supports that are 6-9" wide, to a simple 2" wide belt that fits around the pelvis (the most popular). A removable sacral pad is included (Fig 11-18).

MEASURING INSTRUCTIONS FOR BRACES AND CORSETS

These measurements are approximate only. Each garment must be fitted individually to the patient.

Lumbosacral Corset

• Hip circumference

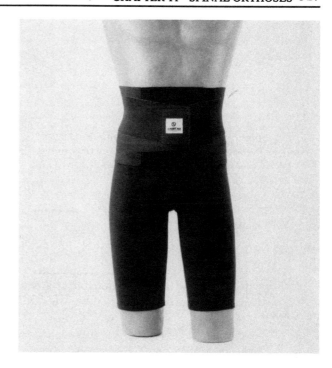

Figure 11-14. Saunders S'port All™ back support.

• Waist circumference (to determine development)

• Height in back from sacrococcygeal joint to lower thoracic area (approximately T10)

• Height in front from angle of hip to comfortable clearance below breasts with patient seated

Chairback Brace-Knight™ Brace, Williams Brace

• Hip circumference

• Height in back to patient's comfort (from approximately mid-sacral to lower thoracic spine)

S'port All™ and Work S'port™ Back Support

• Waist circumference

Sacroiliac Belt

• Hip circumference

Dorsal-lumbar Corset

• Hip circumference

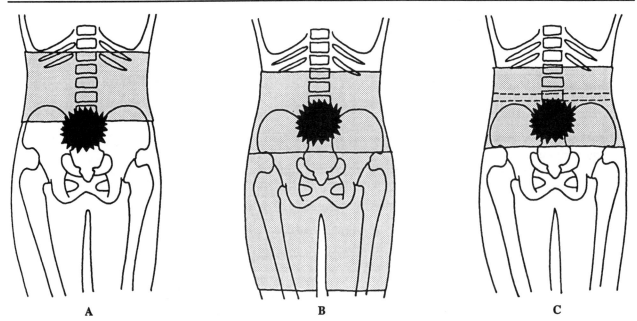

A   B   C

Figure 11-15. A) Many traditional lumbar back supports do not stay in place over the lower lumbar segments; B&C) The S'port All™ and the Work S'port™ are anchored to stay in place over the lower lumbar segments.

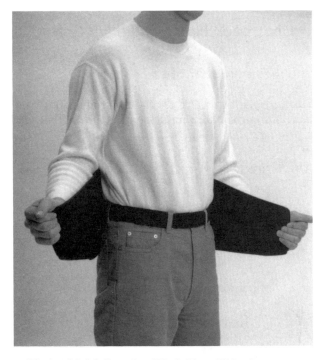

Figure 11-16. Saunders Work S'port™ back support.

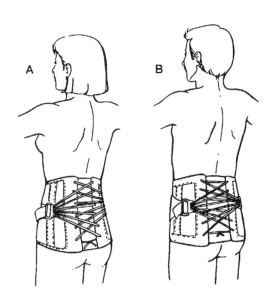

Figure 11-17. Sacroiliac belt - wide style: A) Women's and B) Men's.

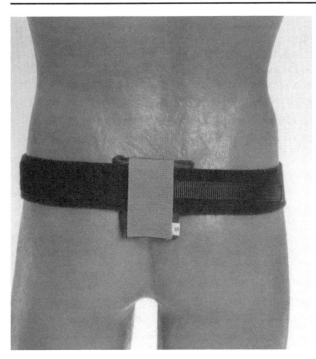

Figure 11-18. Sacroiliac belt - narrow style, including sacral pad.

- Waist circumference (to determine development)

- Height in back from sacrococcygeal joint to one inch below superior angle of scapula

- Height in front from angle of hip to comfortable clearance below breasts with patient seated

Semi-rigid Dorsal-lumbar Braces

- Hip circumference

- Height in back from mid-sacral spine to one inch below superior angle of scapula

Hyperextension Braces

- Height in front from pubic symphysis to sternal notch, less one inch

- Circumference of hips

- Circumference of chest

Cervical Soft Collar-Hard Collar Philadelphia Collar

- Circumference of neck

- Height necessary to position and support head as desired

Two and Four Poster Braces

- Sized small, medium and large according to height and body build of patient

TOTAL MANAGEMENT OF THE SPINAL ORTHOSIS PATIENT

In addition to the sizing information mentioned for each type of spinal orthosis, the following tips for using a spinal orthosis are offered:

1. A spinal orthosis is seldom effective in mechanically correcting posture. Its effectiveness comes from reminding the patient to actively maintain the desired posture. For this reason, small corrections are often possible but one should not expect a brace to hold a patient in a posture that he or she cannot actively assume with some degree of ease. The therapist should have the patient assume his or her optimum posture, then the brace should be fitted to conform to that posture.

2. It is often desirable to explain to the patient the effects of the various braces and supports being considered for his or her condition, then fit each of them to the patient and let the patient make the final selection. In other words, a brace hanging in the closet that the patient will not wear is not going to help.

3. When the patient's condition is acute, he or she may need to wear a support at all times except when recumbent. If this is the case, the support must be put on and taken off while the patient is lying down. The best method of doing this is to roll to the side, place the support against the posterior spine, roll back onto the support and fasten the support in front.

4. Most of the braces and supports described in this chapter are more comfortable with a cotton undershirt or T-shirt worn underneath. This also helps absorb perspiration and keeps the support clean longer.

SUMMARY

Back and neck supports play an important role in the treatment and prevention of low back disorders. While they do not restrict physical mobility effectively (at least in the lumbosacral area) they do provide a beneficial effect by unloading and stabilizing the spine and providing proprioceptive feedback to the wearer. These beneficial effects may also help relieve pain, which helps the patient become active sooner, thus speeding the recovery from a back injury. Back supports can also help prevent injuries. Recent experience with back supports in industry and sports have caused many to rethink the old adage that the use of supports is only for short term management and a clinician should, "Never prescribe a support without a plan to eliminate it." Perhaps the new advice will be to wear a protective back support during potentially stressful activities in the same way an athlete would tape his or her ankles before competition.

Finally, if an individual tries to substitute a back support for exercise, proper posture and good body mechanics, its use is potentially harmful. Therefore, one must always view a back support as an adjunct to treatment and prevention, not as a substitute for any of the other important principles of proper back care.

REFERENCES

1. Ahlgren S and Hansen T: The Use of Lumbosacral Corsets Prescribed for Low Back Pain. Prosteth Orthop Int 2: 101-104, 1978.

2. Bigos S, et al: Back Injuries in Industry: A Retrospective Study II: Injury Factors. Spine 11: 246-251, 1986.

3. Bigos S, et al: Back Injuries in Industry: A Retrospective Study III: Employee Related Factors. Spine 11:252-256, 1986.

4. Colachis S, Strohm B and Ganter E: Cervical Spine Motion in Normal Women: Radiographic Study of Effect of Cervical Collars. Arch of Phys Med Rehab 54:161-169, 1973.

5. Deyo R and Bass J: Lifestyle and Low Back Pain: The Influence of Smoking and Obesity. Spine 14:501-506, 1989.

6. Feeler L: Weight Lifting. In The Spine in Sports. S Hochschuler, ed. Hanley and Belfus, Philadelphia PA 1990.

7. Flemming J: Spondylolysis and Spondylolisthesis in the Athlete. In The Spine in Sports. S Hochschuler, ed. Hanley and Belfus, Philadelphia PA 1990.

8. Holm S and Nachemson A: Variations in the Nutrition of the Canine Intervertebral Disc, Induced by Motion. Spine 8:866-873, 1983.

9. Johnson R, et al: Cervical Orthosis. JBJS 52A:1440-1442, 1970.

10. Kirkaldy-Willis W: Supports and Braces. In Managing Low Back Pain, 2nd edition. W Kirkaldy-Willis, ed. Churchhill Livingstone, New York NY 1988.

11. Million R, et al: Assessment of the Progress of the Back-Pain Patient. Spine 7: 204-212, 1982.

12. Morris J, Lucas D and Bresler M: Role of the Trunk in Stability of the Spine. J Bone and Joint Surg 43A:327-351, 1961.

13. Nachemson A and Lindh M: Measurement of Abdominal and Back Muscle Strength With and Without Low Back Pain. Scand J Rehab Med 1:60, 1969.

14. Nachemson A and Morris J: In Vivo Measurements of Intradiscal Pressure. J Bone Joint Surg 46A: 1077-1092, 1964.

15. Nachemson A, Schultz A and Andersson G: Mechanical Effectiveness Studies of Lumbar Spine Orthosis. Scand J Rehab Med 9(suppl):139-149, 1983.

16. Norton P and Brown T: The Immobilizing Efficiency of Back Braces. J Bone and Joint Surg 39-A (1): 111-139, 220, 1957.

17. Perry J: The Use of External Support in the Treatment of Low Back Pain. J Bone Joint Surg 52A:1440-1442, 1970.

18. Quebec Task Force Study: Scientific Approach to the Assessment and Management of Activity Related Spinal Disorders. Spine 12:7S, 1987.

19. Quinet R and Hadler H: Diagnosis and Treatment of Backache. Sem in Arth and Rheu 8:261-287, 1979.

20. Stamp J, Chock K, and Penrose K: Acute and Chronic Effects Of Pneumatic Lumbar Support On Muscular Strength, Flexibility And Functional Impairment Index. Sports Training Med J 2:121-129, 1991.

21. Walsh N and Schwartz R: The Influence of Prophylactic Orthosis on Abdominal Strength and Low Back Injury in the Workplace. Am J Phys Med Rehab 69: 245-250, 1990.

22. Wasserman J and McNamee M: Engineering Evaluation of Lumbosacral Orthosis Using in Vivo Noninvasive Testing. In Proceedings of the Tenth Southeast Conference of Theoretical and Applied Mechanics. Cincinnati OH 1980.

CHAPTER 12

EXERCISE

INTRODUCTION

Chapter 12 summarizes some of our favorite exercises — the exercises we use virtually every day in the clinic. Some of these exercises are the "old standbys" that every clinician will recognize. Others are exercises that some clinicians may not have "discovered" yet. Still others may be familiar to the clinician, but they have not been used in the same way or in the same combination with other exercises that we describe.

This chapter is not intended to be a complete source of exercises for spinal conditions. Instead, this chapter is meant to provide the therapist with a basic framework of exercises. These are the exercises we consider indispensable in the treatment of spinal patients.

DESIGNING THE EXERCISE PROGRAM TO FIT INDIVIDUAL NEEDS

As discussed throughout this textbook, the therapist should design a program individualized for the patient's needs. No two back injuries are identical, so it is a mistake for the therapist to prescribe the same exercises for every back patient. The physical therapy evaluation thus becomes the most important part of exercise prescription.

Each patient varies in his or her response to exercise. In many cases, a patient can progress quite rapidly. Other patients may not progress to the more aggressive exercises for several weeks or at all. The patient's response to exercise may have very little to do with the original diagnosis. For example, some patients with minor sprain/strain injuries progress much slower than expected, while some patients who initially have severe symptoms and pathology are able to progress quite quickly. Therefore, the therapist's careful reassessment of both subjective and objective findings at each patient visit is very important.

FREQUENCY/INTENSITY/ DURATION OF EXERCISE

The duration of exercises is almost always more important than the frequency or intensity. Patients should be taught early on that they should expect to perform a certain amount of spinal exercise for the rest of their lives. This point is especially true in the case of chronic or recurring spinal symptoms.

The therapist should become skilled at finding out how much each patient is willing to participate in his or her own recovery. If the patient is only willing to invest five minutes per day, a 20 minute exercise program will not be helpful at all. The patient will become impatient and stop performing all of the exercises. The therapist should let such a patient know that only those exercises which are absolutely essential are included in the patient's program. This attitude fosters better patient compliance.

As the patient nears discharge from physical therapy services, the therapist should question the patient about his or her motivation for continuing exercise indefinitely. If the therapist senses that the patient will have trouble maintaining the program after discharge, the therapist should help the patient comply by shortening or prioritizing the exercise list. For example, the patient who has a tendency toward stiffness in extension should know that passive and active extension exercises are the most important items on his or her list.

The frequency of exercise varies depending upon the patient's problem and individual circumstances. If the exercise is designed to increase flexibility or reinforce postural awareness, it should be done very frequently throughout the day (sometimes as often as hourly). Then, as the patient improves, the frequency can be decreased to a maintenance level (as little as a few times per week).

If the purpose of the exercise is to improve strength or conditioning, once or twice daily is often appropriate. Again, as the patient improves the frequency can decrease to three or four times per week. The patient should be told at the beginning that the frequency can decrease later as improvement is noted. This gives the patient a goal toward which to strive.

The intensity of exercise also varies depending upon individual circumstances. Generally, the patient should start out mildly and increase gradually. Stretching exercises are usually done gently and for relatively longer periods of time (20 seconds to a minute or two). It is usually desirable to have the patient perform relatively fewer repetitions more frequently through the day (3-5 repetitions every 1-2 hours throughout the day).

Strengthening or conditioning exercises should usually be performed to fatigue once or twice a day. However, symptom response may prohibit exercising to fatigue initially. Common sense must prevail. Starting with 5-10 repetitions of a moderately challenging exercise is a good rule of thumb for a patient who has moderate symptoms. As the patient improves, 20-30 repetitions may be necessary to achieve the same level of fatigue or symptom response. If the patient can perform more than 20-30 repetitions of a strengthening exercise, the exercise should be

modified to make it more challenging. As more challenging exercises are added, the previous, less challenging ones should be discontinued so that the patient feels he or she has "graduated" to a new level.

Figure 12-1 summarizes general recommendations for the various types of exercise. These general recommendations should be modified at the therapist's discretion to accomplish the goals that have been set for the patient and to fit the patient's schedule/lifestyle.

The therapist must pay close attention to signs and symptoms. Use caution when progressing the patient into any exercise that causes pain to peripheralize, or causes pain lasting longer than a few minutes after stopping the exercise. If the patient does not tolerate the exercise well, the exercise technique should be reevaluated. The exercise may still be appropriate, but the patient should simply perform it with less intensity or fewer of repetitions. There are many alternatives to stopping exercise entirely.

In certain instances, the therapist may decide to proceed cautiously with a more aggressive program even if the patient has continued peripheral pain. The therapist and patient may find that more aggressive exercises do not actually cause the symptoms to worsen dramatically, even though the symptoms peripheralize. The peripheralization may be temporary and non-progressive. If this is the case, the benefit of progressing the exercises may outweigh the drawback of the negative symptom response. On the other hand, progressive neurological deterioration is always a contraindication for exercises that provoke symptoms.

Corrective stretching exercises for conditions involving adverse mechanical neural tension (thoracic outlet syndrome, adherent nerve roots, etc.) can increase symptom peripheralization. Mild to moderate increases in symptoms are acceptable and often necessary, provided the symptoms decrease a few seconds or minutes after the exercise is complete and are not progressive. Since conditions involving AMNT are often highly irritable, the exercise prescription should initially err on the side of caution, progressing to more aggressive stretches as tolerated.

Type of Exercise	# of Repetitions	Hold period	Frequency	Intensity
Stretching/Flexibility	3-5	20 - 60 sec	3-5x/day	Gentle static hold
Strengthening-Power	6-12	N/A	3x/week	Moderate to Heavy
Strengthening-Toning	15-30 or more	5 - 10 sec	1-2x/daily	Light - to fatigue
Conditioning-Aerobic	N/A	20 - 30 min/session	3x/week	At target heart rate

Figure 12-1. General recommendations for exercise. The frequencies for stretching/flexibility and strengthening/toning exercises are beginning guidelines for the individual with an active problem. As the problem resolves, the exercise frequency can decrease to a maintenance level of 3 times per week.

SPECIFIC EXERCISE TECHNIQUES

Neck Stretches

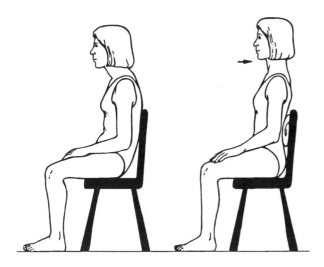

Head Back, Chin In

This is a good stretch to help correct forward head posturing, to stretch tight suboccipital muscles and upper cervical joints, to help correct cervical herniated nucleus pulposus (HNP) and to promote good posture in general. It is important that this stretch be taught correctly. The patient should sit with good lumbar lordosis and sternal elevation, with the scapulæ retracted to neutral. From this position, the patient usually only needs to nod the head slightly to effect the head back, chin in posture. The patient with a flattened mid cervical lordosis should avoid further flattening by excessively retracting the chin. All other cervical exercises should be performed from this neutral starting position.

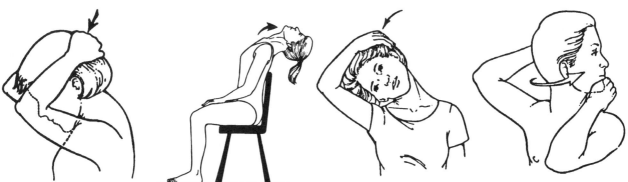

Cervical Flexion, Extension, Sidebending and Rotation

Indicated for soft tissue stiffness, to prevent soft tissue stiffness after injury, to reverse stressful positions and to provide general relaxation or stretching of the cervical musculature. Stretching into end range should be avoided if joint hypermobility, acute joint inflammation or nerve root impingement is present.

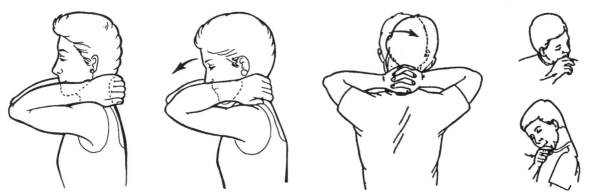

Upper Cervical Flexion, Sidebending and Rotation

Indicated for suboccipital muscle tightness, tension headaches originating from the suboccipital area, tightness of upper cervical joints, forward head posturing, and to reverse stressful positions. These stretches should be avoided if instability of the upper cervical joints is present.

Cervical Extension

Indicated for limited cervical extension mobility, correction of cervical HNP or reversal of stressful positions. Stretching into end range should be avoided if joint hypermobility, acute joint inflammation or nerve root impingement is present. Several variations of cervical extension are shown here. Sitting or supine cervical extension with a chin tuck should be performed when mid and lower cervical extension is desired, yet the therapist wishes to avoid excessive upper cervical extension. Full cervical extension should be performed when general extension stiffness is present.

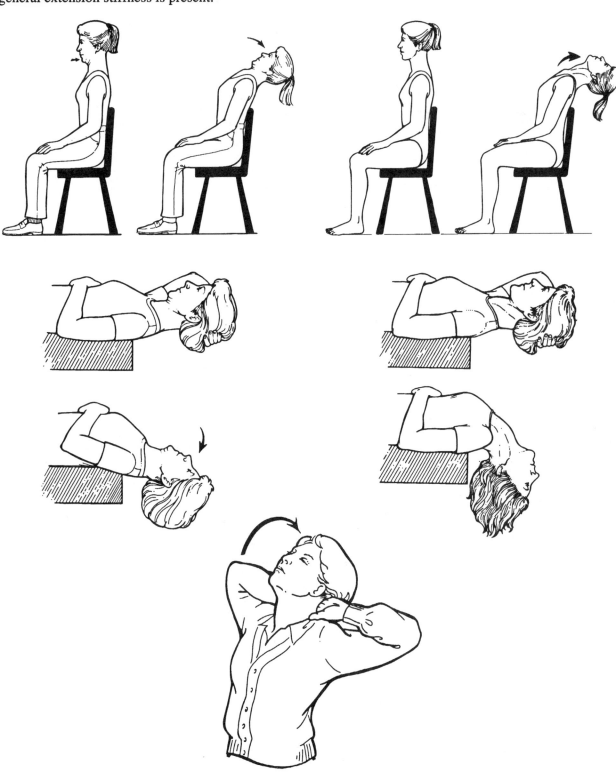

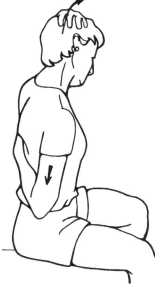

Scalenes Stretch

It is important that the scalene stretch is taught correctly. Shoulder depression should be done first and it must be maintained throughout the stretch. Then the cervical spine is sidebent just enough to effect a stretch to the scalenes. This stretch is important for scalene tightness, thoracic outlet syndrome or upper limb neural tension caused by tight scalenes, forward head posturing, and to reverse stressful positioning. It should be performed gently when irritability of the neural structures is present.

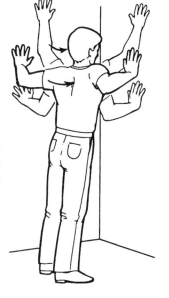

Corner (Pectoralis and Anterior Chest) Stretch

The corner stretch is a good general stretch for the anterior structures of the chest and shoulders. It is useful for treating forward head posturing, thoracic outlet syndrome and to reverse stressful positioning. It can be performed with varying degrees of shoulder abduction to change the location and intensity of the stretch.

Neck Strengthening

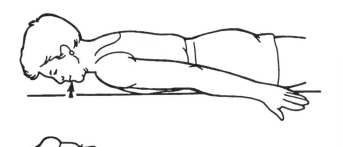

Prone Chin Tucks

Indicated for posterior neck weakness and forward head posturing. This exercise is very useful for forward head, slumped shoulder posturing when done in combination with the prone scapular retraction exercises shown on page 331. This is one of the more important strengthening exercises for most cervical patients.

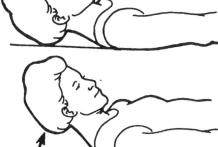

Supine Chin Tucks

This strengthening exercise is performed correctly when the chin is tucked into the chest — not jutting upward. It is indicated for anterior neck weakness or general cervical deconditioning. Caution should be used with acute cervical HNP, but the patient can progress to this exercise in subacute or chronic stages.

Prone Head Raises off Edge of Bed

Indicated for posterior neck weakness and forward head posturing or for general cervical conditioning. The patient should avoid jutting the chin forward when raising the head. The exercise can be made easier by shortening the arc of motion, or more challenging by increasing the arc of motion.

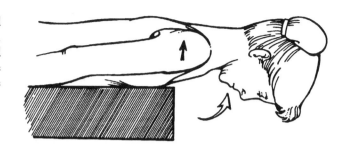

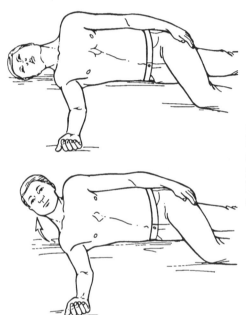

Sidelying Head Raises

Important for strengthening the sidebending muscles of the cervical spine or for general cervical conditioning. Caution should be used with acute cervical HNP, but the patient can progress to this exercise in subacute or chronic stages. Initially, short arcs of motion may be tolerated better, and the exercise can be made more challenging by increasing the arc of motion and even hanging the head off the edge of a bed.

Cervical Rotation, Sidebending, Flexion, Extension with Elastic Tubing

Indicated for strengthening of the cervical spine musculature and general conditioning. The resistance can be varied by changing the arc of motion or adding larger diameter elastic tubing. The patient should be reminded to use slow, smooth movements.

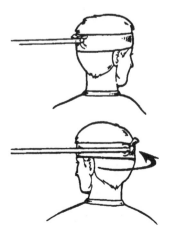

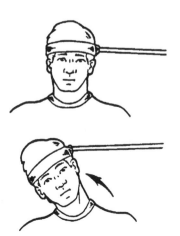

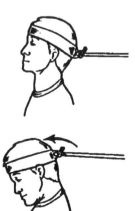

Upper Back Stretches

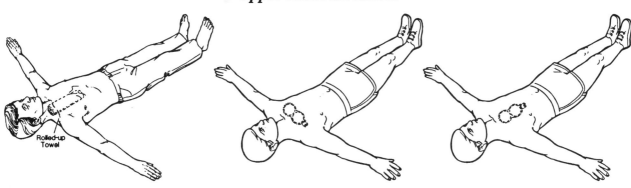

Supine Thoracic Extension
over Rolled Towel

This stretch is useful for general or specific stretching of tight thoracic segments. It is helpful for forward head, rounded shoulder posturing when actual upper back tightness is a contributing factor. Varying degrees of shoulder abduction can be added to stretch tight upper limb neural structures (as in thoracic outlet syndrome). The stretch can be made gentler or more vigorous by varying the size and position of the rolled towel. Tennis balls or racquetballs in a sock can also be used for a more specific or vigorous segmental stretch.

Prone Thoracic Rotation

Useful for general cervical and/or thoracic stiffness, or as a general self-mobilization technique for multilevel rotatory restrictions. This exercise is both a mobility and a strengthening exercise. The patient should be taught to rotate the thoracic spine by raising the posterior shoulder and elbow upward and backward, and not by twisting the cervical spine excessively, especially when cervical hypermobility is present.

Rotation/Sidebending over Rolled Towel

Indicated for unilateral thoracic facet joint or general soft tissue tightness. The tight segment(s) should be on the top. The thickness and position of the rolled towel determine the intensity and location of the stretch.

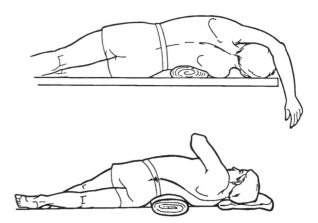

Thoracic Sidebending

The mid thoracic area can be difficult to isolate for stretching into sidebending. Here are two exercises we have found beneficial. They are beneficial for stretching interscapular muscles and trigger areas and for self-mobilizing stiff joints.

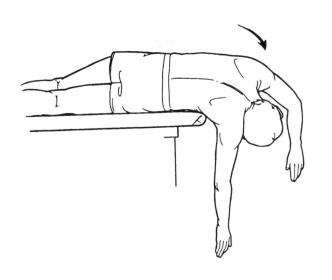

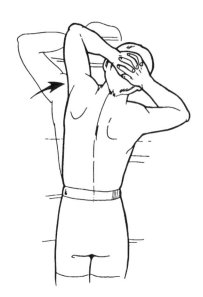

Seated Rotation with Wand

This exercise is appropriate when a vigorous thoracic or thoracolumbar rotational stretch is desired in the more functional position of sitting upright. It does not stretch the cervical spine. Patients should avoid twisting quickly or forcefully. Patients can perform a similar stretch in office or home environments by grasping the back of their chairs to provide the stretch.

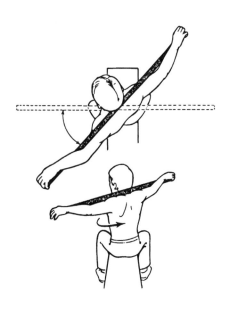

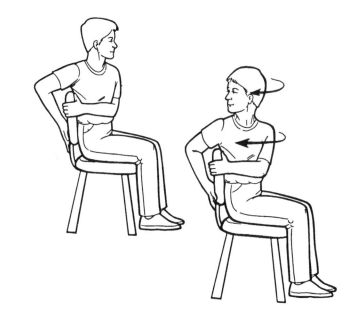

Upper Back/Interscapular Strengthening

Standing Scapular Retraction

Indicated as a postural reminder or gentle strengthening exercise to be performed frequently throughout the day. Scapular retraction also gently stretches the anterior chest musculature. It is appropriate for any condition involving the forward head, rounded shoulder posturing.

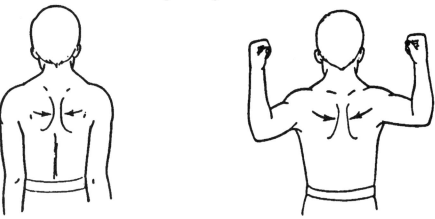

Prone Scapular Retraction Progression

This prone upper back and interscapular strengthening progression is extremely valuable in the treatment of poor cervical or upper back posture, shoulder girdle dysfunction, thoracic outlet syndrome, or general cervical and upper back deconditioning, and to counteract the detrimental effects of prolonged slumped sitting occupations. As the arms are held further away from the body, the exercise becomes more advanced. Hand held weights make the exercise even more challenging. These exercises can also be performed standing with rubber tubing used for resistance.

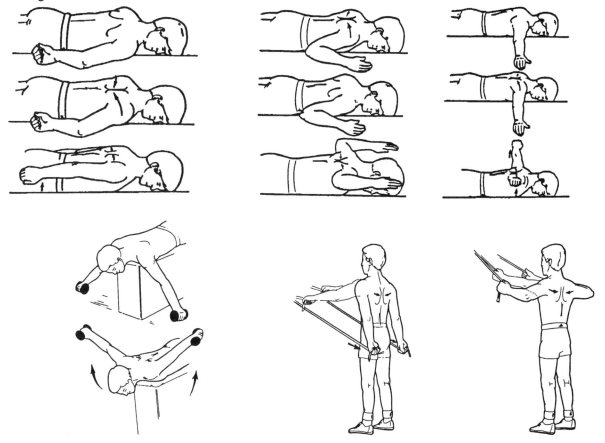

General Upper Extremity Exercise with Tubing

Exercises involving diagonal or horizontal flexion and abduction of the shoulders also strengthen and condition the upper back. Therefore the progression shown here is very helpful for upper back strengthening and conditioning, forward head and rounded shoulder posturing and to counteract the detrimental effects of prolonged slumped sitting occupations.

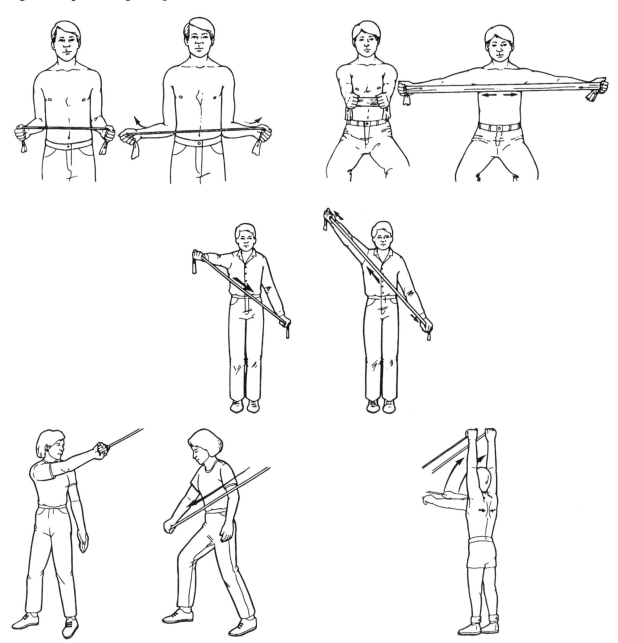

Prone Shoulder Flexion/Upper Back Extension with Wand

A challenging exercise for many patients, prone shoulder flexion with a wand is helpful for shoulder girdle and upper and lower back strengthening and conditioning. As the patient improves, cuff weights can be added to the wand.

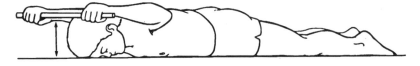

Low Back Stretching

Lateral Shift Correction

Self-correcting an existing lateral shift can be done by performing active and passive lateral shift correction. Often, lateral shift correction is necessary prior to performing the prone extension progression or other exercises. Sometimes the patient must initially learn in prone or against a wall, but then can advance to more functional shift correction as pain relief and increased kinesthetic awareness occurs.

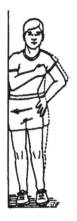 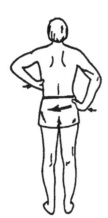

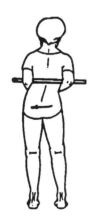

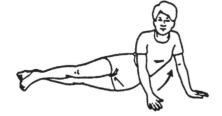

Knees to Chest

The single and double knees to chest exercises are helpful for conditions requiring lumbar paraspinal muscle, spinal interspace or hip flexion stretching. Patients who have a tendency toward excessive lumbar lordosis also benefit. This exercise may aggravate an acute ligament sprain or discogenic back pain, so caution should be used when these conditions are suspected.

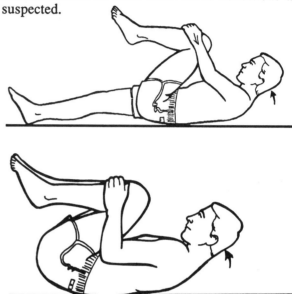

Prayer Stretch

The prayer stretch is an alternative exercise to the knees to chest exercise. Many patients tolerate it more easily because they feel they have more control over the intensity of the stretch. Since this exercise can aggravate an acute ligament sprain or discogenic back pain caution should be used when these conditions are suspected.

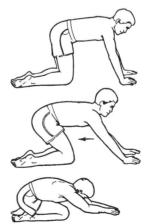

Supine Rotation and Variations

Many variations of supine lumbar rotation are shown here. As a general rule, the further the hips and lumbar spine are flexed, the more superior in the lumbar or thoracolumbar spine the stretch will be felt. If one or both of the knees are extended, a greater force will be felt because of the longer lever arm. If the patient has trouble relaxing when the starting position is supine, the patient can try starting in sidelying, twisting the upper back into supine instead. This will also vary exactly where the rotation stretch is felt along the spine.

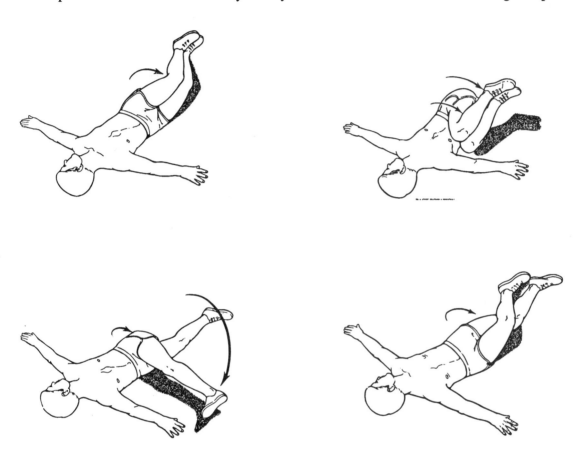

Prone Extension Progression

If the patient has a flat back posture, is stiff in backward bending or has lumbar HNP, the prone passive extension progression is helpful. The patient should be reminded to let the back relax when pressing upward. If a full press up is not tolerated, the hands can be moved further away from the body. The prone on elbows or simple prone position can be a good starting point. This exercise can aggravate a patient with an excessive lumbar lordosis, nerve root impingement, facet joint irritation or a large HNP.

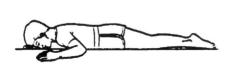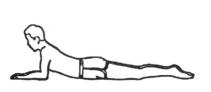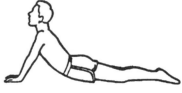

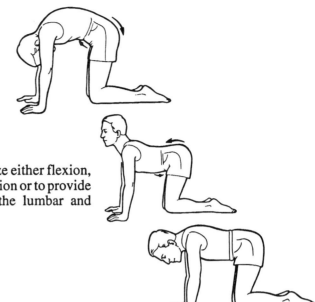

Cat Back

The cat back exercise can be modified to emphasize either flexion, extension or both. It is a gentle way to teach pelvic rotation or to provide a non-weight bearing flexion/extension stretch to the lumbar and thoracic areas.

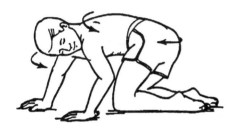

Quadruped "C" Stretch

The "C" stretch is an effective way to provide a gentle non-weight bearing stretch into sidebending. It is helpful for unilateral or bilateral sidebending restrictions or lateral shift correction. It can be effective for thoracic as well as lumbar stretching. As the patient tolerates the stretch better, it should be progressed to kneeling or standing, the more functional positions.

Sidelying with Lower Extremities Off Edge of Bed

Sidelying while hanging the lower extremities off the edge of the bed can provide a non-weight bearing sidebending stretch that is more specific to the lumbar spine. Caution should be used when the patient has acute pain, as this stretch is fairly vigorous because of the long lever arm of the lower extremities.

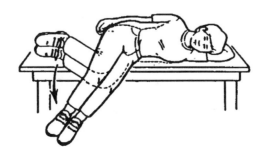

Low Back Strengthening

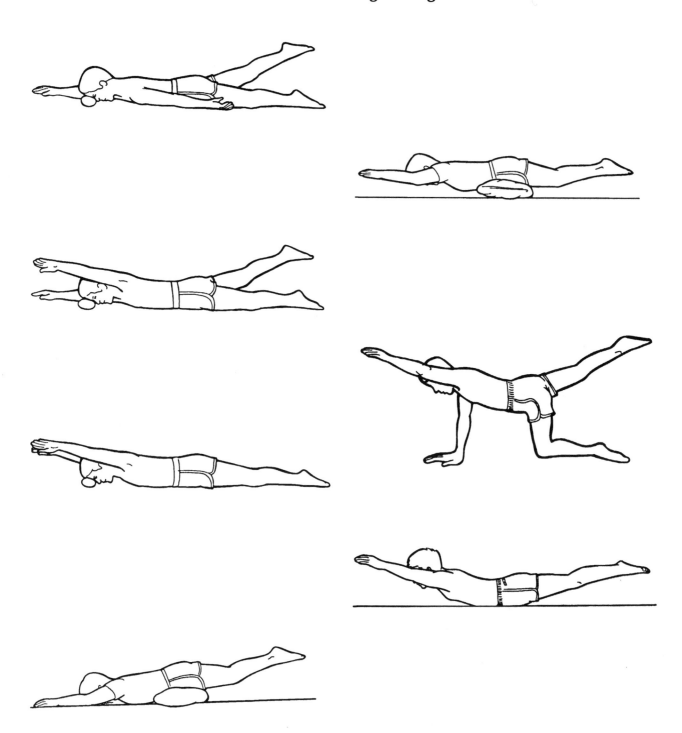

Prone Extension Progression

Indicated for the strengthening and conditioning of the lumbar paraspinals and stability of the trunk. As the patient improves, the exercises can be made more advanced by adding both the arms and legs, decreasing the stability by performing them in quadruped, or adding wrist and ankle weights. If the patient is limited in extension flexibility or end range extension is not desired, a pillow can be used under the abdomen. The patient should isometrically contract the upper and lower extremity musculature and avoid "cheating" during the unilateral variations by bracing with the opposite arm or leg.

Prone Extension Off Edge of Object

A more advanced exercise, prone extension off the edge of a bed, table or chair involves a fuller arc of motion. It can be made more challenging by increasing the arc of motion, extending the arms away from the body or adding wrist weights. A partner, strap or counterweight is required to hold the legs down.

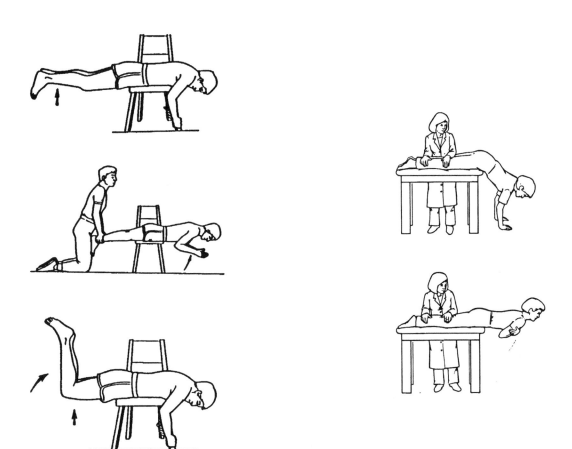

Sidelying with Lower Extremities Off Edge of Bed

This general lumbar strengthening and stabilization exercise is performed in sidelying with the lower extremities hanging off the edge of the bed. The hips are rotated up against gravity and back down to provide the resistance. The patient should be reminded to keep the lumbar spine in neutral flexion/extension and to control the movement carefully. This exercise should not be given to a patient who cannot control the movement well.

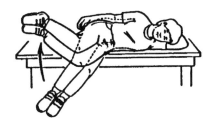

Abdominal Curl Progression

There are many variations of the abdominal curl or "crunch." Variations include raising either the trunk or the legs or both; lengthening or shortening the lever arms by changing the position of the arms or legs; and twisting the trunk to the right or left. Many equally effective variations are not shown here. Abdominal curls are indicated for treating excessive lumbar lordosis, weak abdominal musculature and general deconditioning of the trunk. They can be irritating to an acute lumbar HNP and should be introduced gradually once healing begins.

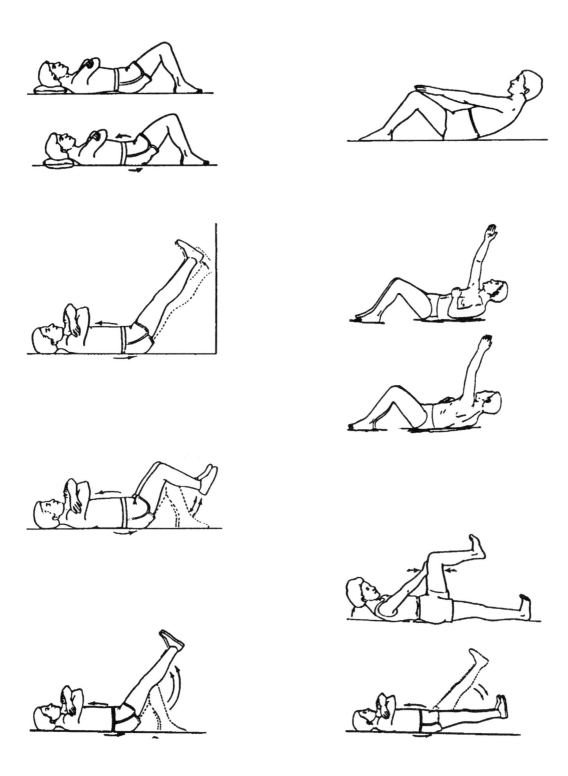

Sidelying Stabilization Progression

The stabilization exercises are helpful for general conditioning and stability of the trunk. With these stabilization exercises, the patient progressively isometrically tightens the ankle, knee, hip, abdominal, upper extremity and neck musculature, without releasing the other muscles. Holding this stable position firmly, an isolated body part (in this case the hip) is moved to an anti-gravity position. As the patient improves, the difficulty of the movement increases by increasing the lever arm or range of movement.

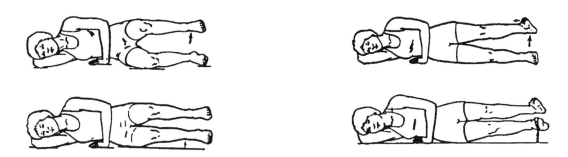

Kneeling Stabilization Progression

The stabilization exercises are helpful for general conditioning and stability of the trunk. With these stabilization exercises, the patient progressively isometrically tightens the ankle, knee, hip, abdominal, upper extremity and neck musculature, without releasing the other muscles. Holding this stable position firmly, an isolated movement is performed (for example, the patient slowly rises from the kneeling position). As the patient improves, the difficulty of the movement increases by increasing the lever arm or range of movement.

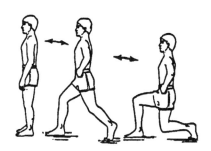

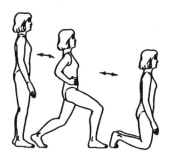

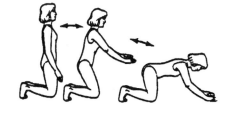

Supine Stabilization Progression (Dead Bug)

The stabilization exercises are helpful for general conditioning and stability of the trunk. With these stabilization exercises, the patient isometrically tightens the trunk musculature. Holding this stable position firmly, isolated body parts (in this case the lower and upper extremities) are moved. As the patient improves, the difficulty of the movement increases by increasing the lever arm or range of movement.

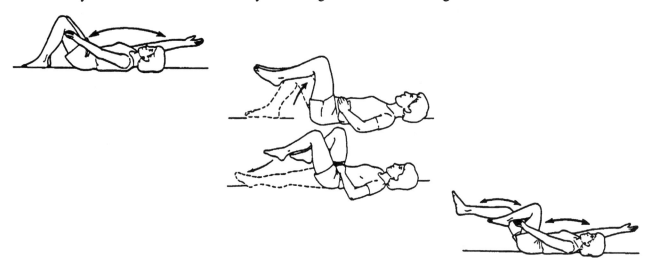

Supine Stabilization Progression (Bridging)

The stabilization exercises are helpful for general conditioning and stability of the trunk. With these stabilization exercises, the patient progressively isometrically tightens the ankle, knee, hip, abdominal, upper extremity and neck musculature, without releasing the other muscles. Holding this stable position firmly, an isolated body part (in this case the lower extremity) is moved to an anti-gravity position. As the patient improves, the difficulty of the movement increases by increasing the lever arm or range of movement.

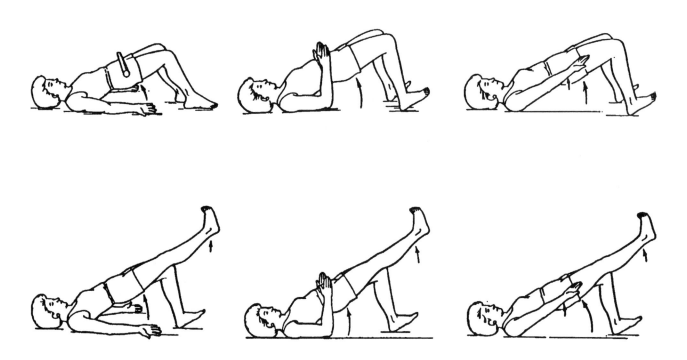

Quadruped Stabilization Progression

The stabilization exercises are helpful for general conditioning and stability of the trunk. With these stabilization exercises, the patient progressively isometrically tightens the ankle, knee, hip, abdominal, upper extremity and neck musculature, without releasing the other muscles. Holding this stable position firmly, an isolated body part (in this case the upper extremity) is moved to an anti-gravity position. As the patient improves, the difficulty of the movement increases by increasing the lever arm or range of movement.

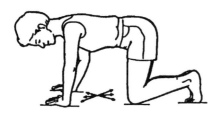

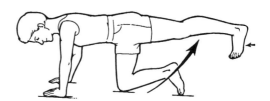

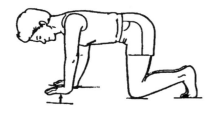

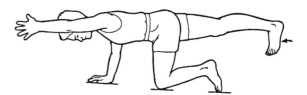

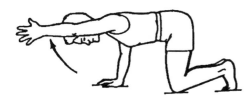

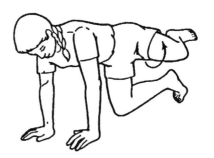

Hip Stretching

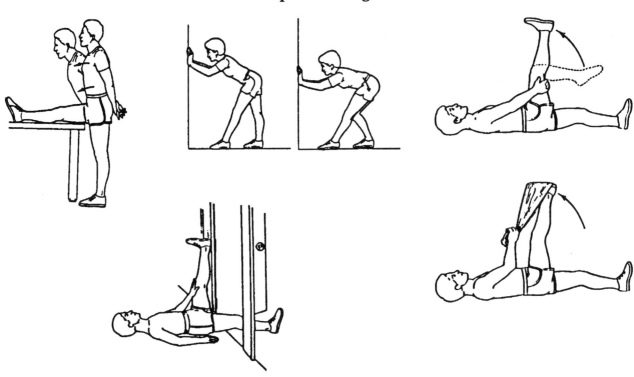

Hamstring Stretches

Many varieties of hamstring stretches are widely used. Hamstring stretching is indicated when tightness exists or when inadequate hamstring length causes the lumbar spine to perform less optimally during functional activities. The hamstring stretches are also indicated for tightness of neural structures such as adherent nerve roots or adverse mechanical neural tension. If a true hamstring stretch is desired, the lumbar spine must be in a neutral, stabilized position during hamstring stretching to avoid transmitting the stretch to the spine. The trunk, head and neck can be flexed, or hip rotation can be added if neuromeningeal stretching is desired. The hamstring or neuromeningeal stretches should be performed gently when an irritable condition exists.

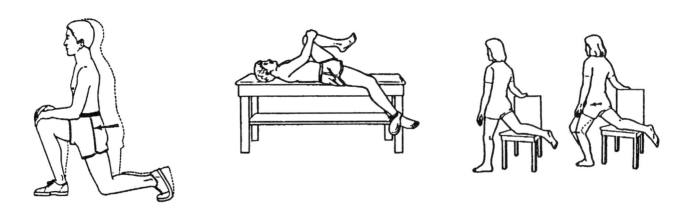

Anterior Hip Stretches

Anterior hip stretching is indicated when tightness of the psoas, rectus femoris, hip joint capsule or other anterior hip structure is present. The patient should be taught to stabilize the lumbar spine to avoid excessive lumbar lordosis, a common substitution pattern with these stretches.

Miscellaneous Hip Stretching

Hip rotation, adduction and abduction stretching is often necessary when tight soft tissues in the hip are interfering with normal lumbar soft tissue or joint mechanics. The patient can vary the degree of hip flexion or extension to isolate and modify the stretch as needed.

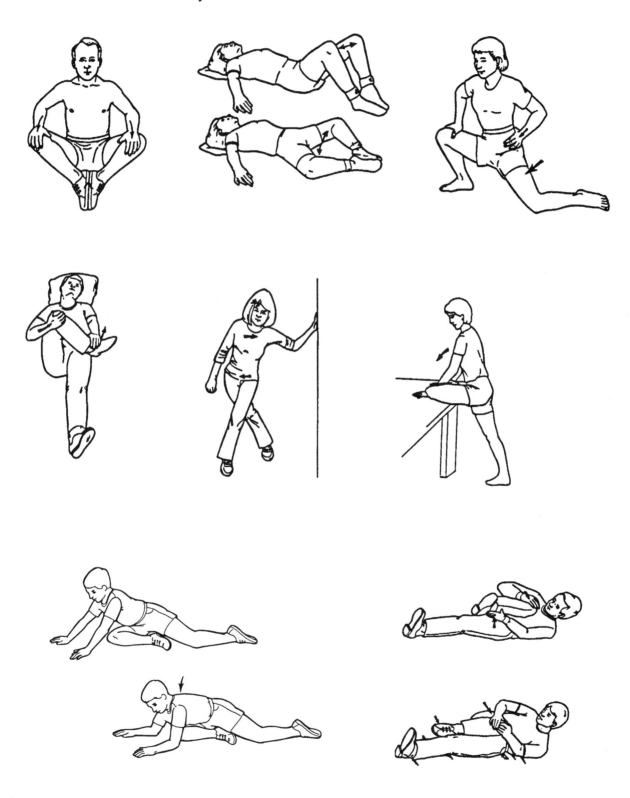

Hip Strengthening and Miscellaneous Strengthening

Wall Slide

The wall slide is a helpful isometric strengthening activity for the quadriceps and hip musculature. It is usually considered less functional than true squatting activities; it is most useful when the patient is too acute to tolerate squatting activities or when his or her functional activities actually require sustained partial squatting.

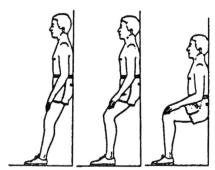

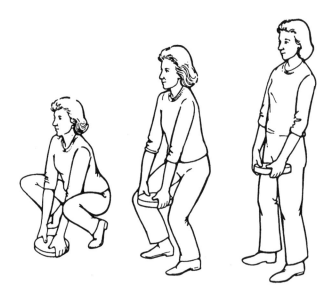

Squats

Full or partial squats are very functional exercises for strengthening the hip and back musculature. As the patient improves, he or she can begin lifting weights or items placed between waist and knee height. As the patient improves further, the weight can be increased and gradually placed lower until the patient is lifting off of the floor.

The "Power Position"

Practicing the "power position" causes increased kinesthetic awareness of lumbar and pelvic positioning and helps stretch the lumbar and hip musculature in a functional position. The therapist can provide verbal instruction by saying, "Now <u>power</u>, now <u>weak</u>," in a variety of problem-solving situations such as lifting out of the trunk of a car, bending to pick up a child, etc., to emphasize further that there is a correct and an incorrect way to do almost any activity.

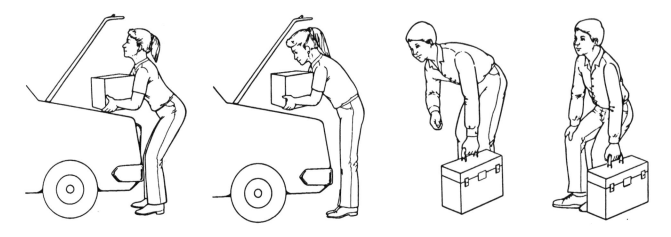

EXAMPLES OF EXERCISE PROGRAMS
FOR COMMON CLINICAL CONDITIONS

Upper Cervical/Anterior Chest Tightness
Interscapular Weakness
Thoracic Outlet Syndrome

Upper Cervical Flexion/Sidebending

Standing Scapular Retraction

Corner Stretch

Prone Scapular Retraction Progression

Scapular Retraction Progression with Tubing

Discogenic Low Back Pain
Low Back Pain Related to Flexion Postures

Lateral Shift Correction

Prone Extension Progression (Stretching)

Prone Extension Progression (Strengthening)

Lumbar Stabilization Exercises

Practice of "Power Position"

Abdominal Strengthening

Facet Joint Pain
Low Back Pain Related to Hyperextension Postures
(Pregnancy, Unstable Spondylolisthesis)

Knees to Chest

Prayer Stretch

Abdominal Exercises

Prone Extension Progression with Pillows (Strengthening)

Lumbar Stabilization Exercises

CHAPTER 13

SPINAL REHABILITATION

REHABILITATION OF ACUTE LOW BACK PAIN

Recent literature has focused much attention on rehabilitation for the chronic back pain patient. Although there are differences of opinion about which equipment and philosophical ideologies work best, authors agree on one point: some sort of active physical exercise is an important component of chronic rehabilitation programs.[9-15, 19, 21-26, 28]

Less attention, however, has focused on aggressive exercise rehabilitation for the patient with acute or subacute low back pain. Some authors do refer to early aggressive rehabilitation for acute disorders.[2, 5, 7, 14, 15, 21, 23] It is far more common, however, to find disagreement in the literature on what treatments work best. Every author describes his or her favorite method for treatment of the low back pain episode, always with favorable results. Yet in a very critical look at the literature supporting these treatments, the Quebec Task Force found the variety of treatments widely used have little scientific basis. This important study found exercise and patient education are the treatments that consistently work in the long-term.[18] Nachemson also criticizes most of the traditional forms of lower back pain treatment.[16]

The Role of Bedrest and a Passive Treatment Approach

Deyo, et. al., compared two days and seven days bedrest for acute low back pain. The study strongly suggests the medical profession is generally too passive and "careful" with the acute back pain patient. His study found patients with shorter periods of bedrest had better long-term results.[4]

Despite the important evidence described above, one still sees bedrest and passive modalities prescribed for several days or weeks for acute low back pain. Then, when the patient does not respond favorably, extensive tests are often performed. If minimal pathology is found, the patient may become suspect in the physician's eyes - maybe the patient is exaggerating the symptoms or doesn't really want to get well. If more significant pathology is found, epidural steroids or surgery may be recommended, "because a trial of conservative care failed." Unfortunately, conservative care in this case has consisted of bedrest and passive treatment. Actually, **active** conservative care (exercise and body mechanics training) has not been tried at all!

Obviously, some patients appear to get better with a very passive treatment approach. In many ways, this is very misleading. The Quebec Study reports approximately 87% of patients who suffer an episode of low back pain recover spontaneously in a short time. However, the recurrence rate for these patients is significantly greater than for those who have never suffered an episode.[18]

So, even when the patient appears to recover from an acute episode, he or she may be at high risk for re-injury. This is often because low back injuries are mistakenly treated as if they are single-event injuries. The fact is, most low back injuries are the results of months or even years of poor posture; faulty body mechanics; stressful living and working conditions; and a general decline of physical fitness. Therefore, most low back injuries, excluding those obviously caused by trauma, should be considered cumulative trauma injuries.

The Case for an Active Treatment Approach

Passive treatment philosophy has not prevented recurrence of back injuries. This poses an obvious question: "If the patient receives a more active treatment approach, focusing on exercise and education, will that patient have less risk of re-injury?" Although the answer seems clear, much research still needs to be performed in this area. Common sense tells us aggressive rehabilitation addressing the causative factors of cumulative trauma should place an individual at lower risk of re-injury. Certainly Lindstrom's study of Volvo workers in Sweden is convincing. Workers who had been off work for 8 weeks were assigned to either a control group or an "activity" group. The control group continued to treat with their own physicians. The others took part in an activation program, consisting of functional capacity testing, a work place visit, patient education and an aggressive physical conditioning program. The results were impressive. On the average, the study group went back to work 5 weeks sooner and had 7.5 weeks less lost time due to back pain over the next two years.[9]

Most clinicians take it for granted a patient should rest an acutely injured ankle, knee or shoulder in a position promoting biomechanical neutrality for a time. The exact period of time required varies depending upon the severity of the injury, but after a day or two, complete immobility is rarely advised. In fact, patients are often warned to avoid letting the body part "stiffen up" and are encouraged to perform active, non-resistive exercise even if it is mildly to moderately painful. If the injury requires several days or weeks of relative inactivity, the patient is always instructed to perform strengthening and/or endurance activities to restore the body part to its pre-injury condition - particularly if high physical demands will be placed on it (sports or work).

Shouldn't this same philosophy apply to all areas of the musculoskeletal system, including the spine? The prescription of bedrest and passive modalities with the advice, "If it hurts, don't do it," can actually cause more harm than good. Consider the following:

First, the patient who rests at home *may not* be placing the injured spine in a position of biomechanical neutrality. A non-supportive bed, a couch or recliner may place the spine in a position of flexion or sidebending for long periods of time. In the case of a

ligamentous sprain or a disc bulge, this is definitely contraindicated. It is analogous to telling a patient with an anterior talofibular ligament sprain to rest the ankle in a plantarflexed and inverted position.

Second, the patient who is told to avoid any movement that hurts is letting his or her spine "stiffen up." Rather, a thorough evaluation should be performed and the patient should be instructed exactly which movements to avoid and how much pain (and what quality of pain) is acceptable. In the case of a discogenic injury, for example, the patient could be told to avoid flexion but to work gently on passive extension, as long as it does not cause sharp pain, or pain that travels down further into the extremity.

Third, the patient who is pronounced "cured" after two weeks of bedrest with no active physical exercise is being set up for failure upon a return to pre-injury activities. The effects of immobilization on soft tissue are well documented.[6, 8] After the patient has experienced two weeks of relative inactivity, the medical practitioner should assume deconditioning has taken place. Active exercise is necessary to restore the spinal structures to their pre-injury condition. This should be a minimum requirement, because often the patient was injured due to preinjury flexibility or strength imbalances. We often see patients who have a history of minor sprains and strains that always "get better," but recur intermittently. The patient will report each episode seems to be more severe and last longer. Yet, the patient persists in thinking of each episode as a separate injury. The patient does not understand each episode is not a distinct occurrence, but a continuance of the original injury, all because normal strength, flexibility and biomechanics were not restored after the condition became pain free.

To avoid turning a relatively straight forward acute back injury into an eventual chronic condition, we must learn to treat the patient using common sense principles based on sound knowledge of physiology. This means we must teach each and every patient how to rehabilitate his or her back.

The operative word here is "teach." Physical therapists do not need to see each patient three times a week for six to eight weeks in the clinic for exercise and rehabilitation. Ideally, many patients can be seen 3-4 times during the first two weeks for pain control and initial exercise instruction. After that, weekly or bimonthly sessions to recheck and progress the patient's home exercise program should take place. These sessions are educational and motivational in nature. After three or four more visits, the patient should have the knowledge and confidence to continue rehabilitation independently.

What about the patient who is not easily motivated and who does not follow through with the rehabilitation plan? Therapists must avoid falling into the role of "babysitter" for such patients. Noncompliance is not a sufficient reason to have the patient come into the clinic for his or her exercise sessions, unless noncompliance comes from a lack of understanding, which should be cleared up in a few sessions.

Implementing an Exercise Program for the Acute Patient

In this section, general exercise and rehabilitation principles will be discussed. Specific exercises are demonstrated in Chapter 12.

Individualizing the Patient's Rehabilitation Program

It is absolutely essential that the therapist design a program individualized for the patient's needs. Every patient's normal daily activities vary, and no two back injuries are identical. Standardized exercise sheets do not help motivate patients. When a patient is given a standard handout of exercises titled, "Exercises for Back Patients," that patient does not feel the exercises have been designed specifically for his or her condition. Professionally drawn or preprinted exercise diagrams can be used, but only if it is clear to the patient the exercise program is special and specific. In other words, if the patient's hamstring muscles are not tight, the therapist should not give the patient hamstring stretching exercises.

The therapist should become skilled at finding out how much each patient is willing to participate in his or her own recovery. If the patient is only willing to invest five minutes per day, a 20 minute exercise program will not be helpful at all. The patient will become impatient and stop performing all the exercises. The therapist should let such a patient know that only those exercises that are absolutely essential are included in the patient's program. This attitude fosters better patient compliance.

The use of special equipment unavailable to the patient elsewhere should be minimized. The therapist should use equipment such as freeweights, mats and elastic tubing, and should emphasize performing aerobic activities that can be continued at home, such as walking. Persistence, not high technology, is the key. Fancy equipment may encourage patients to keep their appointments, but it is not going to keep patients exercising once they have been discharged to a home program.

Even after the initial symptoms have subsided, it is normal for patients to have good days and bad days. It is tempting for the physical therapist to provide electric stimulation or other modalities for pain relief on one of those bad days. The therapist should be wary of sending a mixed message, however. It is better to first try to find an exercise or position that relieves the symptoms. This helps persuade the patient self-management of problems is possible.

The Aggressiveness of the Rehabilitation Program

Each patient varies in his or her response to exercise. In some cases, a patient can progress quite rapidly. The patient with a mild lumbar sprain or strain may be able to progress to vigorous lower back and abdominal strengthening exercises within the first week. On the other hand, a patient with a moderate disc bulge may wait for several weeks to progress to aggressive abdominal exercises that place the spine in a flexed position. However, that patient can begin gentle isometric abdominal exercises and a variety of general strength and conditioning exercises fairly early.

The therapist must pay close attention to signs and symptoms and use caution when progressing the patient into any exercise causing pain to peripheralize or causing pain lasting more than a few minutes after stopping the exercise. If the patient does not tolerate the exercise well, the therapist should re-evaluate the technique. The exercise may still be appropriate, but the patient should simply perform it with less intensity or fewer repetitions. There are many alternatives to stopping exercise entirely. The instances where all exercise is contraindicated are rare and are discussed in Chapter 5.

The Importance of Functional Activities

With the advent of Work Hardening and Work Conditioning programs, the importance of functional, job related activities has become well accepted. Unfortunately, body mechanics training and job simulation training are often left to such programs. Acute care therapists should also be concerned with functional activities.

Physical therapists who treat sports injuries know function must be addressed for the patient to succeed. With the athletic patient, success is usually measured by whether the patient can return to his or her sport.

This should also be the case when dealing with back and neck injuries. Pain relief is not sufficient.

The patient must feel comfortable performing hobbies or job activities. This can only be accomplished through emphasis on functional activities during the rehabilitation.

It is not necessary for the physical therapy clinic to have a Work Hardening facility for the patient to practice those activities essential to daily function. Very early on, each patient should practice activities such as picking an object up off the floor, bending to brush one's teeth, or reaching into the trunk of a car. These standard activities are followed by more specific activities as the therapist learns more about the patient's daily routine and as the patient improves.

REHABILITATION OF CHRONIC LOW BACK PAIN

How Acute and Chronic Rehabilitation Differ

We consider any injury older than 10 weeks a chronic disorder from a treatment standpoint, even though many authors define a chronic disorder as being older than six months. After 10 weeks, assuming no new trauma has taken place, any damaged tissue should be stable. Without severe pathology, the patient's continued pain is probably due to factors unrelated to initial tissue damage - factors such as poor posture; faulty biomechanics; imbalanced flexibility, strength or endurance; or continuing microtrauma resulting from any of the above. It would therefore be a mistake to treat the patient as though he or she has acute low back pain, even though the quality of the pain may feel the same to the patient.

With the acutely painful patient, much of the focus of education is on what caused the injury to occur, how to relieve the current pain, and how to prevent the next episode. The patient with chronic pain must be taught the same principles, but may have other problems as well. The patient may have been to multiple practitioners, many of whom have given him or her conflicting information. The patient is often not interested in preventing the next episode, as a feeling of hopelessness about the current episode may prevail. It is much more difficult to persuade the chronic pain patient to "work through" stiffness and soreness, as the patient may feel *any* pain indicates harm.

With the chronic pain patient, it is extremely important to obtain a detailed history of previous treatment and its effect on the problem. Patients who have seen multiple practitioners are naturally skeptical; such a patient must be persuaded the new therapist's approach is different, and therefore worth putting a renewed effort into it. If the patient has already unsuccessfully tried many of the ideas the therapist has to offer, the prognosis is poor. If, on the other hand, the patient has never tried an active treatment approach, the prognosis is better. Many patients will say they tried exercise programs and they either did not help or made the problem worse. It is important to quiz the patient about the specific exercises, and ask the patient to demonstrate them. If the patient cannot demonstrate them, or if the technique is poor, chances are good the patient has not given exercise an adequate trial. Some patients try exercise once, and quit for a variety of reasons. Either the importance of exercise has not been explained, the patient has not had adequate guidance, or the patient has a lack of motivation. If the exercise program was inappropriate or incomplete, yet the patient was faithful with the program, the prognosis is good for improvement when the correct exercise program is taught.

The patient with chronic pain often suffers from discouragement, anxiety, lack of motivation and even depression. Often, these problems go away spontaneously when the patient begins to succeed in an appropriate physical rehabilitation program. However, sometimes the problems are more deeply rooted and cannot be helped by the physical therapist alone. It is important that the therapist realize this, and be aware of other resources available for such patients. It is irresponsible and detrimental for the therapist to continue to treat the condition as purely physical when the problems that may be interfering with success are nonphysical or only partly physical in nature.

The Role of Work Hardening and Work Conditioning Programs

Definitions

There is quite a bit of confusion regarding specific program definitions. The Commission on Accreditation of Rehabilitation Facilities (CARF) has outlined specific definitions and criteria for Work Hardening programs.[3] The American Physical Therapy Association (APTA) has developed definitions and criteria for Work Hardening and Work Conditioning programs.[1] Some states have used CARF's guidelines for deciding reimbursement issues. For example, some states have adopted legislation restricting payment for Work Hardening services to CARF accredited facilities. Widespread controversy exists about whether CARF accreditation is either adequate or necessary to ensure the quality and consistency of Work Hardening programs.

CARF has defined Work Hardening programs as follows: "Work Hardening is a highly structured, goal-oriented, individualized treatment program designed to maximize the person's ability to return to work. Work Hardening programs are interdisciplinary in nature with a capability of addressing the functional, physical, behavioral and vocational needs of the person served. Work Hardening provides a transition between the initial injury management and return to work, while addressing the issues of productivity, safety, physical tolerances, and work behaviors. Work Hardening programs use real or simulated work activities in a relevant work environment in conjunction with physical conditioning tasks. These activities are used to progressively improve the biomechanical, neuromuscular, cardiovascular/metabolic, behavioral, attitudinal and vocational function of the person served."[3]

The APTA has defined Work Hardening Programs as: "Work Hardening is a highly structured, goal-oriented, individualized treatment program designed to return the person to work. Work Hardening programs, which are interdisciplinary in nature, use real or simulated work activities designed to restore physical, behavioral and vocational functions. Work Hardening addresses the issues of productivity, safety, physical tolerances and worker behaviors."[1]

Despite CARF and APTA criteria, one can visit several Work Hardening programs and see several different types of treatment protocols. For example, some programs use quite sophisticated strengthening and conditioning equipment almost exclusively, with very little job simulation occurring. Others use job simulation exclusively with very little exercise equipment present. Some Work Hardening programs have tools, forklifts, warehouse racking or mini-work stations available so actual work is performed.

Terminology standards are essential. CARF and APTA definitions and standards are appropriate and descriptive of what is widely practiced and accepted. When these authors refer to Work Hardening programs, the reader should assume we are writing of programs following CARF and/or APTA guidelines.

The APTA definition of Work Conditioning is as follows: "Work Conditioning is a work related, intensive, goal-oriented treatment program specifically designed to restore an individual's systemic, neuromusculoskeletal (strength, endurance, movement, flexibility and motor control) and cardiopulmonary functions. The objective of the Work Conditioning program is to restore the client's *physical* capacity and function so the client can return to work."

One important distinction between Work Hardening programs and Work Conditioning programs is that Work Hardening programs must be interdisciplinary and must address the psychological and vocational needs of their clients as well as the physical. Work Conditioning programs may also be less time intensive than Work Hardening programs (less number of hours per day and/or days per week), so Work Conditioning programs are usually less expensive than Work Hardening programs.

Many hospitals and clinics advertise Work Hardening and Work Conditioning programs. The term "program" attached to any term implies a more formal approach. Since a CPT-4 code did not exist for Work Hardening or Work Conditioning programs until January 1993, the way these services are billed still varies greatly. Many hospitals and clinics have adopted a per hour or per day charge. Because billing practices vary greatly, and because there are no universally accepted definitions for Work Hardening and Work Conditioning programs, payors are understandably confused.

It is our strong opinion the terms Work Hardening and Work Conditioning should not be used by therapists unless they are referring to specific programs with specific entrance and exit criteria, specialized staff and the other components described in this chapter. In other words, a "Workers' Comp" patient who is performing "Conditioning Exercises" is not necessarily performing "Work Conditioning." If the patient receives conditioning exercises, body mechanics instruction or job simulation training as a part of his or her physical therapy session, but the patient is not enrolled in a specialized program as described in this chapter, the service should be billed using the standard billing codes describing the individual services (i.e., therapeutic exercise and functional activities). It is not beneficial for the physical therapy profession to create new terms for services that already exist.

The Role of Work Hardening Programs

Work Hardening Entrance Criteria

Work Hardening programs are appropriate when all six of the following criteria are met:

1. The patient is unable to return to his or her optimum level of employment because of pain or dysfunction following an injury or illness.

2. There is a reasonably good prognosis for improved employment capabilities as a result of the Work Hardening program.

3. The patient has a clear, job-oriented goal, and understands the purpose of the Work Hardening program is return to work.

4. The patient's goal is attainable within a maximum of 6-8 weeks.

5. The patient does not have a psychological diagnosis, chemical dependency or symptom magnification that interferes with progress toward the goal.

6. Work Hardening is not medically contraindicated, and the treating physician supports the Work Hardening plan.

The Work Hardening Trial Period

Sometimes patients who do not meet all the above criteria are appropriate for a short trial of Work Hardening. However, if the patient does not meet all six criteria after a two week trial, he or she should not continue in the Work Hardening program. It is possible further medical intervention is needed, or the patient needs further physical conditioning, psychological counseling or other services before initiating the Work Hardening program. Sometimes, the patient's goal is simply unrealistic. In such cases, the goal should be modified.

By the time a patient becomes a candidate for Work Hardening services, many people are involved intimately with his or her case. These people include the patient, the family, the employer, the insurer, physicians and the rehabilitation or vocational counselor. All involved parties must support the Work Hardening goal.

At times, patients begin the program uncertain of their goals. Indeed, they may even be convinced they cannot reach a goal, especially if someone else has set it for them. If the insurance company wants the patient to achieve a higher goal than the patient does, for example, the resulting conflict will undermine the success of the program. Such patients will almost always fail a Work Hardening program.

A one or two week trial is often worthwhile. Patients may gain confidence or communication between all parties may be facilitated, thus causing a better result. In our experience, however, improvement must be seen clearly in the trial period for the program to succeed. Continuing beyond the one or two week trial when the goals are still doubtful is almost always unsuccessful.

Work Hardening Exit Criteria

Work Hardening programs should also have clear criteria for exiting the program. Work Hardening patients should be discharged when any of the following conditions are met.

- The patient meets the goals of the program

- The patient plateaus or stops progressing toward the goals

- The program becomes medically contraindicated

- The patient wishes to discontinue the program

- The patient is noncompliant with the program

A Work Hardening program with clear criteria for entering and exiting the program will have a successful track record. On the other hand, if the program becomes a place to send patients who have "nowhere else to go" or the program indiscriminately takes inappropriate referrals, it will soon gain a reputation for having poor success.

Components of a Successful Work Hardening Program

The Work Hardening Evaluation

A standardized evaluation should be performed at the beginning of the Work Hardening program. The evaluation does need to test baseline functional abilities, but it does not have to be a formal Functional Capacity Evaluation (FCE).

In most cases, it is not necessary to determine detailed endurance capabilities before beginning a Work Hardening program. Therefore, the Work Hardening Evaluation can be less comprehensive and more cost-effective than a formal Functional Capacity Evaluation.

The purpose of the Work Hardening Evaluation is threefold:

1. Establish the appropriateness of the client to participate in the Work Hardening program by addressing symptom magnification, medical condition, musculoskeletal condition and functional tolerance levels

2. Establish a baseline to which progress in the Work Hardening program can be compared

3. Identify other services that may be necessary in addition to or instead of the Work Hardening program

The necessary components of a Work Hardening Evaluation are as follows:

1. <u>Intake Interview</u> - This includes medical history, job history, psychological and vocational assessments.

2. <u>Neuromusculoskeletal Evaluation</u>

3. <u>Baseline Functional Evaluation</u> - The intent is to establish the client's safe maximum tolerance levels for a variety of functional tasks and to determine the limiting factors. This usually includes a standardized list of material handling tasks, as well as static postures and positions and repetitive motion tasks.

At the end of the Work Hardening program, the Work Hardening evaluation is repeated to compare pre- and post-Work Hardening abilities. The client's function as it relates specifically to job tasks should be well documented. In addition to the standardized job tasks, performance of specific job duties important for an individual client should be addressed. The final report should be in a format easily understood by the client's physician, employer, insurer, and vocational or rehabilitation counselor, and its primary purpose should be <u>to specify abilities for return to work.</u>

Work Hardening Program Standards

Consistent methods and standards are essential to the success of a Work Hardening program. The methods and standards established should be described in writing. In addition to outlining entrance and exit criteria, the standards should address such issues as guidelines for written communication (format, content and timeliness), adequate progression in the program, how to identify and address symptom magnification, how often to have patient/staff meetings, how to train new staff, how to evaluate the success of the program, how to ensure quality of the program, and many other issues. Each Work Hardening program will have its own issues that are of greater or lesser importance. The methods and standards will probably evolve as the program grows and develops. The many seminars available on Work Hardening contain valuable information about methods and standards and how to develop them (see Resource List at the end of this chapter).

The Work Hardening Staff

The most important asset of a Work Hardening program is its staff. A staff whose members are experienced, creative, enthusiastic and have good communication skills is essential. A program investing in its staff members will always be successful, even without expensive, sophisticated equipment and a beautifully decorated office. Work Hardening staff members must be specialists. They cannot rotate through various departments in a physical therapy clinic or hospital and still be able to give their patients the consistency needed. Many excellent Work Hardening seminars and workshops are available to train staff in the many issues and techniques unique to Work Hardening programs. Work Hardening staff members should also have a basic understanding of Workers' Compensation law in their state. Often, this understanding comes with experience, but talking with rehabilitation counselors, attorneys and colleagues who work with Workers' Compensation clients is extremely helpful.

For daily exercise and job simulation activities, an appropriate staff to patient ratio is 2:10 (one physical or occupational therapist and one assistant or aide per ten patients) Many programs have only part-time psychological and vocational personnel, because physical therapists, occupational therapists, assistants and aides coordinate most of the daily activities. In some programs, physical therapists' and occupational therapists' roles are very similar; in others, their roles are more clearly delineated, with physical therapists more responsible for exercise, and occupational therapists more responsible for job simulation. This varies widely depending upon the structure of the program. Philosophically, a program may be more psychologically than physically oriented, or vice versa. Staff ratios will therefore vary widely.

Work Hardening Equipment and Space

Work simulation and basic exercise equipment are also a must (Fig 13-1). The exercise equipment does not have to be fancy or expensive, since the patient will not have this equipment available when he or she is discharged from the program. The patient should instead use equipment available at home or in a health club, where the patient will hopefully exercise after discharge. The exercises should be individually designed for each patient's problems and situation.

The work simulation equipment must adequately simulate job tasks. <u>Computerized printouts are less important than real life activities.</u> An unfortunate myth exists regarding the objectivity of computerized

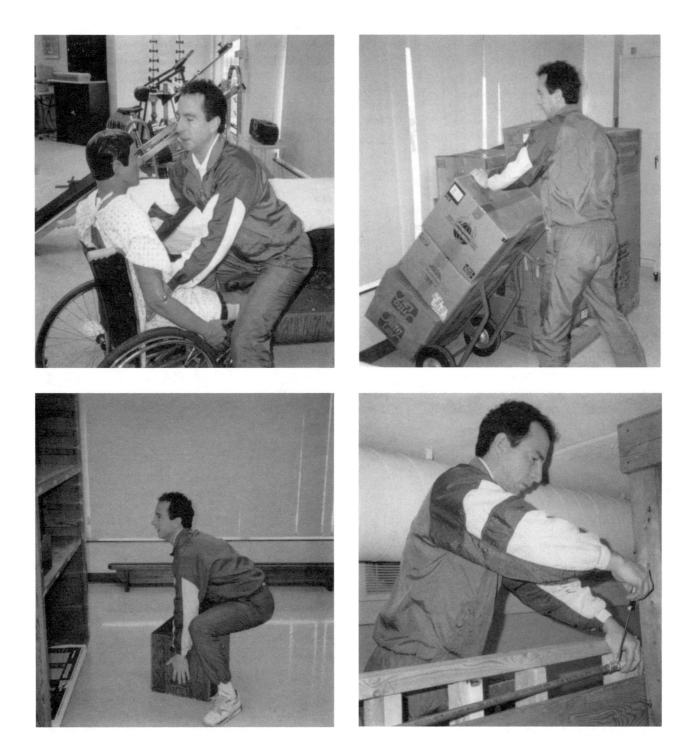

Figure 13-1. Basic work simulation and exercise equipment used in Work Conditioning and Work Hardening programs.

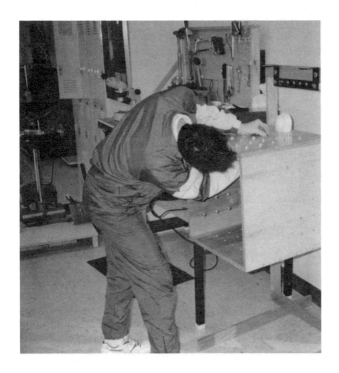

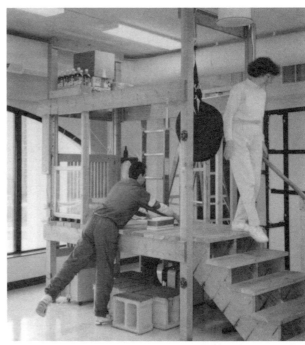

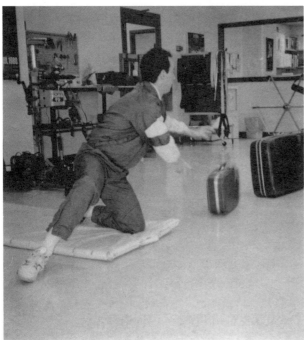

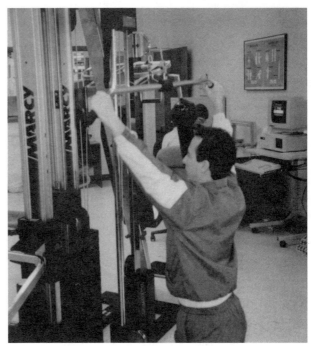

Figure 13-1. Continued.

testing and exercise equipment. Some therapists and referral sources feel they need computer-generated numbers to determine whether patients are improving or whether they are giving forth good effort. This is certainly not true. An experienced therapist can document objective changes in a patient's status without the use of a computer. That same therapist can determine the consistency or inconsistency of a patient's effort by close observation. Effective documentation is the key. Some computer data are actually misleading, because they appear to be objective, yet they are not easily applied to a real situation on the job.

Adequate space is important. The actual square footage required will vary depending upon the caseload. Patients must have enough room to perform their exercise and job simulation tasks. Usually, 2,000-3,000 square feet will accommodate 10-15 patients, depending upon the tasks they are performing.

The Role of Work Conditioning Programs

Work Conditioning Entrance Criteria

The entrance criteria for Work Conditioning programs are identical to those of Work Hardening programs. When, then, are Work Conditioning programs more appropriate than Work Hardening programs? Patients are appropriate for Work Conditioning programs when they do not have the major psychosocial or vocational issues Work Hardening patients often do. Since psychological and vocational issues usually become more complicated the longer the patient is off work, the Work Conditioning patient is usually less chronic than the Work Hardening patient, but not always. CARF guidelines dictate Work Hardening programs should simulate a full day of work activities before a client's discharge.[3] Work Hardening programs are usually 4-8 hours per day, five days per week. Because Work Conditioning clients are often less chronic, the Work Conditioning program may be less time intensive than the Work Hardening program. It is common for Work Conditioning clients to attend for 1-3 hours per day, three days per week.

The Work Conditioning Trial Period

It should be rare that a patient first needs 6-8 weeks in a Work Conditioning program and then another 6-8 weeks in a Work Hardening program. The Work Conditioning Evaluation should attempt to screen out those people who need the more

comprehensive services of a Work Hardening program. If symptom magnification or significant psychosocial or vocational issues are present, the client is likely to benefit more from a Work Hardening program. If the patient is so severely deconditioned that more than 6-8 weeks of conditioning is needed to reach the goals, then he or she is not ready for *either* program. The patient may need to perform general therapeutic exercise to improve his or her condition before taking part in either program. Appropriate client selection is the key to success for both Work Conditioning and Work Hardening programs. When the therapist is in doubt whether a Work Conditioning program will be successful at achieving the goals, a one to two week trial is appropriate. If the client does not make adequate progression toward the goals during the trial period, a Work Hardening program may be more appropriate, or the client may not benefit from either program.

Work Conditioning Exit Criteria

Work Conditioning programs should also have clear criteria for exiting the program. Work Conditioning patients should be discharged when any of the following conditions are met:

- The patient meets the goals of the program

- The patient plateaus or stops progressing toward the goals

- The program becomes medically contraindicated

- The patient wishes to discontinue the program

- The patient is noncompliant with the program

- It becomes clear the patient needs the more comprehensive psychological and/or vocational services of a Work Hardening program

Components of a Successful Work Conditioning Program

The Work Conditioning Evaluation

A Work Conditioning Evaluation must be performed for the same reasons a Work Hardening Evaluation is performed:

1. Establish the appropriateness of the client's participation in the Work Conditioning program

2. Establish a functional baseline against which progress in the Work Conditioning program can be compared

3. Identify other services that may be necessary in addition to or instead of the Work Conditioning program.

For this reason, the components of a Work Conditioning Evaluation are identical to those in a Work Hardening Evaluation. Psychological and vocational screening tests are still important because they identify any needs that go beyond the scope of the Work Conditioning program.

At the end of the Work Conditioning program, the Work Conditioning Evaluation is repeated to compare pre- and post-Work Conditioning abilities. The client's function as it relates specifically to job tasks should be well documented. In addition to the standardized job tasks, performance of specific job duties important for an individual client should be addressed. The final report should be in a format easily understood by the client's physician, employer, insurer, and vocational or rehabilitation counselor, and its primary purpose should be to specify abilities for return to work.

Work Conditioning Program Standards

Work Conditioning Programs should have written methods and standards outlining entrance and exit criteria and other issues as described above in the section on Work Hardening program standards.

The Work Conditioning Staff

A specialized staff for the Work Conditioning program is extremely important. The staff must be just as knowledgeable about return to work issues as the Work Hardening staff. The staff ratio of 2:10 (one physical or occupational therapist and one assistant or aide per ten patients) is the same for both programs. Work Conditioning programs do not have the psychological and vocational staffing requirements unique to Work Hardening programs.

Work Conditioning Equipment and Space

Like a Work Hardening program, the Work Conditioning program should have both work simulation and basic exercise equipment available. Adequate space is also important. Therefore, Work Conditioning facilities and Work Hardening facilities may be identical.

Measuring the Success of Work Hardening and Work Conditioning Programs

Since the main purpose of Work Hardening and Work Conditioning programs is to facilitate return to work, return to work should be the ultimate criteria for success. However, many factors can cloud the issue and make it difficult to determine whether a program was truly successful or not. For example, many clients will not have an immediate job to which they can return. These clients will enter vocational training programs or proceed with job search. They are successfully controlling their symptoms, have stopped medical treatment for their problems, and are ready to "get on with their lives." They may have successfully met their goals, but it may take them time to find suitable jobs. If return to work is the only criterion for success, it appears these cases were unsuccessful.

On the other hand, a temporary, unsuccessful return to work does not indicate success. If a program only keeps statistics about its immediate results, the statistics may be very misleading.

For this reason, the following statistics should be kept. The data should be collected at three months (to give time for case closure) and one year after concluding each client's Work Hardening program.

1. Percentage of clients working, and whether they are working in same job or a different job and with the same employer or a different employer.

2. Percentage of clients involved in job search or vocational rehabilitation.

3. Of those who are not working or involved in vocational rehabilitation, what is the reason?

    A. Increased symptoms from injury or related injury.

    B. Seeking more medical care for injury or related injury.

    C. Unrelated injury or illness.

    D. Unrelated issue (fired, laid off or quit for reason unrelated to injury).

A program can track its true success by carefully analyzing these statistics. The results can then be used to market the program. Individual Work Hardening programs may wish to track additional statistics that apply to issues unique to their settings. The above statistics represent the minimum amount of information that should be considered.

The Role of Functional Capacity Evaluations

A Functional Capacity Evaluation (FCE) is a systematic, comprehensive objective measurement of an individual's maximal work abilities.[27] The idea of functional evaluation is not new, and for years medical and rehabilitation professionals have used functional evaluations to assess an individual's ability to perform activities of daily living. In more recent years, FCE's have evolved as a popular method of assessing work abilities because of the difficult medical-legal issues involved with appropriate return to work after a work-related injury.

There are many different types of FCE's. All major FCE methods (Key, Polinsky, Blankenship, Matheson, Isernhagen, and others) have strengths and weaknesses depending upon individual circumstances. No two evaluations or clients are alike. It is not the intent of this text to advocate or discourage the use of any particular method. This discussion is intended to highlight the purpose and potential uses of FCE's, important components that must be included in an FCE and effective documentation of FCE results. For more information on specific FCE methods, the reader should consult the Resource List at the end of this chapter.

The Purpose of a Functional Capacity Evaluation

A Functional Capacity Evaluation determines work related physical capabilities . Many persons/entities are potentially interested in this information, including the worker's physician, employer, insurance adjuster, rehabilitation or vocational counselor, attorney, family and others. For this reason, the physical therapist who performs FCE's has many potential referral sources.

For every FCE client, there is always a specific reason for the referral. In other words, the referral source always has a specific question he or she wants answered. Depending upon the referral source and the individual circumstances of each client's case, the specific question can vary. A good FCE is structured to specifically answer the referral question. Examples of the referral question can include:

1. What generic, work related activities can this person do? (What is the maximum amount of weight this person can lift, carry, push or pull, and how long can he or she sit, stand or work overhead, etc.?)

2. Can this person do a particular job? (Can this person drive a delivery truck, lift 40 lb frequently and 80 lb maximum from floor level?)

Components of a Functional Capacity Evaluation

An FCE should include:

A. INTAKE INTERVIEW - This includes history, job history and possibly a psychological screening assessment.

B. NEUROMUSCULOSKELETAL EVALUATION - The examination should include Waddell's tests for non-organic source of symptoms[29] or some other way to determine validity, effort level and consistency demonstrated by the client.

C. ASSESSMENT OF MAXIMUM SAFE CAPABILITIES - The intent is to establish the client's safe maximum tolerance levels for several tasks and to determine the limiting factors. The type and number of tests can vary between testing facilities, but should be standardized within a facility. At a minimum, the baseline functional evaluation should include assessment of:

1. Material Handling Tasks
   a. Floor to knuckle level lift
   b. Knuckle to shoulder level lift
   c. Shoulder to overhead level lift
   d. Single hand lift
   e. Lifting into/over obstacle
   f. Bimanual carry
   g. Push/Pull

2. Static Postures and Positions
   a. Kneeling
   b. Overhead work
   c. Balancing
   d. Sitting
   e. Standing
   f. Bending/Stooping

3. Repeated Motion Activities
   a. Stair climbing
   b. Repetitive squatting and reaching or bending
   c. Crawling
   d. Walking

D. ASSESSMENT OF ENDURANCE CAPABILITIES - The intent is to establish the client's safe tolerance levels for repetitive work (endurance capabilities) and to determine the limiting factors. Activities should be structured to answer the referral question and thus can be either generic, specific or a combination of both generic and specific.

Expert opinion varies about how best to assess endurance. Some extrapolate endurance by using a computerized data base, graphs or charts. Others advocate actual endurance testing over a series of several days. Some experts use a combination of extrapolation and actual endurance testing. We feel _actual_ endurance testing is the best method.

Specific activities tested can vary widely depending upon the type of job tasks to be evaluated. When the referral question is whether the client can perform specific job duties, the job should be simulated as closely as possible. It is the therapist's responsibility to determine whether he or she has enough information to simulate a job accurately and if not, to seek a way to obtain the additional information needed. The therapist can decide upon a list of activities to evaluate by considering one or more of the following:

- Verbal report by patient, rehabilitation counselor, employer, insurer, physician or other informed source, preferably a combination of the above.

- A standardized form (used by many states) completed by rehabilitation counselor, employer, insurer or other informed source.

- Previous experience of the job by the therapist.

- Videotape, written job description, or other information relevant to the job tasks, obtained from rehabilitation counselor, employer, insurer or other informed source.

- Actual Job Site Evaluation performed by the therapist

At the conclusion of the FCE, the therapist should feel he or she has performed a sufficient number and variety of generic or specific job tasks to confidently answer the referral question. In addition, however, the evaluation tasks performed must be standardized well enough or documented thoroughly enough to reproduce them in the future. Otherwise, credibility will be lost.

One obvious advantage to the standardized testing methods is their reproducibility. However, they often do not allow for enough flexibility and creativity to answer a specific referral question such as, "Can this person return to work as an ironworker for 8 hours per day?" A more flexible evaluation may answer the referral question better, but the therapist still must have a standardized methodology for performing and documenting such an evaluation.

Regardless of the FCE method used, every clinic performing FCE's must have written methods and standards describing the performance and interpretation of the testing procedure. This is true even of those clinics using an FCE developed in-house. Although in-house FCE's can be extremely effective (we use one), the development of a customized FCE requires considerable experience in the field of industrial testing and rehabilitation. The therapist who is new to industrial rehabilitation and testing would be wise to seek assistance or use one of the standardized methods until he or she has gained more experience.

Effective Functional Capacity Evaluation Documentation

A good FCE report is easy to read and contains enough detailed information to support its conclusions and recommendations. However, the detail must not get in the way of a clearly worded summary of the findings. The referral source should be able to find the evaluator's impressions and specific recommendations easily, and they should usually fit on one page or less for ease of reading.

The FCE report should contain the following components:

Introduction - A standard paragraph explaining the length of evaluation, purpose, and instructions given to the client. Any reasons for a deviation from the clinic's standard evaluation procedure should be clearly stated.

Summary of the Intake Interview - A brief summary of the client's history, job history and results of the psychological screening (if used) should be documented.

Neuromusculoskeletal Evaluation - The results should include the client's response to Waddell's signs (or other special tests) and whether or not inconsistencies in the neuromusculoskeletal evaluation were found.

Results of Maximal and Endurance Capabilities Testing - The results of each functional test should be summarized, along with a discussion of limiting factors for each activity tested.

The therapist should also summarize any specific observations necessary to support the conclusions under the "Impressions" and "Recommendations" sections. Detailed documentation of objective findings should be the goal. The therapist should also comment on whether or not the client's subjective reports correlated well with objective findings.

Impressions - The therapist's general impressions about client's effort and cooperation; consistencies or inconsistencies in presentation of function; and limiting factors are documented here. Any general impression stated here should be supported with specific observations found in the more detailed documentation above.

Recommendations - This section should clearly and concisely provide the answer to any specific referral questions. If therapist was unable to answer the referral question, the reasons should be clearly stated.

SUMMARY

This chapter has discussed various rehabilitation techniques, including Work Hardening and Work Conditioning programs. We have stressed the importance of early intervention and discussed the purpose of FCE's and the necessary components of FCE testing and documentation. It is not the scope of this text to discuss specific evaluation and rehabilitation techniques, as opinion varies greatly among the recognized experts in this field. The resource list below should help the therapist who seeks more specific information than is contained in this chapter.

RESOURCE LIST FOR FUNCTIONAL CAPACITY EVALUATIONS, WORK HARDENING AND WORK CONDITIONING PROGRAMS

Seminars and Training Materials

Advantage Health Inc.
Anne K. Tramposh
920 Main, Suite 700
Kansas City, MO 64105
816-471-8100

Assessment Centers Technology
Dennis Hart
103 Broad Street W, Suite 300
Falls Church, VA 22046
703-536-3190

Educational Opportunities
A Saunders Group Company
7750 78th St. W
Bloomington, MN 55439
800-654-8357.

Employment and Rehabilitation Institute of California
Leonard Matheson
600 S. Grand Avenue, Suite 101
Santa Ana, 92705
714-836-1224

Isernhagen Work Systems
2202 Water Street
Duluth, MN 55812-2145
218-728-6455

Keith Blankenship
American Therapeutics, Inc.
Box 5084
Macon, Georgia, 31208-5084

KEY Functional Assessments, Inc.
1010 Park Ave
Minneapolis, MN 55404
612-333-1191

Roy Matheson and Associates, Inc.
15375 Barranca Parkway, Suite I-111
Irvine, CA 92718

Publications

Bullock M: Ergonomics: The Physiotherapist in the Work Place. Churchill-Livingstone, London 1990.

Demers L: Work Hardening, A Practical Guide. Butterworth-Heinemann, Andover MD 1992.

Isernhagen S: Industrial Physical Therapy. Orthopædic Physical Therapy Clinics of North America 1:1, July 1992.

Isernhagen S: Work Injury, Management and Prevention. Aspen Publishers, Gaithersburg MD 1988.

Isernhagen S: Work Injury. Aspen Publishers, Gaithersburg MD 1994. To be published.

Mayer T, Mooney V and Gatchel R: Contemporary Conservative Care for Painful Spinal Disorders. Lea & Febiger, Philadelphia 1991.

Niemeyer L and Jacobs K: Work Hardening, State of the Art. Slack Incorporated, Thorofare NJ 1989.

REFERENCES

1. American Physical Therapy Association: <u>APTA Guidelines for Programs in Industrial Rehabilitation Programs</u>. American Physical Therapy Association, 1111 Fairfax St N, Alexandria VA 22314. Adopted Fall 1992.

2. Bigos S and Battie M: Acute Care to Prevent Back Disability: Ten Years of Progress. Clin Orthop and Rel Res 221:121-130, Aug 1987.

3. CARF: <u>CARF 1992 Standards Manual</u>. Commission on Accreditation of Rehabilitation Facilities. 101 North Wilmot Road, Suite 500 Tucson, Arizona 85711.

4. Deyo R, Diehl A, Rosenthal M: How Many Days Of Bed Rest For Acute Low Back Pain? N Engl J Med 315:1064-1070, 1986.

5. Deyo R: Conservative Therapy for Low Back Pain: Distinguishing Useful From Useless Therapy. JAMA 250:11057, 1983.

6. Janda V: Muscles, Central Nervous Motor Regulation And Back Problems. In The Neurological Mechanisms in Manipulative Therapy. IM Korr, ed. Plenum Press, New York NY 1978.

7. Kendall P and Jenkins J: Exercises for Backache: A Double-Blind Controlled Trial. Physiotherapy 54: 154-157, 1968.

8. Kirkaldy-Willis WH: The Pathology And Pathogenesis Of Low Back Pain. In <u>Managing Low Back Pain</u>, 2nd edition. W Kirkaldy-Willis, ed. Churchhill Livingstone, New York NY 1988.

9. Lindstrom I, et al: The Effect of Graded Activity on Patients with Subacute Low Back Pain: A Randomized Prospective Clinical Study with an Operant-Conditioning Behavioral Approach. Physical Therapy 72(4):279-293, Apr 1992.

10. Manniche C, et al: Clinical Trial of Intensive Muscle Training for Chronic Low Back Pain. Lancet 1473-1476, Dec 24/31, 1988.

11. Mayer TG, et al: Objective Assessment Of Spine Function Following Industrial Injury: A Prospective Study With Comparison Group And One Year Follow Up. Spine 10:482-493, 1985.

12. Mayer T and Gatchel R: <u>Functional Restoration for Spinal Disorders: The Sports Medicine Approach</u>. Lea and Febiger, Philadelphia PA 1988.

13. Mayer T, et al: A Prospective Two Year Study of Functional Restoration in Industrial Back Injury. JAMA 258:1763-1767, Oct 2, 1987.

14. Mitchell R et al: Results of a Multicenter Trial Using an Intensive Active Exercise Program for the Treatment of Acute Soft Tissue and Back Injuries. Spine 15(6):514-521, 1990.

15. Nachemson A: Exercise, Fitness and Back Pain. In <u>Exercise, Fitness and Health: A Consensus of Current Knowledge</u>. C Bouchard, et al, eds. Human Kinetics Books, Champaign IL 1990.

16. Nachemson A: Newest Knowledge of Low Back Pain: A Critical Look. Clin Orthop and Rel Res 279:8-20, June 1992.

17. Oland B and Tveiten G: A Trial of Modern Rehabilitation for Chronic Low-Back Pain and Disability: Vocational Outcome and Effect of Pain Modulation. Spine 16(4):457-459, 1991.

18. Quebec Task Force Study: Scientific Approach to the Assessment and Management of Activity Related Spinal Disorders. Spine 12:7S, 1987.

19. Rosomoff H and Steele-Rosomoff R: Pain Management Programs for Low Back Disorders. Miami Medicine, Mar 1988.

20. Rosomoff H: Do Herniated Disks Produce Pain? The Clinical Journal of Pain 1:91-93 1985.

21. Saal JA and Saal JS: Nonoperative Treatment of Herniated Lumbar Intervertebral Disc with Radiculopathy-An Outcome Study. Spine 14:431-437, 1989.

22. Sachs B, et al: Spinal Rehabilitation by Work Tolerance Based on Objective Physical Capacity Assessment of Dysfunction: A Prospective Study with Control Subjects and Twelve-Month Review. Spine 15(12): 1324-1332, 1990.

23. Sikorski J: A Rationalized Approach to Physiotherapy for Low-Back Pain. Spine 10(6): 1985.

24. Tollison D and Kriegel M: Physical Exercise In The Treatment of Low Back Pain Part I. Ortho Rev 17(7): 24-29, July 1988.

25. Tollison D and Kriegel M: Physical Exercise In The Treatment of Low Back Pain Part III. Ortho Rev 17(10), Oct 1988.

26. Tollison D and Kriegel M: Physical Exercise In The Treatment of Low Back Pain Part II. Ortho Rev 17(9):917-23, Sept 1988.

27. Tramposh A: The Functional Capacity Evaluation: Measuring Maximal Work Abilities. In <u>Occupational Medicine: State of the Art Reviews</u>, Vol 7, No 1, Jan-Mar 1992. Hanley & Belfus, Inc., Philadelphia PA 1992.

28. Waddell G: A New Clinical Model for the Treatment of Low Back Pain. Spine 12:632-644, July 1987.

29. Waddell G: Non-Organic Physical Signs in Low Back Pain. Spine 5:117-125, Mar/ Apr 1980.

SECTION 4
Prevention

CHAPTER 14

INDUSTRIAL BACK AND NECK INJURY PREVENTION AND MANAGEMENT

INTRODUCTION

The severe economic problems caused by the rapid increase of industrial back and neck injuries have led American companies to ask consultants to help them understand the problems and implement positive solutions. The concepts presented in this chapter are for the industrial consultant.

Back injury prevention consultants can come from many different backgrounds, including fitness, medical, ergonomics and business. The most qualified consultant, however, is one who understands the answer to the back injury problem does not lie in any one specialty area. Medical providers can be very effective consultants, as long as they take the responsibility to become competent in the areas that are traditionally non-medical, or direct their clients to resources that can help them develop a comprehensive prevention and management strategy, of which the medical provider is only a part.

Back injury prevention strategies encompass four major areas that overlap: 1) Management Practices; 2) Ergonomics; 3) Education and Training; and 4) Fitness. If a prevention consultant addresses any of these areas without considering the other areas, he or she has provided the client with a short-term solution at best, and has caused new problems at worst. For example, if employees are given ergonomics awareness training without making sure management is willing to make changes in the workplace, frustration or even open hostility may result.

Management practices are of great importance. If management personnel do not support the prevention process, attempts to take proactive steps in the other areas will be futile. Therefore, strategies to help management develop a comprehensive, prevention-oriented philosophy and a way to handle injuries when they do occur are paramount. Three main management issues will be discussed: 1) Administrative Management; 2) Medical Management; and 3) Claims Management.

Ergonomics is also crucial, because providing a safer, more productive workplace is important in the overall prevention process. As do all the other areas, ergonomics, education and management practices overlap significantly. For example, training employees in proper body mechanics often makes them aware of needed ergonomic changes, but it will not be possible to implement the changes successfully unless management provides the means to do so.

Education and training spans all the other areas. It is the vehicle used to provide information necessary to implement effective back and neck injury prevention. Everyone in the company – hourly employees, supervisors and upper management – must be part of the educational process. The information on management policies and attitudes is just as important to present as the traditional back and neck injury prevention program for the hourly employee, and must not be forgotten.

Both the *method* and the *content* of education and training are critical to its effectiveness. This chapter will not discuss the content of educational programs in detail. There are excellent training resources available to the educator that provide the needed content, including actual presentation materials.[1,3,10] This chapter will focus instead on the method and process of delivering information to the appropriate personnel in an organization, including the basic information that must be presented to the management team.

Finally, a serious look at fitness is important to overall preventive strategy. No matter how well a company performs in all other areas, injuries will still be a problem if the members of the work force is not fit to perform the critical physical demands of their jobs. Fitness is often a difficult area to address because how well individuals take care of themselves is usually outside company control. However, there are many things employers can do to facilitate on-the-job fitness and to motivate and educate individuals to practice healthier lifestyles away from the job.

PROOF THAT THE INJURY PRE-VENTION PROCESS REALLY WORKS

There is much controversy about the effect injury prevention programs can have on back and neck injuries. The earliest, most often cited study of back school effectiveness was that of Bergquist-Ullman and Larsson.[4] In this study, an educational program resulted in a 30% reduction in the time required to return to work, and a 50% decrease in the time required for recovery (14.8 days for the back school group and 28.7 days for a placebo group). Johnson[27] reported a 70-90% reduction in injury costs and incidence rates at PPG Industries two years after injury prevention training. Tomer, et. al.,[29] stated 67% and 70% abatement in back liability claims and lost workdays, respectively, after introducing the back school concept at Lockheed Missiles and Space Company. In a massive undertaking at Southern Pacific Transportation Company, 39,000 employees participated in a back school. The low back injury rate decreased 22% and there was a concomitant

43% decrease in lost workdays two years after training was initiated.[25] Three years after introducing a training program at American Biltrite, Fitzler and Berger[11,12] claimed a 90% reduction in back injury claims, a 50% reduction in lost workdays and a ten-fold reduction in workers' compensation costs. In her study of eight different industries, Melton[18] reported a decrease in lost work days with associated reductions in medical insurance premiums. Although an increase in the reports of lower back pain was noted, those reporting showed an 86% reduction in lost time days. Hultman, Nordin and Ortengren[14] observed the effect of training upon postural changes observed at the worksite. Their results showed a 74% increase in the time spent in "safe" postures and a 54% reduction in time spent in "risky" postures at three months post training.

Our own consulting experience has been very positive. Figure 14-1 shows the results of implementing a comprehensive back injury prevention process for several of our clients.

Some studies show that back and neck injury prevention training has no effect on injury statistics. However, these studies contain questionable standardization of methods, make faulty basic assumptions and contain flaws in the experimental design.[8,15,24,25,28]

In any case, the effectiveness of back and neck injury prevention programs can be difficult to assess because of the wide variety of subjects the various training programs emphasize. For example, some programs emphasize training in exercise, rest postures, first aid and body mechanics, while others concentrate on management training to effect attitudinal and administrative changes. As stated before, it is our experience that in most cases, a comprehensive process - one addressing the four components of management practices, ergonomics, education and training, and fitness - is necessary to effect the greatest and most lasting positive change.

BACK AND NECK INJURY PRE-VENTION AND MANAGEMENT STRATEGIES

Management Practices

Administrative Management

In this section, we will discuss the various actions that a company's upper management must take to create the environment in which active and effective

ADC Telecommunications, Inc., Minneapolis, MN

69.2% reduction in recordable back injuries with days away from work.

37.5% total reduction in OSHA recordable back injuries.

Gross Given Manufacturing Company, St. Paul, MN

Reduction • 13% in recordable injuries.
  • 22% in lost days.
  • 43% in lost time injuries.
  • 19% in company incident rate.

Demonstrated experience mod decrease from 1.58 to 1.26, with decrease in insurance premium.

Naval Air Systems Command
–Pensacola, FL

21.7% reduction in lost work days.

–Jacksonville, FL

60% reduction in recordable cumulative trauma disorders.

Rural Nursing Home, Rural, MN

1989: 824 lost employee work days due to back injuries.

1990: 705 lost employee work days due to back injuries.

1991: After intervention, only 39 lost employee work days due to back injuries.

Fig 14-1. Positive results for companies with whom we have worked.

injury prevention can thrive. Not all the actions discussed are easy to implement. Many companies may initially resist the consultant's efforts to take a serious look at the effect management policies and attitudes have on their workers' compensation costs. Many companies want a "quick fix," such as a body mechanics training session or an ergonomic analysis.

It has been our experience that successful injury prevention involves detailed consultation with management about a comprehensive plan to decrease the incidence and severity of injuries, which may require a willingness to change the way the company operates.

It is not the scope of this chapter to describe the following items in detail. Instead, we will list some of the more common steps that progressive employers are taking to decrease their injury and severity rates and the effect injuries have on their bottom lines.

1. Job Rotation - Employees "trade" jobs with other employees, which increases variety and reduces exposure to repetitive actions or sustained, awkward positions.

2. Job Enlargement - Employees perform more and different tasks in the manufacturing process, which again promotes variety, reducing exposure to repetitive actions or prolonged positions.

3. Job Enrichment - Employees are given job goals, but are allowed more choices in how to accomplish those goals. This promotes teamwork, problem-solving, shared responsibilities and increased control over pace.

4. Reduced Pace - Employers reduce the required production pace.

5. Work Place Exercise - Stretch breaks or exercise breaks are incorporated into the work day.

6. Disability Accommodation - Employees with disabilities or injuries are truly accommodated and become productive members of the workforce.

7. Encouragement of Early Injury Reporting - Employers need to know about symptoms early, when they are easiest to treat.

8. Modified Duty Programs - Productive, temporary jobs that encourage early return to work.

9. On-the-job Work Hardening Programs - Progressive return to work programs that gradually ease the injured worker into unrestricted duty while maintaining co-worker relationships and support.

Gaining Support

For back and neck injury prevention to be successful, management must support it. This fact seems simplistic, but often companies need to be persuaded that they really can influence the rate and severity of work related injuries. It is frequently necessary to convince them that a proactive, organized effort on their part will pay dividends.

Top management is motivated by bottom line profit. If they can be convinced injury prevention will increase the profitability of the company, they will support it. There is good evidence that back and neck injury prevention procedures, as described in this chapter, *can* reduce workers' compensation costs. It will be necessary to present this information to the management team members to help them make the decision to implement effective interventions.

Getting department managers and supervisors to buy into the program may be a different story. Often, managers and supervisors live within their own departments and have somewhat misguided ideas of their ultimate role with the company. A production manager or engineer, for example, may think his or her job is to produce a certain product as quickly and efficiently as possible. If a new assembly line design or work procedure improves efficiency by 5%, he or she will, of course, think it is a good idea and want to implement it as soon as possible.

What if the new design or procedure also increases the risk of back and neck injuries?

The question really gets down to who pays for what. The improved efficiency will add to the bottom line of the production department. But who will pay for the injury? If the production department manager is held accountable to a safety or workers' compensation budget, he or she will immediately see that improving efficiency that simultaneously creates another expense is not necessarily a good idea. On the other hand, if the health and compensation department at corporate headquarters pays for the injury, the production department manager may not see the same bottom line effect that the company president would. Of course, one of the goals of this program is to get department managers and supervisors to see the same bottom line as top management. A good start is to charge the workers' compensation costs back to the individual departments where they originated. They become an expense item, the same as raw materials. This way they will be factored into the efficiency formula and department managers and supervisors will see that health and safety issues are production issues.

Top management support must come by way of approval of funding and clear communication of policies, including written directives.

Above all, however, all levels of the management team must be vocal and visible in their efforts to decrease and manage injuries. In other words, management cannot simply give "lip service" to injury reduction, but must be seen as an active champion and facilitator of the entire prevention process.

Providing Authority

In addition to supporting the back and neck injury prevention process, top management must provide authority for implementation, establish accountability and delegate responsibility to appropriate team members to put into effect the recommended policies and procedures.

This may require a major shift in the current corporate culture. However, if management has done a good job of selling the program to department managers and supervisors, then establishing accountability and creating new responsibilities for certain team members can be a smooth process.

Changing Attitudes Toward Work Injuries

Making the department managers and supervisors accountable for the injuries occurring in their departments will go a long way to change all employees' attitudes from reactive to proactive. The direct supervisor's attitude in particular should be addressed because he or she is the most visible representative of management in the injured worker's environment. If the supervisor has misconceptions about the cause and effect of back and neck injuries, misunderstandings can easily occur and undermine the success of upper management's policies.

For example, many back and neck injuries occur gradually without any definite precipitating incident. However, if a supervisor is not informed about the nature of back and neck injuries and is not aware of the implications of his or her attitudes, an atmosphere of suspicion can develop when such an injury is reported. In a work environment where the supervisor and employee do not have mutual trust and respect, and the supervisor has negative opinions or experiences with back and neck injuries, the following thoughts may cross his or her mind:

1. Why wasn't the injury reported when it happened?

2. How do I know this injury didn't occur at home?

3. How do I know the employee isn't trying to get out of work?

4. How do you know a back or neck injury is real? I can't see any evidence of harm.

5. Doesn't everyone's back hurt at one time or another? Mine sure does, but I don't miss work because of it.

Verbal and nonverbal communication may convey to the injured employee that he or she is not trusted and that the supervisor does not care about his or her welfare. Without support and training, this supervisor may turn a minor problem into a major confrontation that will eventually cost the company a lot of money and will start the injured worker down a long path that will eventually lead to disability. In the end, everyone will lose.

To avoid the above situation, supervisors must be taught to do the following:

1. Eliminate problem workers before they have an injury. The workers' compensation system sometimes pays for the mistakes made because an effective employee evaluation system is not in place. Workers who take advantage of their employers by demonstrating low productivity, poor quality work, and high absenteeism can be expected to take advantage of the workers' compensation system, too. Companies with an effective employee hiring and evaluation system eliminate many of these problems before they become major workers' compensation cases.

2. Understand the nature of back and neck injuries, how they occur, and what causes them, so that they can be leaders in preventing injury.

3. Convey a positive attitude when injury does occur. Supervisors should treat injured workers with the same respect they would expect if they were injured. Helping find solutions is everyone's responsibility.

4. Solicit employee involvement. This will help develop a positive attitude. Employees should be involved with the safety committee and the injury prevention team. Supervisors should routinely seek suggestions and ideas from the workers so they feel they are a part of the solution. Ask employees to critique the back and neck injury training programs and the prevention process in general. Employees need to know that their concerns are heard.

Establishing Work Procedures and Rules

During the investigative process, problems contributing to injury and possible solutions to them will surface. It is imperative that each of these specific problems and solutions be documented and that someone has the authority and responsibility to communicate the resolutions to all personnel. All companies have work rules and procedures, but they are not always fully understood or enforced. It is essential to clarify safety rules and work procedures, to gain consensus and support, and to make sure everyone understands what is expected.

Medical Management

Business and industry can rapidly improve their work injury statistics through medical management. Much of this change can be accomplished simply by teaching the workers themselves about back and neck injuries and what effective and non-effective treatment consists of. This same information, of course, will help management and supervisors as they counsel the injured worker to make sure he or she is receiving proper care and support from the organization in a timely fashion. However, equally important is the active involvement of management with the medical providers who actually treat the injured employees. Management can be proactive in the following ways:

1. Encourage early, aggressive treatment of reported injuries

When an individual reports an injury or the first symptoms of a cumulative trauma problem, management should encourage early, aggressive conservative care. Acute injuries are easier to treat than chronic ones.

2. Find Competent Physicians and Therapists

A company must find competent physicians and therapists with whom to work if they are going to implement an effective medical management program. They must actively seek physicians and therapists who practice the principles of treatment and management described in this textbook (an emphasis on exercise and education). Then, they must make clear to these medical providers their expectations of them.

3. Encourage Employees to See Designated Medical Providers

Employers cannot afford to allow their employees to be treated by physicians and therapists who do not support their injury prevention and management philosophy. Workers' compensation laws vary from state to state and a company does not always have total control over this situation. Our experience has shown that companies with an organized, positive, proactive medical management system are able to direct most injured workers to the providers selected.

4. Provide Modified Duty and On-the-Job Work Hardening and Make Sure Medical Providers Understand It

It is essential that the company's medical providers do everything possible to return the injured workers to appropriate work. Some experts believe return-to-work is the single most effective thing that can be done for the injured worker.[21] There is considerable evidence of the cost effectiveness of early return-to-work programs.[7,17,20,22,23] Management and all employees must understand that return-to-work is a treatment issue not a production issue. Returning injured workers is cost effective even if little or no productive work is accomplished.[7,17,20,22,23]

A common mistake that has been made with return-to-work programs is that they have been used in isolation as the only method of treatment or rehabilitation. In such cases, the injured worker is likely to stay in a status quo situation for weeks or months at a time. One should never think of return to modified duty as the sole means of treatment or rehabilitation. The return-to-work process should always involve patient education and an exercise or Work Hardening program. It should always have time limits and involve weekly or bi-weekly reassessments and updates by the physician and therapist. An appropriate on-the-job Work Hardening program is preferred to a clinical Work Hardening program.

5. Make Sure Medical Providers Consider Ergonomic Factors in the Treatment Plan

The medical provider must have a basic knowledge of the interaction between the work setting and the employee's abilities. An ergonomic change may be the most important "treatment" of all. Even if the patient has symptom relief, return to the same job without ergonomic changes may cause the problem to recur.

Claims Management

A corporate claims management philosophy should emphasize the following objectives:

1. Regular contact with an injured employee

2. Effective communication with medical providers

To accomplish the above, companies should have specific, written claims management policies. The policies should outline clearly a sequence to be followed every time there is an employee incident that may result in a lost time injury. The following list is an example of an acceptable claims management policy.

1. When an accident happens, the supervisor determines the severity of the injury. If the injury cannot be treated by in-house first aid, the injured employee is provided transportation to the medical provider the company has selected. A standardized form is sent along with the employee. The form is to be used by the treating provider to list clearly the employee's restrictions and their time frames.

2. Once the initial treatment has been completed, the company's standard form is completed by the treating provider and returned with the employee. Transportation is provided for the employee to return to the workplace.

3. The employee and supervisor meet to discuss the incident or injury and the restrictions, if applicable. They determine how long the employee is going to be off work, if at all. If the case is complex or appears it will involve extensive lost time, the supervisor and appropriate management personnel will be involved immediately to plan a return-to-work program.

4. If the employee must miss work, the supervisor or management representative will explain his or her employee benefits and rights under workers' compensation law. Complete details about his or her weekly wage, when it will be received, who will be sending it, and how payment will be arranged are discussed.

5. The supervisor contacts the employee regularly during the time he or she is off work. These contacts are to make sure the employee is receiving benefits and adequate medical care, and to let him or her feel like an important part of the organization. Whenever a contact is made, the discussion will always include mention of when the employee will return to work and what will be available when he or she returns.

6. A specific return-to-work plan will be developed for any employee who will be off work two weeks or more. It is the manager's and supervisor's responsibility to determine precisely what jobs are available for the employee within the restrictions that have been set forth by the treating physician. Part of this determination involves establishing a plan and submitting the plan to the treating physician for review.

7. Once the physician accepts the return-to-work plan, the supervisor meets with the employee to discuss the details and inform what work will be available and when.

8. When the employee and the physician have agreed upon the return-to-work program, the plan is submitted to the insurance adjuster.

9. The facility's manager, the departmental supervisor and appropriate management personnel will monitor the employee's work load if he or she is on modified duty. They will be certain the employee

is performing tasks within the restrictions. Progress toward release to full-time duty is discussed periodically with the employee.

Injured workers need to be managed as well as treated. The medical providers treat the individual, but the company manages the case. It is no longer appropriate to rely entirely upon the doctor's opinion about the injured worker's care and management. Obviously, the workers' compensation insurance company will be involved in case management to some degree, but it is still necessary for company management to know medical management principles (if for no other reason than to make sure their insurance carrier is doing a good job).

Injured workers must not be allowed to continue ineffective treatment. If progress is not being made with a certain treatment approach, the Claims Manager must be proactive and ask the treating physician if other methods of treatment and rehabilitation should be considered.

Eventually, the injured worker will achieve maximum benefit from medical treatment. Too often, cases go on and on from one physician to another, with very little, if any, progress. If the employee has had adequate evaluation and appropriate treatment and rehabilitation; has had multiple medical opinions; and an unusual amount of time has lapsed since injury, he or she has probably achieved maximum benefit from available medical care. The case should be settled. The employee may return to a permanent job within his or her restrictions at the present employer, or may have to be placed outside the company. Even so, the case should be settled because keeping a case open that is not progressing and has no end in sight is damaging for both the employee and employer.

Another case that must be settled is the uncooperative employee. When the employee refuses to cooperate with the treatment and rehabilitation plan, the case must be moved to a conclusion. Good communication between the company, the insurance adjuster and the medical providers is critical to identify and manage these cases.

The key to long-term success in managing injured employees is developing a positive, open line of communication between the supervisor and injured worker. If the employee genuinely feels that management cares about his or her well-being, it is more likely that he or she will cooperate. A positive atmosphere is extremely important. The objective is to make the employee feel secure and welcome. Without this feeling, an employee is far more likely to seek legal counsel, which will only result in higher costs and increased frustration.

Ergonomics

Introduction

Ergonomics is the science of designing workplaces, machines and tasks with the capabilities and limitations of the human body in mind. By applying the basic principles of ergonomics, the company and its employees can take many steps toward a safer, more productive work environment.

The best ergonomist is the employee doing the job. Therefore, a major part of an ergonomics program is educating the workers and front line supervisors about the basic principles of ergonomics. Once these basic principles are understood, the employees can return to their workplace and recommend needed corrections.

Worksite evaluation and redesign can also be performed by experts who are trained in industrial engineering and ergonomics. If specific problems are found that cannot be corrected by application of the basic principles of ergonomics, a company may want to hire an ergonomic consultant to redesign a particular job or machine. However, even if major worksite redesign is impractical, simple and inexpensive modifications can often be made to greatly reduce the risk of back and neck injury.

When conducting the ergonomic survey, it is important to note good examples as well as bad. Most of the information gathered in the ergonomic survey will be incorporated into the education sessions later. Positive information will be just as important as negative information as the process unfolds.

Purpose of Ergonomic Survey

A worksite evaluation or ergonomic survey of the work area is important to perform early when undertaking back and neck injury prevention. It is done for two purposes: 1) to familiarize the prevention team with the work tasks and work procedures so that any educational programs presented can be customized to address the specific problem areas and 2) to identify problem areas that can be redesigned or modified to prevent injuries.

It is important for the prevention team to be familiar with the company's injury records before the worksite evaluation begins. This helps focus attention on possible problem areas.

Performing an Ergonomic Survey

Some basic design principles must be understood before performing a worksite evaluation. With these principles firmly in mind, the worksite evaluation should begin by reviewing an activity or job believed to be more physically stressful than others. All the jobs in the work area should then be carefully reviewed. Examine the positions employees assume or maintain as work is performed.

Back pain can result from many different sources. Be sure to consider more than just the heavy lifting jobs. Potential problem areas include:

1. Work too low

If the work is too low, an employee will be forced to stand or sit with the head and neck forward, shoulders slightly rounded, and the low back in a forward bent position. Try to find ways to reduce the need to bend forward. Can the work be raised or tilted toward the worker? Ideally, the work station should be adjustable. The right work height also depends on the type of work. Regular work should be at elbow height; light, precision work above elbow height; and heavy work below elbow height. If the work level is not adjustable, the fixed work height should be biased toward taller individuals ($\approx$36" for regular work). This may be accomplished simply by placing boards under the legs of a table.

2. Work too high

Continuous working at or above shoulder level can be very stressful. Look for tasks that cause the elbows to exceed a 45° angle away from the sides or front of the body, and attempt to lower the work height or raise the worker. This can often be accomplished by using raised work platforms, rearranging storage areas or by providing stair platform ladders that are safer than step ladders.

3. Work too far away.

Regardless of whether the worker is standing or sitting, repetitive forward reaching at arm's length is very stressful. All work should be performed in a manner allowing efficient use of the arms and shoulders, without creating a long lever arm that transfers excessive force to neck, arms and back. The least stressful work position involves working between shoulder and waist level, with the elbows at a 90° angle and angled <45° away from the sides or front of the body.

4. Work activities in confined areas or jobs which require twisting.

If there is limited space for employees to maneuver and move objects, they will often twist to accomplish the task. Repetitive twisting is one of the most damaging movements for the back. Try to provide enough floor space so the employee can pivot the feet when lifting or moving an item. In some cases, it helps to place some items far enough apart that the employee must turn and step, rather than twist. Swivel chairs help workers who are sitting. Conveyors, chutes, slides and turntables can be used to change the direction of material flow. Always allow for proper clearance through doorways and down aisles.

5. Prolonged standing on hard, concrete surfaces.

The muscles of the low back significantly help maintain the standing position. Without occasional relief, these muscles become fatigued. A foot rail, box or stool allows the worker to slightly elevate one foot and reduce stress. Rearranging the work so the employee alternates between standing and sitting tasks, or allowing a brief stretching break periodically throughout the day may also reduce fatigue effectively. Rubber floor mats; Viscolastic™ cushioned shoe inserts; shoes with leather uppers designed for work; and cushioned soles and heels also reduce the strain on the legs and the back.

6. Sitting or standing in a static position for prolonged periods of time.

When work requires intense concentration or does not allow movement, the back and neck can become fatigued or tense. It is important to provide some movement to relieve the stress that occurs. Jobs that provide a variation between sitting and standing activities have less stress because they increase the normal joint and muscle movement.

7. Sitting with the back unsupported.

Sitting is even more stressful if the worker slouches forward to complete his or her work. A high stool with no back or foot support is a common example of a work station that encourages the employee to assume a slouched position (Fig 14-2). Sitting jobs should be designed so that 90° angles can be maintained at the elbows, hips and knees. Chairs and stools should provide support for the lower back and allow the feet to rest on the floor or a foot support comfortably. The head, shoulders and hips should all be aligned in an erect, well-balanced position. Ideally, the chair should be able to be easily adjusted from the sitting position. The back support should be easily adjusted from the sitting position. The back support should be easily adjustable up and down and forward and backward. It should be curved to support the lower back in its neutral inward curve. The height of the seat should adjust easily from the sitting position and the seat should tip slightly forward or backward to accommodate variations in the work tasks. The chair

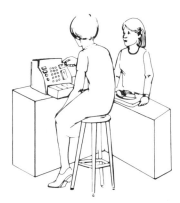

Fig 14-2. A workstation that encourages slouching.

should roll and pivot easily and have arms and other special features if needed (Fig 14-3). If the back support of the chair is flat, a rolled towel or small pillow or cushion can be used to fit the inward curve of the low back. A variety of cushions and back supports are available for office chairs and automobile and truck seats. Recently, some truck and automobile manufacturers have made an effort to improve the seats in their cars and trucks. Truck seats that are mounted on shock absorbers; are fully adjustable; and are contoured to provide support to the lower and mid back are readily available.

8. Frequent manual material handling.

Even when proper body mechanics are used, any time employees lift and carry objects there is potential for a problem. Manual tasks should be reduced or eliminated by using lift tables, lift trucks, hoists, work dispensers, conveyors and similar mechanical aids when possible. To eliminate the lifting and reaching tasks completely, materials can be delivered to the worker by roller ball caster tables, automatic conveyor systems or other means. Follow three principles of task design for manual material handling: 1) minimize the weight or bulk; 2) minimize the vertical and horizontal lifting distances; and 3) provide sufficient time for stressful tasks.

Many items used by companies today can be packaged in smaller boxes or containers. This should be considered when ordering supplies. Boxes and bags of materials can be broken down and placed into tote containers with handles. This not only lightens the load, but also eliminates lifting from the floor. Shelves should be arranged so that the heavier, more frequently used items are between shoulder and waist height, which is a more convenient height for lifting. The lighter, less frequently used items are placed higher. The rarely used items should be on the lowest shelves. Another idea uses baskets or storage pallets

What to look for in a chair:
1. Hydraulic controls
2. Seat back adjusts up/down
3. Seat back pivots forward/ backward
4. Seat pan tilts
5. Five caster-easy roll base
6. Seatback supports natural lumbar curve
7. Seat height adjusts
8. Waterfall seat front
9. Seat back and seat pan appropriate size for user

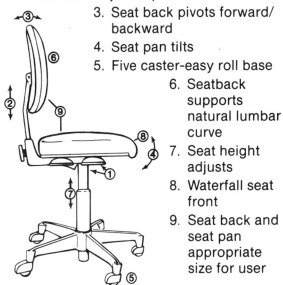

Fig 14-3. A chair with excellent ergonomic design.

that can be tipped for easier access. Side opening baskets also help avoid excessive bending.

9. Awkward or oversized loads.

Manual handling of an awkward or oversized load can be a dangerous task if not performed properly. Employees should be encouraged to ask for help or use an assistive device if they are unsure of their ability to handle a load safely. If a load is oversized and is being handled manually, repackaging the material, using mechanical assistance or performing a team lift should be considered.

10.   Miscellaneous hazards.

Pieces of metal, paper and liquid spills on the floor are all potential hazards for trips, slips and falls. One should always note these conditions on an ergonomic survey. Is proper non-slip footwear being used? Is absorbent material readily available if there is a spill?

Education and Training
Education for Employees

As stated before, almost all aspects of effective back and neck injury prevention involve education and training. Effective dissemination of information is essential if policies addressing ergonomics, fitness and management are to succeed. There is, however, basic background information about back and neck injuries with which everyone must be familiar so that all education is enhanced.

All participants of a back and neck injury prevention program, whether they are managers, employees or patients who already have a back problem, must first have a basic understanding of certain back facts, the common causes of back problems, what to do when an injury occurs, and the importance of a healthy lifestyle, good body mechanics, ergonomics and fitness.

Although an educational program must be flexible and meet the individual needs of companies and institutions, a standard or model program should be developed. The basic program should consist of two to four hours of instruction by a qualified and experienced instructor. Ideally, a maximum of 30 participants should be included in each course. Instruction should be carried out by means of an audio-visual program, instructor demonstration and active class participation. Open discussion should be encouraged.

The session should start with a summary of the contents of the whole course. Common misconceptions about the way back injuries occur must be abolished at the outset. Back and neck injuries have been so difficult to prevent and to treat in the past because of two incorrect assumptions: 1) Assuming back and neck injuries are caused by a single event such as lifting a heavy weight (the back "going out"); and 2) assuming that when there is no pain, there is no problem. Before proceeding with the rest of the training session, it must be understood that 1) back problems are seldom caused by a single event, injury or incident; and 2) one can have a "back problem" without having back pain (Fig 14-4)

The participants should be instructed in anatomy and function of the back and results of research and studies on the back. The mechanical strain in different positions and during different movements should be discussed, and the relationship between the center of gravity and strain on the back should also be explained. The function of the muscles and their influence on the back should be demonstrated. Unfavorable working postures should be analyzed in detail.

The pathology of back and neck injury (muscle, ligament, disc and joint) should also be discussed in relation to the above-mentioned stressful postures. Various methods of treatment should be talked about and the body's natural capacity for healing should be emphasized.

The program should teach individuals what to do when a back or neck injury occurs. Participants should be taught that what they do to manage their injuries is almost always more important than what their physician or therapist does.

Even when a company makes every effort to eliminate stressful, repetitive or prolonged positioning and heavy material handling, there will still be times when the employee's choice of technique will make a big difference. Therefore, employees must be educated about proper technique and safe work practices as well as how to reverse stressful activities through positional changes and exercise.

Many workers recognize how to lift and carry properly but they do not take proper work procedures seriously. Instruction should be directed strongly toward attitudes, forcing the worker to recognize his or her obligation to perform work tasks properly.

The participant should be encouraged to review his or her personal standards of fitness, nutrition and stress control. The harmful effects of smoking and its relationship to back pain should be emphasized.[9,16] Participation in various types of physical activities and sports should be encouraged to improve psychological and physical tolerance to pain and stress. The participant should be informed that proper nutrition is a foundation of good health. Overweight people tend to have a vicious cycle going on within their bodies. Increased weight leads to greater wear and tear on joints, which can make them irritated and painful. This increased discomfort forces a person to become less and less active, thereby favoring further weight gain. It should be pointed out that stress directly affects emotions and muscle tension. The participant should be told how relaxation exercises can be helpful in stressful situations.

At the conclusion of the program, the participants should actually participate in a flexibility and strength evaluation and should practice an exercise program that will help them maintain a healthy back. Participants should also practice proper body mechanics and posture techniques. Each participant should receive a booklet or pamphlet outlining the main points of the course. The booklet should also contain a section of general flexibility and strengthening exercises for the spine. Each of the exercises should be demonstrated and discussed in the class.

Education for Management

Many concepts regarding management's role in overall prevention have already been discussed. A company should never present a back or neck injury prevention program to hourly employees without

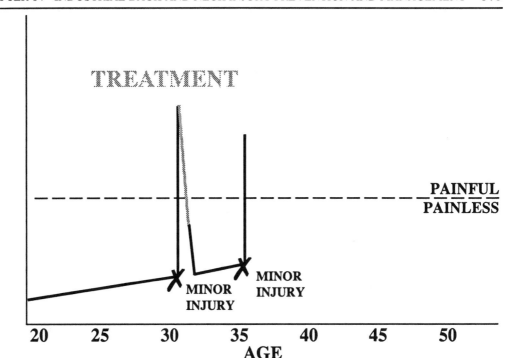

BACK PROBLEMS
(Risk Factors)
• **Poor Posture**
• **Faulty Mechanics**
• **Ergonomic Problems**
• **Soft Tissue Stiffness**
• **Muscle Weakness**
• **Smoking**
• **Static Positions**
• **Traumatic Injury**
• **Repetitive Wear/Tear**
• **Fatigue**
• **Poor Fitness**
• **Overweight**
• **Congenital Defects**
• **Unequal Leg Length**
• **Emotional Stress**
• **Poor Attitude**
• **Inadequate Diet**
• **Lack of Rest**
• **Other Factors**

Fig 14-4. The relation between back problems and back pain. The list on the left represents risk factors for back problems. The problems can be slowly worsening with time but the individual does not yet have pain. A minor incident occurs that causes pain. Treatment directed toward pain relief effectively alleviates the pain. However, if the treatment does not address the risk factors, the back problem is still present and may continue to worsen, eventually leading to a major disorder.

making sure management's issues are addressed concurrently, and management personnel have received aggressive training in needed areas.

Additionally, all management personnel should take part in the same program that is presented to hourly employees. This will make sure that everyone in the company is receiving consistent information, and will also underscore management's commitment to injury prevention. The management team is then seen as active participants and facilitators of prevention rather than passive observers.

A representative from the company's workers' compensation insurance carrier should participate in any educational programs presented to management and employees so that the insurance adjusters handling the company's claims are well-informed about company philosophy and policies.

Fitness

Introduction

Many stressful or repetitive movements will be unavoidable. If the worksite cannot be modified, workers can be taught specific stretches to counteract stressful movements or positions. These stretches can

be performed during short breaks that take place naturally in most jobs.

There is considerable evidence to indicate that people who are in poor physical condition and who practice other unhealthy lifestyles are at a greater risk of back and neck injury. [2,5,6,9,16,19] Therefore, it seems logical that one important aspect of a back and neck injury prevention program would be to help individuals identify deficiencies and attempt to help them improve their level of physical fitness, thus reducing their risk of injury. It is important to emphasize that many work situations are like athletic events: they require a certain level of physical fitness, strength and flexibility. Many people attempt to work at jobs that require considerable physical labor and involve stressful positions, but they make little or no effort to keep their bodies in the physical condition required to do these jobs.

It is true that most individuals work hard at their jobs and it is sometimes difficult for them to think that they should exercise when they are already tired from work. However, hard work and exercise are not always accomplishing the same thing. In most work situations, we get too much of one type of activity or exercise and usually not enough of another. Many people work hard all day, yet are still very stiff and are in poor cardiovascular condition. An exercise program should emphasize the type of exercise that is lacking at work. For example, if an employee spends a lot of time flexing (forward bending) at work, he or she should emphasize extension (backward bending) exercises at home and during breaks at work.

Business and industry have a lot of options when it comes to fitness. On one hand, the importance of exercise and other healthy lifestyles can be incorporated as a part of a back and neck injury prevention educational program.

A certain number of individuals will indeed be motivated to exercise on a regular basis through such a program. However, it is unrealistic to expect that every employee will be motivated enough to participate on their own in a home exercise program. Therefore, a company can take the issue of fitness much further than simply teaching about it in an educational program. Some companies are encouraging on-the-job exercise programs.

On-the-job exercise as an important component of the total injury prevention process is just beginning to create interest in industry. Many companies begin by helping start voluntary programs. In such cases, the company may provide a place to exercise and then hire an instructor to organize and lead the exercise sessions. Once a group gets started, participants from the group often volunteer to lead the sessions and the paid instructor is no longer needed. Voluntary exercise classes are usually offered before or after working hours or during break times. Exercise classes during lunch are often popular, and companies sometimes extend break times or the lunch hour a few minutes longer for participants. On-the-job strength and flexibility exercise programs can be very effective if offered three to five times per week in 10-20 minute sessions.

Mandatory exercise during work is attracting some interest at this time. Companies are trying mandatory exercise programs on a limited or experimental basis. If these programs prove to be effective, mandatory exercise during work hours may become a popular and effective way to reduce back and neck injuries. The obvious advantage to mandatory exercise is that those who are in poor physical condition and lack motivation to exercise on their own can be required to participate. It is often easier to get these people to participate willingly after they have attended an educational session or gone through an individualized strength and flexibility assessment program. Perhaps one of the most effective uses of mandatory exercise is to require those who have had previous back problems and those who score poorly on strength and flexibility assessment tests to participate. Mandatory

exercise programs may prove to be a major step toward solving the back and neck injury dilemma in the future. In the meantime, supervisors can organize warm-up exercises before starting work and require change of pace and movement activities throughout the work day.

However, a mandatory exercise program can backfire if it does not have the grassroots support of the employees. Companies should move with caution if they plan to implement a program of this sort without emphasis on participation in the decision making process.

Individualized Strength and Flexibility Assessment

The strength and flexibility assessment that we use provides the employee with an objective determination of his or her strengths and weaknesses and imparts the necessary knowledge and encourages responsibility to correct any problem that may be found.

In limited instances, strength and flexibility assessment may be used to determine job placement. Assessment used in this way is controversial since some say that it may be used unfairly to discriminate against weaker or less flexible workers. Physical testing to determine work qualification should test *specific job tasks*; the more generic strength and flexibility assessments as described here should normally be used only as an informational or motivational tool.

General strength and flexibility assessment can, however, be used for a pre-placement exam if it has been validated to the specific job in question. Validation requires a longitudinal study that shows that individuals with certain strength and flexibility deficiencies do indeed have significantly greater back and neck injuries in a specific job than their stronger and more flexible counterparts.[2,13]

To achieve widespread acceptance of back strength and flexibility assessment and exercise training programs, they must be practical, easy to use, and affordable. Another requirement of a back strength and flexibility assessment and exercise training program is that it is comprehensive enough to involve several areas of strength and flexibility. It is common to find people who are strong or flexible in one direction, yet weak or stiff in another. These strengths and weaknesses are usually job related or may even be related to the type of exercise program in which an individual is participating (i.e., too many low back flexion activities and not enough emphasis on extension strength and flexibility). Back testing protocols that test only one or two movements will usually miss these out-of-balance individuals.

Above all, a back strength and flexibility assessment and exercise training program should be functional and biomechanically sound. Many back testing devices or machines are promoted as more objective or "scientifically based" than the simple assessment exam advocated here. One must be wary, however, of devices that assess strength and range of motion in nonfunctional or unacceptable biomechanical positions. For example, measuring total flexion/extension range of motion is of little value since many people will have excess mobility in one direction (e.g., flexion) and limited mobility in the other direction (e.g., extension). Such people would score "normal" on a machine only measuring total range of motion.

Lifting with the legs straight and the back in a forward bent position is biomechanically unsound. *Testing trunk flexion strength in the standing or sitting position requiring a concentric contraction of the abdominal muscles is also unsound.* Industrial workers should not be tested in this manner for safety and practicality reasons. Only strength and flexibility assessment tests readily converted into a corrective exercise easily performed at home or at work should be used.

Normal standards for range of motion and strength are lacking. Opinion varies about normal and abnormal range of motion and strength. Some opinions expressed in the literature are based on scientific studies, while others are based on experience and the particular bias of the author. For this reason, we recommend that the tester make an effort to objectify acceptable levels of flexibility and strength within reason, without becoming too technical.

The list of strength and flexibility tests we recommend and a brief summary of a satisfactory response follows (Fig 14-5 to 14-16).

The strength and flexibility assessment we recommend can be done at the worksite, and it requires less than one hour of each employee's time. One evaluator can assess and train six to eight people per hour. No expensive equipment is involved. The test positions easily convert into exercises that can be done at home. The basic rule of thumb is that any exercise on which an employee's performance is less than satisfactory should be incorporated into that employee's overall fitness program.

Test	Satisfactory Response
1. Lumbar Flexion (Fig 14-5)	Lumbar spine flattens to neutral during sitting toe touch
2. Lumbar Extension (Fig 14-6)	Ability to achieve test position with smooth lumbar curve
3. Lumbar Rotation (Fig 14-7)	Ability to achieve test position
4. Hamstring Flexibility (Fig 14-8)	Ability to achieve test position with 80-110° hip flexion
5. Hip Flexor Flexibility (Fig 14-9)	Ability to achieve test position with knee (on side of extended hip) flexed to 80°
6. Hip Joint Flexion Flexibility (Fig 14-10)	Ability to achieve test position with hip (on side of flexed hip) flexed to 125°
7. Squat to Stand Strength and Flexibility (Fig 14-1)	Ability to achieve test position and repeat correctly 10 times
8. Shoulder Girdle Strength and Flexibility (Fig 14-12)	Ability to achieve and maintain test position (stick 9" off floor) for 30 seconds
9. Back and Hip Extension Strength (Fig 14-13)	Ability to maintain test position for 60 seconds
10. Abdominal Strength (Fig 14-14)	Ability to maintain test position for 10 seconds (repeat with right and left twist)
11. Abdominal Strength (Fig 14-15)	Ability to maintain test position for 10 seconds
12. Anterior Thigh Strength (Fig 14-16)	Ability to maintain test position for 60 seconds

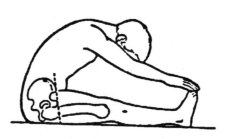

Fig 14-5. Lumbar flexion test position

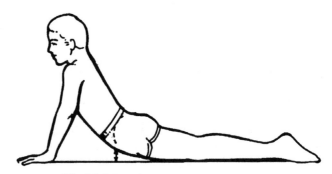

Fig 14-6. Lumbar extension test position

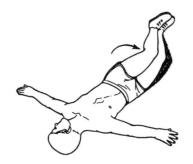

Fig 14-7. Lumbar rotation test position

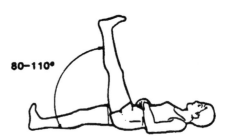

Fig 14-8. Hamstring flexibility test position

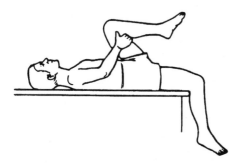

Fig 14-9. Hip flexor flexibility test position

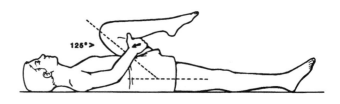

Fig 14-10. Hip joint flexion flexibility test position

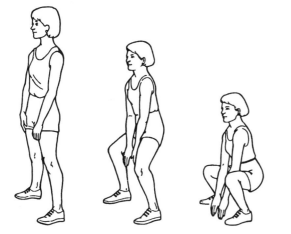

Fig 14-11. Squat to stand strength and flexibility test position

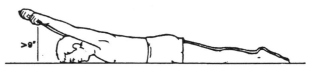

Fig 14-12. Shoulder girdle strength and flexibility test position

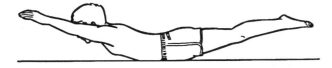

Fig 14-13. Back and hip extension strength test position

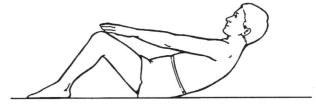

Fig 14-14. Abdominal strength test position

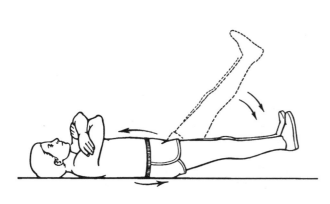

Fig 14-15. Abdominal strength test position

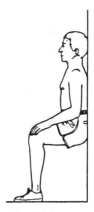

Fig 14-16. Anterior thigh strength test position

CASE STUDY

Introduction

The following case study illustrates the need to take a comprehensive look at the factors affecting a company's injury rate and the financial impact of those injuries.

XYZ Nursing Home is a typical 120 bed, long-term care facility in rural Minnesota. The workforce of 137 individuals is mostly young to middle-aged females. For many years, they had a back injury rate that was consistently above the workers' compensation average for their category. The high injury rate was causing a morale problem because the "healthy" nurses had to do most of the heavy work and at least two young nurse's aides had suffered considerable pain and disability from back injuries.

The administration and board of directors of XYZ expressed a genuine concern about the welfare of their employees, not to mention that their workers' compensation insurance carrier had given them notice that their injury record had to improve or they would be transferred to the high risk insurance pool. Being transferred to the high risk pool would double, or even triple their workers' compensation insurance rates, which would pose a real threat to the existence of the home as a viable business. The nursing home administration described it as a crisis. It was under these rather dire circumstances that the board of directors and management team decided that they must undertake whatever measures were necessary to effectively reduce the number and severity of their back injuries.

One of the authors (HDS) was selected as an injury prevention consultant to evaluate the situation, make recommendations and implement total injury prevention.

The nursing home had established a Risk Management Task Force consisting of a member of the board of directors, the nursing home administrator, the director of nurses and the controller. I met with members of the Task Force to be apprised of their perceptions of the problem. I then presented the Task Force with a written proposal that outlined the process that came to be called the "Save Your Back Program." The Task Force then understood the comprehensive nature of the program, the costs, the time commitment and their individual responsibilities.

My first recommendation was to form a committee with which I would work as we implemented the "Save Your Back Program." This was done by simply expanding the Task Force to include front line supervisors, workers and representatives from departments that would be significantly affected by the process. In the case of this nursing home, it involved the physical therapist, the nurse responsible for employee training and education, and the Workers' Compensation Claims Manager from the Human Resources Department. In addition, several hourly employees were members of the committee. This was necessary to get first hand information from the people who were actually doing the work. It was also important for the hourly employees to feel involved with the program and know that they had input into the process as it developed.

My first task was to make a short presentation to the newly formed "Save Your Back Committee" to discuss, in a general way, the four areas (Management, Ergonomics, Education, and Fitness) that would be involved as the process unfolded. During this meeting, I was trying to listen and learn from all the individuals involved to find out what they thought their problems were. I soon had a good idea of the extent of their problems. For example, many of the employees disliked their return to work program; there was considerable difference of opinion of the quality of training and supervision of the staff; and most injured employees were receiving passive treatment, without any rehabilitation or education.

Following this preliminary orientation and information gathering, I was ready to do a one day on-site evaluation. One of the nurses from the Task Force accompanied me. Our mission was to find out all we could about ergonomics, work rules, education and training, staff responsibilities, and management of the injured workers. The on-site evaluation revealed major problems in all areas (see section below, Problems Found During the On-site Evaluation).

In most cases, after the on-site evaluation, I would have presented the findings; made recommendations to the Task Force; obtained a consensus of actions and directions to take; and prepared and presented a customized comprehensive training and education program for all the staff (supervisors and employees).

In this particular case, however, it was felt that because of the unusual lack of interest and understanding of the supervisory staff, it was necessary not only to present our findings and recommendations to the Task Force, but to involve all the supervisory staff. This was necessary to determine if the supervisory staff could, in fact, be educated and persuaded to support and carry out all the changes essential for a successful program.

This was done in a very serious, sometimes tense training session for all the management and supervisory staff. These training sessions were not merely a presentation of back care information, but also included determination of policies and procedures and establishment of various individuals' priorities, responsibilities and authority. Everyone knew the importance of the "Save Your Back Program" when these sessions were concluded.

Following the management and supervisory staff training session, I developed and presented customized training sessions to the entire staff. These training sessions encompassed the educational principles found earlier in this chapter. Other actions taken are summarized in the section, Solutions.

Problems Found During the On-site Evaluation

Management Problems

Administrative Management

Probably the greatest disappointment of the day was the supervisors lack of understanding of the responsibility they had toward back injury prevention. This was evident from the top down. When we arrived in the morning, the director and assistant director of nurses were told that we wanted to meet with them sometime that day at their convenience. They were told that we would be on the floor doing our worksite visit and could be interrupted at any time. When late afternoon arrived, I inquired about them and found that they both had gone home.

We could only conclude that they did not understand the importance of injury prevention and the very important role that they and their supervisory staff had. I believe the supervisors perceived their role to be primarily that of patient care and did not understand their role in personnel health and safety.

There was no continuity in what we were told about general or specific patient handling and transfer rules. On separate occasions, I asked three supervisors where to find specific transfer instructions for a particular patient. I was given three different explanations of where the information was to be found. In fact, complete, organized information on specific patient transfers did not exist.

Medical and Claims Management

The nursing home had a modified duty program that most of the employees disliked and did not feel

was working. Two common mistakes are often made with return to work programs and these were being made here. When an injured worker was returned to work with a lifting restriction, he or she was nevertheless assigned a full patient schedule and was told not to do any heavy lifting, but to get help. Of course, this meant that the healthy nurses had double duty - their own heavy lifting and that of the modified duty nurse. This, of course, caused considerable resentment and confusion for the staff.

Another mistake they were making with the return to work program was that there was no time limit and there was no rehabilitation program being done parallel to the return to work program. How was the injured nurse ever to get stronger so that he or she could get back to regular duty?

The five primary care practitioners in the community were very busy and had very little time to communicate with the claims manager at the nursing home. The three chiropractors appeared to be practicing traditional manipulative techniques with little or no evidence of patient education, functional training or exercise. The two medical doctors were prescribing rest and medication followed by modified duty return to work without time limits. Physical therapy, or any form of rehabilitation (patient education and exercise), was not being used except in a couple of cases when employees had been off work for several months before it was initiated. Several of the injured workers reported to me that they did not like to go to the "nursing home doctor" (MD) because it usually meant waiting one or two hours and then, without being examined, they were given medication and rest or modified duty. These individuals said that they preferred to go to the chiropractor who could see them in less than ten minutes and actually did something.

Ergonomic Problems

We found problems with wheelchair locks, bed locks and side rails that were difficult to manipulate. Beds were arranged in ways that made it difficult to transfer patients and adjust the beds. There was a need for more electric beds for the difficult care patients. There was no clear understanding of when and how to use the mechanical assist devices.

Education and Training Problems

I usually like to give examples of both good and bad body mechanics. In this case, I finished the day with a lot of poor examples and hardly any good examples. It was soon evident that there was simply no regard for proper body mechanics or proper patient transfer techniques. When a few basic ideas were demonstrated to the nurse's aides on the floor, it became evident that they had not had adequate training.

The apparent disregard for proper technique was present even though the nursing home had a physical therapist on staff who was interested in and willing to be involved with employee training and with rehabilitation of injured employees as they returned to work. She had conducted some in-service classes on body mechanics and patient transfer, but attendance was voluntary and involved only a few new employees. No supervisors attended.

Fitness Problems

No one was performing exercises on the job to reverse the stressful positions that are inherent in the nurse's or nurse's aide's daily routine.

Solutions

To Administrative Management Problems

1. The nursing home administration and supervisors took more responsibility for improved communication. A critique system was initiated so all employees had input into the injury prevention process. Policies were clearly communicated in writing.

2. Policies were established concerning who had responsibility to evaluate new patients and determine each patient's transfer and handling needs. Supervisors and employee representatives had input into the policy formation. Policies were then documented and were easily accessible.

3. Supervisors assumed more responsibility for observing the nurse's aides as they do their work. They became more proactive, helping the aides with suggestions and individualized training. It became the supervisor's responsibility to make sure the aides in his or her department were trained and are performing properly.

To Medical and Claims Management Problems

1. Written policies and procedures for dealing with injured employees (medical management) were established.

2. We met with the medical providers, asked for, and received, their cooperation in implementing an early return to work program that included a physical therapy evaluation and on-site rehabilitation. XYZ

Claims Managers and supervisors became more aggressive about asking for clarification and suggestions from the medical providers.

3. The employee on an early return to work program was carried as an "extra" and was not assigned to patients who required care that was beyond his or her restriction.

4. Employees on early return to work were evaluated by the medical providers on a regular basis and their duties updated by the physician and physical therapist.

To Ergonomic Problems

1. A regularly scheduled maintenance program for all equipment was instituted.

2. A member of the board of directors who had attended the two sessions found 35 electric high-low beds in storage at a nearby hospital that had closed a wing. These were purchased at a good value and used for some of the difficult patients.

To Education and Training Problems

1. Proper body mechanics and patient transfer techniques were taught to all employees, and the supervisors were to see they were carried out.

2. Personnel were taught exactly how and when to use assistive devices.

3. Regular in-services and review sessions were scheduled for all nursing personnel regarding body mechanics, patient transfer and other back care principles.

To Fitness Problems

A class on exercise was conducted to show individuals how to evaluate their own need for exercise. Demonstration and practice time for exercises was allowed. Each employee was given an exercise manual and they were encouraged to do certain exercises on their own time. Additionally, employees were taught activities that reverse stressful positions and were taught relaxation stretches to perform intermittently to control fatigue.

Results

The XYZ Nursing Home ended 1990 with 705 lost employee work days. This dropped to 39 in 1991.

SUMMARY

A complete back and neck injury prevention process involves more than a body mechanics training program. The four areas that must be addressed are: 1) Management Practices; 2) Ergonomics; 3) Education and Training; and 4) Fitness.

The consultant's tasks include the following:

1. Gain management support.

2. Perform worksite evaluation, recommend interventions, and use information gained to customize a training program.

3. Perform management training. Emphasize giving authority and facilitating the prevention process.

4. Perform supervisor training. Emphasize openness to communication, facilitation and enforcement of preventive principles.

5. Perform employee training. Emphasize communication, body mechanics and exercise.

6. Help the company implement administrative policies that support the prevention process (i.e., behavior modification, reward structures, job rotation, and exercise breaks).

7. Help develop case management and medical management policies.

8. Help develop of an employee feedback system, complete with an ongoing program of prevention awareness.

REFERENCES

1. American Back School, 5936 Swanson Dr, Ashland KY 41102

2. Anderson C: Physical Ability Testing as a Means to Reduce Injuries in Grocery Warehouses. International Joul of Retail and Distribution Management 19(7):33-35, Nov/Dec 1991.

3. Back School of Atlanta. 1465 Northside Dr. NW #217, Atlanta GA 30318

4. Bergquist-Ullman M and Larsson U: Acute Low Back Pain in Industry: A Controlled Prospective Study With Special Reference to Therapy and Confounding Factors. Acta Orthop Scand 170: 1-117, 1977.

5. Biering-Sorenson F: Physical Measurements as Risk Indicators for Low Back Trouble Over a One-Year Period. Spine 9:106-119, 1984.

6. Cady L et al: Strength and Fitness and Subsequent Back Injuries in Firefighters. Joul of Occ Med 21:269-272, 1979.

7. Centineo J: Return-To-Work Programs: Cut Costs and Employee Turnover. Risk Management 44-48, December 1986.

8. Dehlin O, Hedenrud B, Horal J: Back Symptoms in Nursing Aides in a Geriatric Hospital. Scandinavian Journal of Rehabilitative Medicine 8:47-53, 1976.

9. Deyo R and Bass J: Lifestyle and Low Back Pain: The Influence of Smoking and Obesity. Spine 14:501-506, 1989.

10. Educational Opportunities, A Saunders Group Company. 7750 W. 78th St, Bloomington, MN 55439

11. Fitzler S and Berger R: Chelsea Back Program: One Year Later. Occupational Health and Safety 52:52-54, 1983.

12. Fitzler SL, Berger RA: Attitudinal Change: The Chelsea Back Program. Occupational Health and Safety 35:24-26, 1982.

13. Gilliam T: A Two Year Prospectus: Pre- Employment Physical Capability Testing. Injury Reduction Technology, Inc., 110 Streetsboro St W, Suite 2A, Hudson OH 44236. Unpublished study.

14. Hultman G, Nordin M, Ortengren R: The Influence of a Preventive Educational Programme on Trunk Flexion in Janitors. Applied Ergonomics 15(2):127-133, 1984.

15. Linton SJ, Kamwendo K: Low Back Schools: A Critical Review. Physical Therapy 67(9):1375-1383, 1987.

16. McFadden J: Smoking May Be Significant Risk Factor in Failed Back Surgery. Back Pain Monitor 4:41-52, Apr 1986.

17. McReynolds M: Early Return to Work. Clinical Management 10:10-11, Sept/Oct 1990.

18. Melton B: Back Injury Prevention Means Education. Occupational Health and Safety 52:20-23, 1983.

19. Nachemson A: Newest Knowledge of Low Back Pain: A Critical Look. Clin Orthop and Rel Res 279:8-20, June 1992.

20. Nachemson A: Work for All: For Those With Low Back Pain as Well. Clin Orthop and Rel Res. 179:77-85, Oct 1983.

21. Quebec Task Force Study: Scientific Approach to the Assessment and Management of Activity Related Spinal Disorders. Spine 12:7S, 1987.

22. Ratzliff J. and Grogrin T: Early Return to Work Profitability. Professional Safety 11-17, Mar 1989.

23. Ritzel D. and Allen R: Value of Work. Professional Safety 23-25, Nov 1988.

24. Scholey, M: Back Stress: The Effects of Training Nurses to Lift Patients in a Clinical Situation. International Journal of Nursing Studies 20(1):1-13, 1983.

25. Snook SH, Campanelli R, Hart J: A Study of Three Preventive Approaches to Low Back Injury. Joul of Occ Med 20(7):478-481, 1978.

26. Snook SH, White AH: Education and Training. In Occupational Low Back Pain. MH Pope, J Frymoyer, G Andersson, eds. Praeger Scientific, Philadelphia PA 1984.

27. Snook SH: <u>The Control of Low Back Disability: The Role of Management</u>. American Industrial Hygiene Association, San Francisco CA 97-101, 1988b.

28. Stubbs DA, et al: Back Pain in the Nursing Profession: The Effectiveness of Training. Ergonomics 26(8):767-779, 1983.

29. Tomer GM, Olson C, Lepore B: Back Injury Prevention Training Makes Dollars and Sense. National Safety News (Jan)36-39, 1984.

Index